SPORTS AND ATHLETICS PREPARATION, PERFORMANCE, AND PSYCHOLOGY

AN ESSENTIAL GUIDE TO SPORTS PERFORMANCE

Sports and Athletics Preparation, Performance, and Psychology

Additional books and e-books in this series can be found on Nova's website under the Series tab.

SPORTS AND ATHLETICS PREPARATION, PERFORMANCE, AND PSYCHOLOGY

AN ESSENTIAL GUIDE TO SPORTS PERFORMANCE

DANIEL CASTILLO ALVIRA, PHD
AND
JAVIER RAYA-GONZÁLEZ, PHD
EDITORS

nova
science publishers
New York

Library of Congress Cataloging-in-Publication Data

Names: Castillo Alvira, Daniel, editor. | Raya-González, Javier, editor.
Title: An essential guide to sports performance / Daniel Castillo Alvira and Javier Raya-González, editors.
Description: Hauppauge, New York : Nova Science Publishers, 2020. | Series: Sports and athletics preparation, performance, and psychology | Includes bibliographical references and index. |
Identifiers: LCCN 2020008325 (print) | LCCN 2020008326 (ebook) | ISBN 9781536176087 (hardcover) | ISBN 9781536176094 (adobe pdf)
Subjects: LCSH: Sports--Physiological aspects. | Soccer--Physiological aspects. | Human mechanics.
Classification: LCC RC1235 .E76 2020 (print) | LCC RC1235 (ebook) | DDC 613.7/1--dc23
LC record available at https://lccn.loc.gov/2020008325
LC ebook record available at https://lccn.loc.gov/2020008326

Published by Nova Science Publishers, Inc. † New York

CONTENTS

PREFACE

This collection investigates hot topics related to sports performance, that is, the match analysis, the training loads, the physical performance, the anthropometric characteristics and the recovery strategies in outfield and goalkeeper soccer players. In addition, this book analyzes the influence of contextual variables and initial players' level on the athletes' performances. Thus, coach staff could find relevant information and practical approaches to include in the soccer training processes. Furthermore, a systematic review of how periodize the training loads troughout a mycrocicle is written to understand the training process substantially. Additionally, this collection focuses on the methodology of muscle force of volleyball players as well as a relevant topic, which could apply to any sports modality, such as the flexibility interventions and protocols to optimize the athletes'' sports performance. Thus, physical trainers of different sports could learn some strategies to enhance the sports performance of their athletes. Finally, considering that cycling is one the most practiced sports around the world, two chapters are prepared to bring both the amateur and professional practioners towards novel sport perspectives. Therefore, one chapter is based on leisure cycling and women's participation in Scotland, and another chapter is developed to improve the saffle height configuration of cyclists to achieve better performance.

Chapter 1 – The match analysis has been particularly increasing and improving their practical applications and the overall body of knowledge. The purpose of this chapter is to present the most recent approaches in match analysis and reveals their practical implications to adjust the training process and also to help coaches to make decisions. The chapter will present a brief review of the observational methodology, tactical analysis, temporal patterns, network analysis and computational measures of collective behavior that have been used in soccer. Each topic will reveal different evidence, measures and practical implications aiming to summarize the main benefits of each approach for practice. All the sections will be focused on an evidence-based approach, thus presenting the main evidence and results observed in the last years

Chapter 2 – The knowledge of the technical demands encountered by goalkeepers during match-play is crucial to design specific soccer training tasks. The aim of this investigation was to examine the influence of situational factors on technical performance indicators of elite goalkeepers competing at the First Spanish Division (*La Liga*). Twenty goalkeepers, who completed a total of 344 matches during the 2018-19 season in the First Spanish Division, participated in this investigation. Technical performance measures, such as goals conceded, goal attempts, saves, clear-outs, successful short passes, successful long passes, and game restarts were registered. The situational variables introduced for the analysis were: game location (home and away), quality of the opponent (Champions League, UEFA, intermediate, and low-level) and match outcome (winner, drawer, and loser). The results provide a more thorough understanding of goalkeeper's performance profiles, what allows to design novel approaches for the goalkeepers' training and development process.

Chapter 3 – Soccer performance is dependent on a multitude of factors and is a multifaceted sport, in which success depends on several physical, technical, and tactical factors. The aims of this investigation were to determine the differences in anthropometric, acceleration, vertical jump and change of direction ability among amateur and professional senior soccer players and describe differences in the anthropometric characteristics and physical performance among playing position. Forty-six male soccer players were divided into 2 groups according to their competitive level and into 6 groups according to their playing position. The evaluation sessions consisted of anthropometric measurements, vertical jump, acceleration and change of direction ability tests. No statistically significant differences were observed between groups in anthropometrics characteristics in means parameters, vertical jump height and change of direction ability. The professional group showed significant better results than the amateur group in 5 m, 15 m, and in vertical jumps. According to position, significant differences were found in both groups in comparison to goalkeepers in 10 m, 15 m and 20 yards tests. The acceleration capacity appeared to distinguish professional and amateur players, reflecting as a discriminate reason according to the competition level and the acceleration capacity (10 and 15 m) and 20 yards change of direction ability test appeared to distinguish among goalkeepers and others playing positions.

Chapter 4 – High-intensity actions in soccer occur mainly during decisive moments of the match-play, pointing out the the key role of high-intensity activities to achieve a great on-field performance. The aim of this study was to analyze the differences in power performance attending to sprint capacity and asymmetry level in young elite soccer players, using a median split analysis to separate faster and slower athletes and players with higher and lower asymmetry scores. Thirty-one young elite male soccer players participated in this study and completed the following physical tests: countermovement jump (CMJ), Abalakov jump (ABK), 30-m linear sprint test, and change of direction sprint test. Faster soccer players performed better in all the speed-power tests, without differences in change of direction deficit (CODd) in comparison to slower players. These findings show the importance of separating young soccer players by their speed performance to identify its specific training needs, as well as to reduce the inter-limb asymmetries to improve the capacity to efficiently change direction.

Chapter 5 – Heart rate recovery (HRR) is the rate at which the heart rate (HR) decreases (i.e., the time taken for HR to recover) following a moderate-to-heavy exercise in response to a combination of parasympathetic activation and sympathetic withdrawal. The aim of this study was to check if soccer players with better aerobic fitness have better recovery (both after maximum efforts in laboratory and field tests, and after submaximal efforts at progressive intensities in a field test). Eighty (n=80) young soccer players took part in this study. All players performed a laboratory ergoespirometric maximal test on a treadmill (LabTest) and an incremental intervallic intermittent field test (TIVRE-Soccer© test). Soccer players with better aerobic capacity ($VO_2max \geq 60$ ml/kg/min) present significantly ($p = 0.039$) better HRR after the 30 s laboratory test and significantly ($p = 0.028$) better HRR in recovery stages after the anaerobic threshold in the TIVRE-Soccer© test. It is possible that soccer players with better aerobic fitness could better adapt to maximal or submaximal efforts and, therefore, present a better HRR.

Chapter 6 – In competitive soccer, the organization of the weekly training load (TL) should warrant peak performance in the official match The aim of the study was to review the weekly TL that players are exposed to during in the competitive period while playing one-match a week. Three electronic databases (Pubmed, SPORTdiscus and ProQuest Central) were searched for research articles published up to February 2018. Articles were considered when one-match weekly TL quantification included training and match loads and players′ participation level on both sessions were specified during the regular competitive period in male soccer players. TL arising from the match represented 38% of the weekly differentiated sRPE-TL, being almost the exclusive source of weekly high-speed and sprinting (90-97%) in professional soccer players. The number of weekly training sessions carried out by the team does not seem to influence weekly TL in both professional and young soccer players. TL progressively increased up 4 days after the previous match (i.e., 3 days before the next match) to get reduced up to the day before the competition in professional soccer players, but a clear trend for weekly TL distribution was not apparent for young soccer players. Finally, inter-players training, match and weekly TL variability was lower for young soccer players in comparison to professional soccer players.

Chapter 7 – Successful performance in volleyball often depends on the ability of the individuals to perform high enough high jumps, a good spike and a good landing. The aim of this study is to discover the mechanisms of muscle force generation in spike and to determine the methodology of its development in the training course of the elite volleyball players. Biomechanical and functional analyses of muscle force generation in isometric and dynamic muscle working mode were performed. The study was conducted on a sample of 21 top volleyball players. During the vertical-landing jumps the elite volleyball players synchronize up to 94.7% of the leg extensors motor units. The greatest impact on the enormous increase in muscle force along with the shortening time of its generation in reversible contractions in service is attributed to the disinhibition process at all levels. In accordance with the results of the analysis a muscle force development methodology is suggested in which, in addition to mastering the disinhibition process, the whole set of required parameters is devised, on which the level and muscle force generation velocity depend, on a daily, weekly, monthly and annual basis, applying the appropriate resources and methods for each particular parameter. Within the proposed methodology, a mathematical model of managing training changes in the domain of force is defined.

Chapter 8 – Psychology has increasingly become interested in the study and training of mindfulness and compassion. This chapter focus on the increase interest in mindfulness-based interventions in sport psychology as a way to improve the performance of elite athletes and also in interventions more closely based on compassion, acceptance and commitment approach that want that athletes have a different perspective on their thoughts and feelings, resist attempts to control or suppress them, and engage in behaviour's consistent with desired sport performance and efforts. This approach encourages mindful present- moment acceptance and willingness to be in contact with internal experience, self-compassion, and full engagement of attention and behaviour on valued activities. Overall findings indicate positive and promising results of a Mindful-Compassion and psychological flexibility-based interventions in increasing the dispositional flow state (indirect measure of performance evaluation), and relief from psychological distress associated with competitive tasks and periods of high workload. These approaches appear to be effective in increasing perceived performance measured directly by the athletes and their coaches.

Chapter 9 – This chapter aims to investigate overriding factors that prevent female participation in leisure cycling. There has been little written about the influence of individual attitudes and perceptions of bicycle use and even less has been written about female attitudes. There is a general gap in research in terms of cycle tourism. However, there is even less research that looks at issues related to female constraints in leisure cycling. Shaw (1994) recognized the need to "remove constraints and to encourage increased opportunities for participation," in terms of LTPA. This research combines literature on LTPA gender constraints, cycle tourism and cycling in general to contribute to the limited existing knowledge concerning female cycling constraints. Moreover, in contrast to other papers it considers personal attitudes, as well as objective constraints that previous research has been lacking (Raymore 2002). This paper intends to expose constraints in leisure cycling to better prepare governments and organizations to serve the female market that has a desire to cycle for leisure.

Chapter 10 – An optimal bicycle configuration is crucial to maximize performance and minimize injury risks for both recreational and elite cyclists. The aim of this work was to compare self-reported cycling comfort in recreational cyclists pedaling under three different saddle height configurations. Ten recreational cyclists were asked to self-report their comfort after pedaling under four different saddle height configurations defined by: i) cyclists' self-selected saddle height (Self-selected); ii) anthropometric measures (Anthropometric), iii) static measurement of knee flexion angle (Static); iv) dynamic measurement of knee flexion angle (Dynamic). The highest self-reported comfort was found to be paired with pedaling under saddle height configured based on a dynamic measurement of knee flexion angle. Moreover, comfort reported for pedaling under self-selected saddle height was significantly larger than for Anthropometric and Static conditions. Based on the positive association reported for pedaling discomfort and musculoskeletal problems, our results lead to the suggestion that recreational cyclists should configure their bicycle's saddle height based on dynamic measurement of knee flexion angle in order to avoid injuries.

In: An Essential Guide to Sports Performance ISBN: 978-1-53617-608-7
Editors: Daniel Castillo Alvira et al.

Chapter 1

MATCH ANALYSIS AND ITS APPLICATIONS FOR SOCCER TRAINING

Filipe Manuel Clemente[1,*], Hugo Sarmento[2] and Gibson Praça[3]

[1]Escola Superior Desporto e Lazer, Instituto Politécnico de Viana do Castelo, Rua Escola Industrial e Comercial de Nun'Álvares, Viana do Castelo, Portugal

[2]Research Unit for Sport and Physical Activity, Faculty of Sport Sciences and Physical Education, University of Coimbra, Coimbra, Portugal

[3]Centro de Estudos em Cognição e Ação/UFMG Soccer Science Center, Departamento de Esportes, Escola de Educação Física, Fisioterapia e Terapia Ocupacional, Universidade Federal de Minas Gerais, Belo Horizonte, Brazil

* Corresponding Author's Email: Filipe.clemente5@gmail.com.

ABSTRACT

The purpose of this chapter is to present the most recent approaches in match analysis and reveals their practical implications to adjust the training process and also to help coaches to make decisions. The chapter will present a brief review of the observational methodology, tactical analysis, temporal patterns, network analysis and computational measures of collective behavior that have been used in soccer. Each topic will reveal different evidence, measures and practical implications aiming to summarize the main benefits of each approach for practice. All the sections will be focused on an evidence-based approach, thus presenting the main evidence and results observed in the last years.

Keywords: association football, performance, observational methodology, temporal patterns, social network analysis, tactics, collective organization

INTRODUCTION

The match analysis can be defined as a sub-area of performance analysis that aims to observe, determine, characterize and analyze the individual behavior and the collective organization and dynamics of sports (Sarmento et al. 2014; 2018). In the context of soccer, the match analysis has been particularly increasing and improving their practical applications and the overall body of knowledge (Barreira et al. 2014; Tenga, Mortensholm, and O'Donoghue 2017). Such fact is closely associated with an increase of approaches, techniques, and methodologies that have been applied in match analysis, thus not limiting the process to the common and more traditional observational methodology and notational analysis (Duarte et al. 2012; Travassos et al. 2013; Sarmento et al. 2018).

Globally, match analysis may consider analyzing the individual performance of players and their tactical behavior, the collective organization, and patterns within the team and the inter-personal dynamics that emerge within the team and against the opposite players (Araújo, Silva, and Davids 2015). To analyse all those aspects, there is not a single technique or method that can be used in match analysis. Based on that, it is important to briefly present and describe the opportunities of different techniques and methods that may allow sports scientists and practitioners to apply the more appropriate approaches to answer to their individual and specific questions in the context of their team.

Therefore, the purpose of this chapter is to present the most relevant approaches, techniques, and methods in the match analysis and their possible opportunities for who works in the context of match analysis. The chapter will be organized in (i) observational methodology; (ii) analysis of the tactical behavior; (iii) temporal patterns; (iv) network analysis; and (v) computational metrics. Within each section will be briefly described the principal approaches and scientific evidence. Moreover, some practical examples will be provided aiming to bridge the gap between theory and practice.

OBSERVATIONAL METHODOLOGY

The use of observational methodology for studies in sports has grown exponentially over the past few years. The preference for the use of this methodology is natural, since they are investigations focused on contents in which perceptible behaviors predominate, which are an essential element in this methodology (Anguera 1999; Sarmento 2012). The observation process in sports context implies the realization of objective and reliable procedures in order to give a scientific character to this process. Notwithstanding the enormous diversity of events that happen simultaneously and consecutively in the collective sports games end up hindering the observation registration process (Sarmento 2012). Therefore, in the sense of a closer approximation of the objectification of the observed actions in the scope of this type of games, based on the "bond" or invariance, on the one hand, and by the chaos and variations or disorder (i.e., by the randomness and variability that characterize it), on the other hand, it is of fundamental importance the definition and precise delineation of models to guide the observation (Lopes 2007).

Thus, it becomes clear that behavior will only become the object of scientific investigation if its recording and quantification are done objectively and actively. It should be noted that in many situations the only way to study behavior without distorting it excessively is to observe it as it occurs spontaneously in context (Sarmento 2012). By the way, Anguera (Anguera 2009) states that observation in sport needs a clear definition of its scope of activity, particularly in two areas: content, and process, or methodology.

It is in this context that the observational methodology exposes its full potential, since the multiple characteristic variables of the behaviors in a competitive situation, the interaction that takes place between them and the difficulty in controlling the contextual variables, never identical in the various situations, recommend the use of this methodology, which, from the point of view mentioned above, opens the door to the description and analysis of socio-driving dynamics from the logic of scientific research (Egaña et al. 2005).

The observational methodology that develops in natural contexts (e.g., a football match), consists of a scientific procedure in which the occurrence of perceptible behaviors in context stands out, to proceed with its organized registration and its analysis, both qualitative and through the use of an appropriate instrument based on suitable criteria and parameters, enabling the detection of the diverse relationships between them and an evaluation of them. These behaviors, due to the spontaneous or habitual form in which they occur, will reveal all the elements that will need to be highlighted to achieve their proper objectification (Anguera 2003). In the context of collective sports games, the possibilities of application of this methodology are massive, being able to focus as much on the nature of the events of the game as on the dynamics of their interaction, contemplating a perspective that can be group or individual (Anguera 1992).

Research in the field of match analysis has traditionally focused on analyzing quantitative rather than qualitative data. Nevertheless, over the last few years, studies that propose innovative methodologies in order to increasingly highlight qualitative processes have proliferated (Sarmento et al. 2016; Anguera et al. 2017) which reliably allow coaching and data analysts to represent the regularities that emerge from the chaotic nature of the game. Such studies are based on the use of specific observational methodology and software such as SDIS-GSEG and Théme.

Specifically in the context of football, the proliferxation of studies that use the observational methodology to investigate the game's contents has focused mainly on the offensive process analysis, and fewer on the defensive process or on the goalkeeper analysis. Networks (see Figure 1). In order to carry out these investigations, the authors mainly used sequential analysis, polar coordinates or T-patterns analysis as stated in the review published by Sarmento and colleagues (Sarmento et al. 2013).

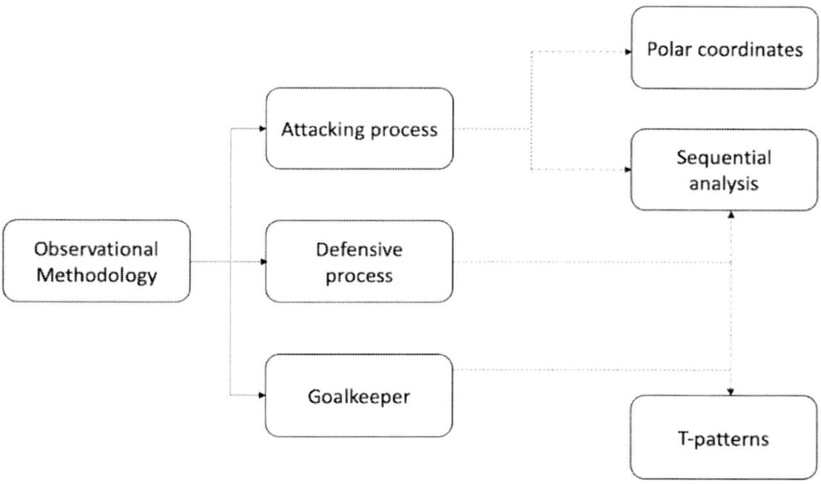

Figure 1. Categorization of game analysis studies according to methodological design and type of variables analyzed (adapted from Sarmento and colleagues (Sarmento et al. 2013)).

Interestingly, it has been found that most of the studies published in this field have been carried out by a community of Portuguese and Spanish authors. However, progressively, these methodological issues have also received attention from scientific communities in other countries, and their use by Brazilian, Italian, Icelandic authors, among others.

Considering the potential of this methodology, the development of studies in this field seems to be fruitful, and it is desirable that the investigations develop in this area include, in their analyzes, the situational variables, namely the match location, match status, match half, quality of opposition, among others which, with few exceptions, have not been included in studies of this nature (Sarmento et al. 2013).

Analysing the Tactical Behavior

In a soccer context, players constantly face problem-solving situations, in which the processes of option-generation and decision-making are demanded (Serra-Olivares et al. 2015). At this point, it seems mandatory to include, during the training process, situations in which these decisional processes are emphasized in order to develop players' ability to make the right choices in game-based situations (Práxedes et al. 2019), which is understood as a tactical behavior. The correctness of these actions (understood here as behaviors) is comprehended as the tactical performance (Praça et al. 2017a). Considering the relevance of the tactical actions within a soccer context, the assessment of players' tactical behavior and performance during both training and competition is important to provide coaches with qualified information that may be used to better systematize the training process. The richest is the information about players' tactical behavior, the more specific may be designed the training tasks, which increases the effectiveness of the whole training process.

A frequent problem faced by researchers and coaches when looking for analyzing players' tactical behavior and performance in soccer was the lack of validated and specific instruments considering the internal logic of the soccer. Historically, this analysis was based on instruments that were validated for team sports in general, such as the Game Performance Assessment Instrument (GPAI) (Memmert and Harvey 2008; Oslin, Mitchell, and Griffin 1998) or the Team Sport Assessment Procedure (TSAP) (Gréhaigne, Godbout, and Bouthier 1997). These instruments provide important information about players' tactical skills, mainly for the ones in the initial process of deliberate practice, when only general structures of knowledge are developed. Both GPAI and TSAP were largely used in the literature, although they lack specificity for soccer context, which is more evident when talking about top-level players and those in older youth academies, which are supposed to have a good level of knowledge about general tactical principles measured by these instruments. On the other hand, the System of Tactical Assessment in Soccer (FUT-SAT), which has been recently proposed in the literature (Costa et al., 2011), provides information about the knowledge about specific concepts of soccer, called "core tactical principles". By adopting this instrument, the previously presented problem of specificity of the instruments is supposed to be overcome.

Table 1. Core tactical principles and its definitions (Costa et al. 2011)

Sub-categories	Variables	Definitions
Offensive	Penetration	Movement of player with the ball towards the goal line
	Offensive coverage	Offensive supports to the player with the ball
	Depth mobility	Movement of players between the last defender and goal line
	Width and length	Movement of players to extend and use the effective play-space
	Offensive unity	Movement of the last line of defenders towards the offensive midfield, in order to support offensive actions of the teammates
Defensive	Delay	Actions to slow down the opponent's attempt to move forward with the ball
	Defensive coverage	Positioning of off-ball defenders behind the "delay" player, providing defensive support
	Balance	Positioning of off-ball defenders in reaction to movements of attackers, trying to achieve the numerical stability or superiority in the opposition relationship
	Concentration	Positioning of off-ball defenders to occupy vital spaces and protect the scoring area
	Defensive unity	Positioning of off-ball defenders to reduce the effective play-space of the opponents

The FUT-SAT is characterized as an observational tool, used to assess players' behavior and performance in regard to tactical principles (Table 1). Tactical principles may be understood as the general rules that guide players' decisions during the game (Garganta and Pinto 1994). The core tactical principles proposed by the FUT-SAT can be divided into offensive and defensive ones. The box below presents the definition for all of them. This instrument may be applied in two different contexts: a standardized field test, in which players may be tested for their tactical skills and compared in-between; and an observational set of principles, which may be used to understand the impact of different training contexts with Small-sided and Conditioned Games (SSCG) on players' behavior. The macro category of the FUT-SAT comprises three different dimensions: the tactical principles, the place of the action in the game field, and the action outcome (Costa et al., 2011). For the purpose of this chapter, we will discuss the use of the first category in different scientific-based contexts.

FUT-SAT Field Test

The standardized field test of the FUT-SAT is a game-based task, played in a 3vs3 format, in a field of 36x27 with small goals (6x2m). All the official rules of the modality must be applied. This field test allows researchers and coaches to easily compare players (for example, from different positions), and, most importantly, to analyze the long-term effect of the training process by applying regularly the same format throughout a season, for example. In fact, this later example has been demonstrated recently in the literature (Praça et al., 2017), and results showed three interesting issues regarding the tactical development of youth soccer players: this development is not a linear process, so decreases may be expected because, for example, maturational processes; there are differences in the development when comparing different categories, so coaches must adapt the training process for each group of athletes; and, finally, a large inter-subject variation is expected, what increases the importance of individually adjusting training contents.

Another issue that has been extensively investigated by the use of the FUT-SAT field test is the influence of playing position on players' tactical behavior. At this point, an interesting result that is consensual in the literature is that, although the 3vs3 small-sided game represents a non-specific context for positional decisions (i.e., players are demanded to act irrespective to their positional status in the formal game), players' tactical behavior is position-specific. This indicates that the knowledge about the game constrains players' actions even in less-specific scenarios. Specifically, it has been shown that midfielders are the most prominent players in offering defensive coverage (Praça et al. 2018), which is also expected in official matches. Also, defenders and midfielders performed more delay actions than forwards (Praça and Greco 2019), which is also in line with the specificities of official matches. Besides, few differences between positions were observed when young players (U-13) were evaluated (Padilha, Moraes, and Teoldo 2013), although more differences were observed in older players, such as U-17 (Praça, Pérez-Morales, and Greco 2016). This reinforces the rationale that the knowledge about acting as a defender or as a midfielder (just as examples) is developed as a result of the long-term training process, not an innate issue. In summary, a coach may use the data provided by the FUT-SAT to assess the development of specific tactical skills regarding the different playing positions.

Finally, FUT-SAT has been used to compare the tactical behavior of different ages. At this point, it has been shown that the tactical performance of the players, which is calculated by the percentage of successful tactical actions, increases from U-11 to U-17 (Américo et al. 2016; Borges et al. 2017). This increased tactical performance may be associated with better management of the space by the players, resulting from the knowledge acquired during the years of practice. The better tactical management of the space of the game is also confirmed by the higher incidence and percentage of successful actions of width and length performed by the older players (Costa, Almeida, and Teoldo 2015; Américo et al. 2016). Considering all these results together, the FUT-SAT seems sufficiently sensitive to capture the long-term changes in regard to players' tactical skills, which confirms its usefulness for talent identification and development in soccer youth academies.

Tactical Behavior in Different SSCG

Considering the observational characteristic of the FUT-SAT, it has been extensively used in the literature to investigate whether changing the small-sided and conditioned game rules, pitch size and number of players impact players' tactical behavior and performance. In general, these researches are justified by the need to provide the coach with enough information to adequate choose between format A or B for each training aim. For example, imagine that your session aim is to develop players' ball circulation skills, a skill strongly based on their ability to create passing possibilities in width, reducing the possibility of the defending team to create a numerical superiority situation. Which SSCG would you choose: a 1-floater format, in which the same floater is used by both teams, inside the pitch, or a 2-floater format, in which each team has its own floater, who starts its action when the team recovers the ball possession always from the own midfield? These situations are represented in the Figure 2.

This specific problem has been recently investigated using the FUT-SAT observational items (Praça et al. 2019). The authors compared the incidence of each core tactical principle between these two formats. Results indicated a higher frequency of width and length actions in the 2-floaters format. This result may be explained by the facility created by the presence of the floater starting the offensive process from the own half, always with a clear passing line, that allowed the teammates to move in-width more frequently. So, as a coach, you should prefer the 2-floater format to develop players' ball circulation ability instead of the traditional 1-floater format.

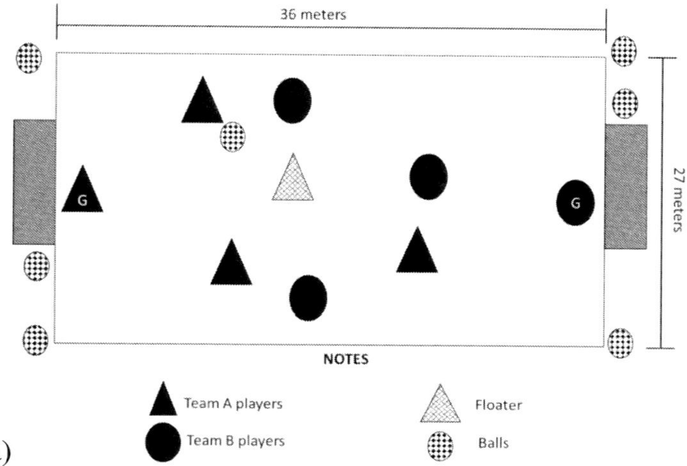

(a)

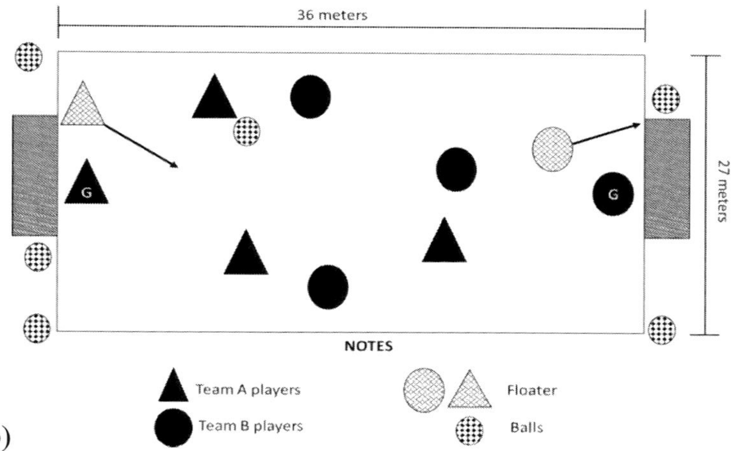

(b)

Figure 2. 1-floater SSCG (a) and 2-floater SSCG (b).

Another format of SSCG that was previously investigated in the literature was the numerical superiority. Contrary to the use of floaters, the numerical superiority condition is characterized by a situation in which one of the teams, often the one in the attack, has a higher number of players than the other, often the one in the defense, and all players with the team with more players are allowed to score points. The use of offensive numerical situations is expected to increase players' zonal marking skills since the man-to-man marking is not enough when the opposing team has more players them my one. In a study that compared the tactical behavior of the players between the 3vs3 and 4vs3 formats, it was found that the numerical superiority situation increased the incidence of offensive unity and depth mobility, which are principles that often occur far from the game center while increasing the frequency of defensive coverage actions (Praça and Greco 2019). These results indicate that the team with a higher number of players adopted a more exploratory behavior, trying to unbalance the defending team, which, in turn, tried to support the player in a delay action, which indicates a more collective defending style.

The influence of the team composition criteria has also been investigated using the FUT-SAT. A study compared the percentage of successful tactical actions when teams were balanced by three different criteria: players' aerobic power, speed performance, or tactical skills (Praça et al. 2017b). Results showed that when teams were composed considering the tactical skills, all players (including those with a lower general tactical skill) increased their tactical performance. This indicates that playing with teammates with a similar tactical level is a more "familiar" context, which may be explored by coaches in order to facilitate the comprehension of tactical principles during the training process.

Another recently investigated issue was the influence of the limitation of ball touches allowed per possession on players' tactical behavior and performance. At this point, the authors conducted two different SSCG: free-play and 2-touches SSCG (Sousa et al. 2019). The most interesting result was the increased defensive tactical performance observed in the 2-touches condition in comparison to the free-play. Coaches usually adopt the 2-touches condition with specific aims to the offensive phase, often related to stablish a ball circulation pattern. However, the adoption of this rule has also impacted the defensive performance, facilitating the decisional process of the players since it has reduced the number of available options for the players with the ball. Therefore, coaches must adopt this rule also when the complexity of the session is higher for the players on the defensive side, creating a pedagogical suitable environment for tactical development.

Finally, the influence of pitch size on players' tactical behavior has also been investigated in the literature (Costa et al. 2011). At this point, the authors have investigated the incidence of core tactical principles in two different pitch sizes: 36x27m and 27x18m. The most interesting result was the higher frequency of defensive coverage actions in the smaller pitch (a difference of 73.34%). Apparently, larger pitches increase the difficulty for the players to offer support to the player that realizes a delay action because of the distance that needs to be covered. So, a pedagogical progression for teaching the principle of defensive coverage should be characterized by a systematic increase in the pitch size, since the larger is the pitch, the harder it is to support the players.

In summary, the FUT-SAT has been proved as a reliable and specific instrument for analyzing players' tactical behavior and performance in soccer. Coaches are encouraged to adopt this instrument in two different situations: firstly, it should be used to systematically test players' tactical skills, which can be useful to adapt training contents to the current needs of the players. Besides, coaches can use this instrument to create a training catalog with different SSCG used in his/her specific team, so he/she can easily choose between the various available formats which one has, at a specific moment, the most adequate level of difficulty for the players and which one emphasizes the tactical principles that are aimed for each training session.

Temporal Patterns

Investigation in football match analysis was substantiated mostly through studies which focused on the description of activity profile, or in the quantification of performed actions in an attempt to quantify the football players' activity. These types of studies, which have been based on the analysis of the frequency of various performance indicators, provide useful information for coaches and practitioners, enabling advances in training processes. Nevertheless, football is characterized by great complexity, which makes it difficult to objectify its observation and analysis (Anguera 1999).

In this sense, and with the purpose of overcoming usual limitations found in strictly qualitative investigations, an increase in the amount of research on game action in football has been observed, based on observational methodology and through various methodological procedures, such as sequential analysis or T-pattern analysis. Notwithstanding the fact that soccer is an arbitrary game and partially determined by chance, this kind of analysis, when it is focused in the sequence of events, allows for the detection of behaviour sequences (play patterns), which have higher probabilities of occurrence than mere chance (Sarmento 2012).

Trying to predict future performance in football on the basis of previous performances is an important goal for those who intend to catapult your team/athlete's performance levels to another level. Typically, the basis for any prediction model is that performance is repeatable, to some degree. In other words, events that have previously occurred will occur again in some predictable manner. As stated by James (2006) this type of prediction is based on the principle that any performance is a consequence of factors like prior learning, inherent skills, and situational variables. In order to detect regular structures of behaviour, sequential analysis and T-pattern analysis has already been used to establish playing patterns in football. The basic premise here is that the interactive flow or chain of behaviour is governed by structures of variable stability which can be visualized by detecting these patterns (Sarmento 2012).

Of the previously mentioned, one promising area of research that has been recently employed at investigating common movement patterns in team sports is T-pattern analysis (Borrie, Jonsson, and Magnusson 2002). The possibility of studying hidden regular structures of behaviour emerged after Magnusson study of the existing methods and software and running into their limitations regarding the analysis of naturally occurring behaviour as complex real-time processes, set out to develop new structural concepts and tools and in particular for the discovery of hidden patterns of behaviour (Magnusson 2000). The detection algorithm used in the software Theme allows the detection of repeated temporal and sequential structures in real-time behaviour records that cannot be fully detected through unaided observation or with the help of statistical methods (Jonsson et al. 2006). A temporal pattern can be defined as a combination of events, which occur, in the same order with temporal distances between each other, which remain relatively invariant in relation to the null hypothesis that each component is independent and is distributed randomly in time (Camerino et al. 2012). As stated by Magnusson (Magnusson 2000) “that is, if A is an earlier and B a later component of the same recurring temporal pattern then after an occurrence of A at t, there is an interval [t+d1, t +d2] (d2≥d1≥d0) that tends to contain at least one occurrence of B more often than would be expected by chance”.

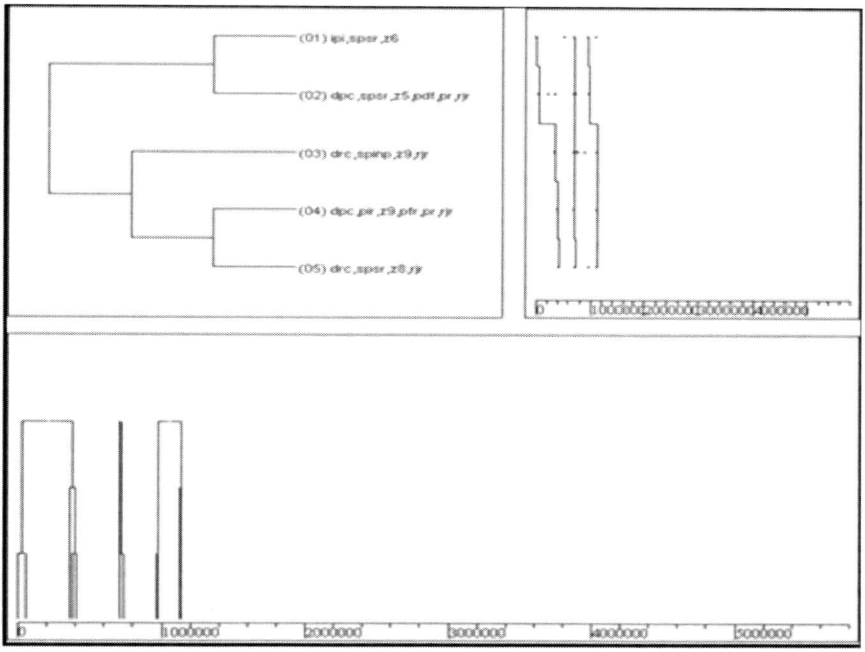

Figure 3. Diagram of the T-Pattern 1 – F.C. Barcelona (adapted from Sarmento and colleagues (Sarmento et al. 2014)).

In order to demonstrate how this type of analysis can help coaches in detecting regular structures of behavior, we present an example of a study developed with top level football teams, more specifically, in the actions of counter-attack of the F.C. Barcelona and Manchester United Football teams (Sarmento et al. 2014). In this study, 24 games (12 per team) from the sporting season 2009/2010 of the F.C. Barcelona and Manchester United teams were analyzed. The matches were analysed through systematic observation by using a specific instrument to observe the offensive process (Sarmento 2012). For the detection of temporal patterns, the software THÈME 5.0 was used, and the following criteria established: the minimum number of times a pattern must occur to be detected was set at 3 and the level of significance was set at 0.05. The data analysis revealed the existence of 787 different T-patterns in the team of the FC Barcelona, ranging from a minimum of 1 level to a maximum of 6 levels and a minimum of 2 events to a maximum of 9 events. For this chapter, we selected 1 t-patterns to present the diagrams an how analyze the information that allow us to elaborate the visual presentations of this pattern of play in the field of the game (Sarmento 2012).

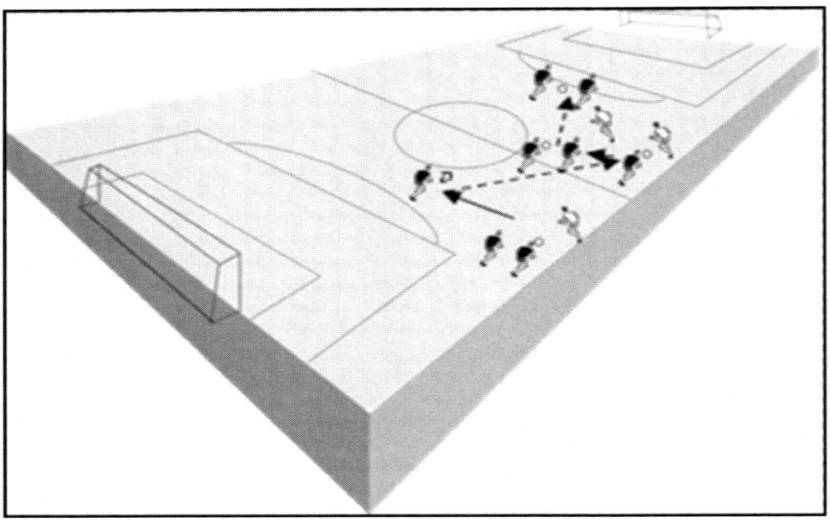

Figure 4. Visual representation of T-Pattern 1 – F.C. Barcelona (adapted from Sarmento and colleagues (Sarmento et al. 2014)).

The pattern of play (Figures 3 and 4) represents an incomplete T-pattern (it does not include the end of the offensive process) in relation to the start of a counterattack sequence (this pattern occurred three times). This counterattack: 1) was initiated by an interception of the ball in the left corridor (zone 6) in an interaction context of numerical superiority, 2) followed by a short pass (diagonally forward) in the central defensive midfield (zone 5) in a context of numerical superiority; 3) a player performed the reception/control of the ball (zone 9) in a interaction context of numerical equality, 4) and then, the sequence developed through a short pass (diagonally forward) performed in zone 5 (numerical inferiority); 5) this pass is followed by a reception/control of the ball by a colleague in zone 8 (numerical superiority).

The results of this study published by Sarmento and colleagues (Sarmento et al. 2014) show that many temporal patterns exist in football, namely in the studied teams. The number (787, 188, respectively), frequency (at least three repetitions for each of the previously mentioned patterns) and complexity (ranging from 1 to 6 and 1 to 5 levels, respectively) of the identified patterns indicate that sport behavior is more synchronized than the "human eye" can detect. Thus, this type of analysis allows coaches, players and practitioners to know and to characterize the regular structures of offensive sequences in football teams. The T-patterns detected in these successful teams allowed us to know how that process is developed in an effective way. This information can be relevant, on the one hand for the team itself because it makes it possible to design training exercises in order to increase this efficacy, and on the other hand it allows, for example, that the opponent coaches can training specific strategies to prevent that the Barcelona and Manchester United teams perform these transitions effectively (Sarmento et al. 2014).

Network Analysis

The application of social network analysis (SNA) in soccer has been growing, in particular, since ten years ago (Duch, Waitzman, and Amaral

2010; Grund 2012; Clemente et al. 2013; Clemente et al. 2015; Clemente et al. 2019). SNA uses concepts from graph theory to determine and characterize the properties of a group, sub-group or agents within a network (Barnes and Harary 1983). The use of SNA is extended to different field of knowledge, namely sociology, psychology or biology (Mason and Verwoerd 2007; Nieminen 1974; Cummings and Cross 2003). In the case of sports, there are different applications namely in the study of collective organization and leaderships in a sociological point-of-view (Bourbousson et al. 2010; Lusher, Robins, and Kremer 2010), sports tourism (Wäsche 2015) or match analysis (McHale and Relton 2018; Clemente 2018; Ramos et al. 2017).

Despite different approaches or conceptions about the topic, it can be organized the use of SNA and their associated measures in three types of levels of match analysis (Clemente, Martins, and Mendes 2016): (i) micro level or centralities; (ii) meso level of inter-dependencies; and (iii) macro level or characterization of the group. Each of the levels of analysis depends on the way how the measures are used and, for that reason, it is our aim to briefly present the more commonly used in the context of soccer analysis.

Network Centralities

Within the micro level of analysis or centralities, it is very common to use the indegree and outdegree measures (Wasserman and Faust 1994). The outdegree measure (also called by degree centrality) represents the level of participation of a player in to establish connections with remaining teammates, thus globally representing that higher levels of degree centrality means that the player was very active in to pass the ball from his teammates (Clemente, Martins, and Mendes 2016). Some studies have been compering the degree centrality levels of different playing positioning during official matches (Clemente et al. 2015; Clemente et al. 2019; Peña and Touchette 2012; Duch, Waitzman, and Amaral 2010). Usually, when considering the overall match (all the passing sequences of a team) the midfielders and the external defenders are the most prominent players in to pass the ball, however in the cases that the analysis is split in moments it is possible to observe that the level of degree centrality varies namely in situations of counter-attack (Malta and Travassos 2014). The degree centrality was also tested aiming to identify the most active regions in the pich from which the passing sequences that resulted in scored and conceded goals started (Clemente, Martins, and Mendes 2016). In that study, it was found that the last third of attacking and the zones immediately before the penalty-box were the regions in which the greater number of passes started in sequences that resulted in scored goals (Clemente, Martins, and Mendes 2016).

The indegree centrality (also known as degree prestige) is another very typical measure used in the context of match analysis. This measure represents the number of "nominations" that a given player has from its teammates, thus in the context of passing sequences represents the balls received. Considering the studies that analyzed the overall passing sequences, it is possible to observe that midfielders and external defenders have the greater levels (Clemente et al. 2015; Peña and Touchette 2012). However, this varies in circunstances of balance or unbalance score, namely forwards increases the degree prestige in favorable unbalanced scores (Clemente et al. 2019). Moreover, strikers and wingers are the players with greater degree prestige in passing sequences counducted in counter-attack situations (Malta and Travassos 2014) or during passing sequences that only resulted in goals (Clemente, Martins, and Mendes 2016). A study that also researched the regions of the pitch with greater degree prestige found that the center of attack midfield and the middle of penalty-box were the most prominent in passing sequences that resulted in scored goals (Clemente, Martins, and Mendes 2016).

Two other inresting measures commonly used in the studies about SNA in match analysis are the clustering coefficient and the betweenness centrality. The betweenness centrality quantifies how often a player lies between other teammates within the network, possibly acting as a "mediator" or a link between their colleagues (Clemente, Martins, and Mendes 2016). The clustering cofficient identify how close a player and its temmates may become a sub-group, thus representing a small-world network within the team (Clemente, Martins, and Mendes 2016). Usually, greater levels of betweenness can be observed in midfielders or lateral defenders. Such fact was reported in a study conducted in the FIFA World Cup 2010 in which the greater values were observed in Van Bommel (The Netherlands, midfielder) and Schweinsteiger (Germany, midfielder), Capdevila (Spain, lateral defender) (Peña and Touchette 2012). In the same study (Peña and Touchette 2012), Xavi (Spain, midfielder), Van Bronckhorst (The Netherlands, lateral defender) and Trochowski (Germany, attacking midfielder) were the players with greater clustering coefficients. Such fact, indicates that, generally, midfielders and lateral defenders are the players that intermediate the passing sequences in the teams and that may creat small-groups within the team during those passing sequences.

In a practical perspective, match analysts or sports scientists within a match analysis department may use these easy-to-use and interesting measures to determine the centralities within a team, namely considering specific moments of the match. Naturally, an analysis of all passing sequences may not provide specific information for coaches. However, a split by attacking moments (positional attack based on passing sequences or counter-attack) or critical moments (goals scored, goals conceded, shots, attacks with success) may provide interesting information about the most prominent players in the specific moments and possibly provide information to coaches to make decisions about which players should play in specific contexts or how to built drills to promote changes in the dynamics of the team.

Inter-Dependencies

Relationships between teammates within the match can be also quantified by using SNA (Li and Horvath 2007). Despite that, there is few examples of the applications in the context of soccer (Clemente et al. 2014). In a study that used five matches as proof-of-concept, it was possible to observe an application of the topological overlap measure and the topological inter-dependency to identify the connections between pairs of teammates (Clemente et al. 2014). The topological overlap, briefly, represents the pair of temmates that cooperates with the same players even in cases of no participation in the same unit of attack (passing sequence) (Clemente et al. 2014). Moreover, the authors (Clemente et al. 2014) also proposed a new measure designated as topological inter-dependency that, birefly, identifies the dependencies between teammates.

In the above mentioned study (Clemente et al. 2014) it was possible to observe that the most independent players (with fewer dependence levels from their teammates) were the midfielders, thus suggesting that these players can connect with any other player easily than other playing positions. On the other hand, external defenders and strikers were more dependent from their teammates to participate in the attacking units, thus revealing that both positions may depend from the "link" players that connect the defensive and attacking lines of the team (Clemente et al. 2014).

One different measure that may be also introduced in a meso-level of analysis is the scaled connectivity (Horvath 2011). This measure can be used to provide information about the level of a given player in interact with the most of his temmates (Clemente et al. 2014). Using this measure, it was possible to observe that the most "connected" players were the external defenders and midfielders in a context of a small sample of five matches analysed (Clemente et al. 2014). On the opposite way, strikers and central defenders presented the lower values of scaled connectivity.

One more measure that can be used in the context of soccer analysis is the reciprocity (Squartini et al. 2013). This measure quantifies the level of dyad reciprocity in the fraction of pair of players that have reciprocited ties over all pairs of players that have any established link (Clemente, Martins, and Mendes 2016). In a study that tested the matches of the FIFA World Cup 2018 it was possible to observe that the mean level of reciprocity varied between 11 and 14% (Filipe Manuel Clemente 2018).

Depiste of the very few examples of studies (Clemente et al. 2014; Clemente 2018) conducted with an inter-dependency level of analysis, it may be really interesting for practical contexts use these concepts namely because may quantify the players that may be independent and the ones that need more connections from their teammates to participate in the units of attack.

General Network Measures

Some general network measures have been used to characterize the level of overall interaction between teammates. Among others, the total links, network density, network heterogeneity or network centralization are the most commonly tested in the case of soccer and match analysis (Grund 2012; Clemente et al. 2015; Clemente et al. 2015; Clemente 2018).

The total links is a simple key concept that, briefly, represents the maximal number of bideiractional interactions among the teammates within a network (Clemente, Martins, and Mendes 2016). This measure, despite simple, is positively correlated with the goals scored and shots on goal and, in a comparison between succeded and non-succeded teams in FIFA World Cup 2014, it was found that more succeded teams also present higher values of total links (Clemente et al. 2015). This measure may also be useful in practical context to compare the variations within the team during periods of the match or between matches.

The network density is also a well-known measure that represents the proportion of the maximum possible lines (passes) present between nodes (players) (Clemente et al. 2015). In two studies conducted in the FIFA World Cup tournaments (Clemente 2018; Clemente et al. 2015) it was possible to observe small and moderate positive correlations between network density and total shots. Despite that, winners seems only have small increases of network density comparing to losers (Clemente 2018).

Two other key concepts in general network measures are the network heterogeneity and centralization (Clemente et al. 2015; Grund 2012). Concisely, the network heterogeneity is closely related to the variation of connectivity among the players and quantifies the possibilities of a team constitute sub-groups within the group (Clemente et al. 2015). The network centralization provides information about the variation of centralities within a team, representing the possibilities of a team be more homogenous in the centralities of the players or more heteregoneus (Clemente et al. 2015). Both, heterogeneity and centralization concepts are, therefore, closely related.

In a study conducted in some English Premier League soccer teams it was possible to observe that increases in the network centralization lead to decrease in team performance (Grund 2012). However, some caution should be made regarding the inferences to the practice, because a team is, in nature, heterogenous and relatively centralized considering the tendencies of moving forward and dynamics that make to emerge specific positions. Therefore, more than compare between teams, the general network measures should be used to compare the variations of the same team in different playing scenarios and matches. Possibly, some specific training drills can be also tested, namely using some variations in the squad or dynamics to understand the effects in the overall capacity to optimize specific collective behaviors.

Computational Metrics

The use of tracking systems (e.g., global positioning system, multicamera tracking system, radio frequency identification) alowed to get information about the specific position of players in a cartesian plane (Memmert, Lemmink, and Sampaio 2017). Such fact, contributed to increase the possibilities in match analysis, namely aiming to use the position data to analyse the collective organization of the teams in specific moments of the match (Duarte et al. 2012; Clemente et al. 2014).

Different position data-based measures have been proposed in the last decade, however we can organize them in the following categories (Clemente et al. 2017): (i) metrics to measure the center of the team; (ii) metrics to measure the dispersion of the players; and (iii) metrics to identify the tactical behavior of the players.

Geometrical Center of the Team

The metrics that aim to analyze the center of the team are mainly focused in to identify the geographical middle point of the team considering that the teams are constituted by different players positioned in the pitch. One of the first proposals, known as geometrical center, was based on the Euclidian distance of the players (Yue et al. 2008). This measure excluded the goalkeepers and fundamentally was used in further studies to analyse the oscillations of the middle point of the team during the matches or in specific moments of the match (Bartlett et al. 2012) or to analyse the inter-team coordination tendencies in temporal series (Frencken et al. 2012). A different approach, with the same objective, was conceived by Clemente et al. (2014) adjusting the relevance of each player for the team centroid/geometrical center based on his distance to the ball. Generally, both approaches identify the center of the team and ultimately are mainly focused in to understand the dynamics of the geometrical center during the match and its relationships with the opponents. Also using the concept of geometrical center it was also proposed the measure of longitudinal and lateral inter-team distances that, essentially, calculate the difference between the positions of the geometrical centers of both teams (Frencken et al. 2012). One more approach using the concept of geometrical center was purposed to test a cross-correlation between the movement of the two teams in the match, being observed that, usually, both teams are synchronized for most of the match time (Silva et al. 2016).

Dispersion of the Team

Measuring the dispersion of the teammates during the match and identify how the spaces are created is also one of the concerns from who wants to use the computational metrics to analyze the match. One of the first concepts was the stretch index that, briefly, is calculated based on the average distance of the players to the geometrical center (Bourbousson, Sève, and McGarry 2010). A derived measure was also proposed by

Clemente et al. (2013) adjusting the distance to the weighted geometrical center of the team. Both measures can be used to quantify how stretch are the players from their geometrical center of the team.

Also aiming to quantify the dispersion of the players, the concept of surface area was proposed, essentially consisting in to define the area of the polygon generated by the positioning of the players in the pitch (Frencken et al. 2011). This measure allows not only to represent how stretch are the players, but also to quantify the area covered by the players in a specific moment (Bartlett et al. 2012). The surface area was also used in a study to determine the typical space covered by a team and translate such information for small-sided games design (Caro et al. 2019; Fradua et al. 2013).

Using easiest but also interesting concepts, the team length and the team width and the length per width ratio were introduced aiming to measure the most advanced and rear players for the length and its rightmost and leftmost players for the length (Clemente et al. 2017). These concepts may help to characterize the mobility of the team and the longitudinal and lateral dispersion on the pitch in a easy-to-use fashion (Duarte et al. 2013; Folgado et al. 2014).

Tactical Behavior

The concept of tactical behavior may not be easily associated with the use of computational metrics. However, some actions associated with the behaviors can be quantified by using position-data.

The teams' separateness was proposed by Silva et al. (2016) to calculate the sum of the distances between each of the team's players and their closest opponents. This measure can be useful to identify which kind of formats of play or pitch sizes should be used for specific situations, namely to test the possibilities of creating more or less distance in relation to the opponents (Clemente et al. 2017).

Considering the relationships between players within the team, it is possible to highlight the intra-team coordination tendencies that have been suggested to calculate the percentage of time spent in-phase between pairs of teammates to identify the levels of synchronization (Folgado et al. 2014). This measure can be really useful to control the capacity of the players to coordinate their movements within the team in pursuit of a common goal (Clemente et al. 2017).

A basic concept was proposed by Clemente et al. (2014) to analyze the organization of the teammates by sectorial positions (i.e., defensive, midfield and forward sectors). The sectorial lines measure classifies the players by their sector and runs a line within the sector using a first degree polynomial that minimizes the Root Mean Squared Error between the polynomial and the players positions (Clemente et al. 2014). Interestingly, the study that proposed the concept (Clemente et al. 2014) was possible to observe that the lines between sectors act in an independent fashion suggesting that the sectors may act independently from each other. Such fact will vary from the specific moments analyzed and the contexts of data visualization.

Aiming to defined the region occupied by each player (or with the theoretical dominance), the concept of dominant region was proposed using the Voronoi-cells (Taki and Hasegawa 2000). This approach may help to characterize the regions with greater predominance of a player and interpret how the spaces are created or occupied by specific players or playing positions. This can be really interesting in the context of match analysis and to conceive new drills for training context, as well.

Also centering the analysis in the players, the major ranges measure was proposed (Yue et al. 2008) to define an ellipse center considering the average position of a player in the pitch in which the axes are defined by the standard deviation of the player's movements (Clemente et al. 2017). This measure can be particularly interesting to compare the effects of different formats of play or pitch sizes on the division of labor between players or to identify the positioning patterns of player within a match.

Conclusion

This chapter allowed to introduce a set of techniques, methods and instruments can be used by coaches and sports scientists in the daily practice or in more advanced match analysis protocols. Ultimately, the strategy adopted by the staff should be congruent with the vision of the coach and the reports should be easy-to-understand aiming to translate the evidence into the practice. From the observational methodology to the more advanced position-data methods to analyze collective behaviors, the best strategy will be centered on the quality of the information and not in the range or size of the data.

References

Américo, Henrique B., Felippe S. L. Cardoso, Guilherme Figueiredo-Machado, Marcelo O. Cabral de Andrade, Elton Ribeiro-Resende, and Israel T. Costa. 2016. "Analysis of the Tactical Behavior of Youth Academy Soccer Players." *Journal of Physical Education* 27: 1–9. https://doi.org/10.4025/jphyseduc.v27i1.2710.

Anguera, Maria T., Oleguer Camerino, Marta Castañer, Pedro Sánchez-Algarra, and Anthony J. Onwuegbuzie. 2017. "The Specificity of Observational Studies in Physical Activity and Sports Sciences: Moving Forward in Mixed Methods Research and Proposals for Achieving Quantitative and Qualitative Symmetry." *Frontiers in Psychology* 8. https://doi.org/10.3389/fpsyg.2017.02196.

Anguera, M. Teresa. 1992. *Metodología de La Observación En Las Ciencias Humanas*. [*Methodology of observation in the human sciences*.] Madrid: Ediciones Cátedra Teorema.

Araújo, Duarte, Pedro Silva, and Keith Davids. 2015. "Capturing Group Tactical Behaviors in Expert Team Players." In *Routledge Handbook of Sport Expertise*, edited by Joseph Baker and Damian Farrow, 209–20. Abingdon: Routledge.

Barnes, J. A., and Frank Harary. 1983. "Graph Theory in Network Analysis." *Social Networks* 5: 235–44.

Barreira, Daniel, Julio Garganta, Julen Castellano, Joao Prudente, and Maria T. Anguera. 2014. "Evolución Del Ataque En El Fútbol de Élite Entre 1982 y 2010: Aplicación Del Análisis Secuencial de Retardos." ["Evolution of Attack in Elite Soccer Between 1982 and 2010: Application of Sequential Analysis of Delays."] *Revista de Psicología Del Deporte* 23: 139–46.

Bartlett, Roger, Chris Button, Matthew Robins, Aviroop Dutt-Mazumder, and Gavin Kennedy. 2012. "Analysing Team Coordination Patterns from Player Movement Trajectories in Football: Methodological Considerations." *International Journal of Performance Analysis in Sport* 12: 398–424.

Borges, Paulo Henrique, José Guilherme, Leandro Rechenchosky, Luciane Cristina Arantes da Costa, and Wilson Rinadi. 2017. "Fundamental Tactical Principles of Soccer: A Comparison of Different Age Groups." *Journal of Human Kinetics* 58: 207–14. https://doi.org/10.1515/hukin-2017-0078.

Borrie, Andrew, Gudberg K. Jonsson, and Magnus S. Magnusson. 2002. "Temporal Pattern Analysis and Its Applicability in Sport: An Explanation and Exemplar Data." *Journal of Sports Sciences* 20: 845–52. https://doi.org/10.1080/026404102320675675.

Bourbousson, Jerome, Germain Poizat, Jacques Saury, and Carole Seve. 2010. "Team Coordination in Basketball: Description of the Cognitive Connections Among Teammates." *Journal of Applied Sport Psychology* 22: 150–66.

Bourbousson, Jerome, Carole Seve, and Tim McGarry. 2010. "Space-Time Coordination Dynamics in Basketball: Part 2 The Interaction between the Two Teams." *Journal of Sports Sciences* 28: 349–58.

Camerino, Oleguer Foguet, Javier Chaverri, M. Teresa Anguera, and Gudberg K. Jonsson. 2012. "Dynamics of the Game in Soccer: Detection of T-Patterns." *European Journal of Sport Science* 12: 216–24. https://doi.org/10.1080/17461391.2011.566362.

Caro, Oscar, Asier Zubillaga, Luis Fradua, and Javier Fernandez-Navarro. 2019. "Analysis of Playing Area Dimensions in Spanish Professional Soccer." *Journal of Strength and Conditioning Research*, August. https://doi.org/10.1519/JSC.0000000000003226.

Clemente, Filipe. M., Fernando. M. L. Martins, and Rui S. Mendes. 2016. "Analysis of Scored and Conceded Goals by a Football Team throughout a Season: A Network Analysis." *Kinesiology* 48: 103–14.

Clemente, Filipe. M., Fernando. M. L. Martins, Del P. Wong, Dimitris Kalamaras, and Rui. S. Mendes. 2015. "Midfielder as the Prominent Participant in the Building Attack: A Network Analysis of National Teams in FIFA World Cup 2014." *International Journal of Performance*.

Clemente, Filipe M., Micael S. Couceiro, Fernando M. Lourenço Martins, Rui Mendes, and António J Figueiredo. 2013. "Measuring Tactical Behaviour Using Technological Metrics: Case Study of a Football Game." *International Journal of Sports Science & Coaching* 8: 723–39.

Clemente, Filipe M.. 2018. "Performance Outcomes and Their Associations with Network Measures during FIFA World Cup 2018." *International Journal of Performance Analysis in Sport* 18: 1010–23. https://doi.org/10.1080/24748668.2018.1545180.

Clemente, Filipe M., Micael S. Couceiro, Fernando M. L. Martins, Monika Ognyanova Ivanova, and Rui Mendes. 2013. "Activity Profiles of Soccer Players during the 2010 World Cup." *Journal of Human Kinetics* 38: 201–11. http://www.pubmedcentral.nih.gov/articlerender.fcgi?artid=3827759&tool=pmcentrez&rendertype=abstract.

Clemente, Filipe M., Micael S. Couceiro, Fernando Manuel Lourenço Martins, and Rui S. Mendes. 2014. "Using Network Metrics to Investigate Football Team Players ' Connections: A Pilot Study." *Motriz* 20: 262–71. https://doi.org/dx.doi.org/10.1590/S1980-65742014000300004.

Clemente, Filipe M., Fernando M. L. Martins, Dimitris Kalamaras, Del P Wong, and Rui S. Mendes. 2015. "General Network Analysis of

National Soccer Teams in FIFA World Cup 2014." *International Journal of Performance Analysis in Sport* 15: 80–96.

Clemente, Filipe M., Fernando M. L. Martins, and Rui S. Mendes. 2016. *Social Network Analysis Applied to Team Sports Analysis*. Netherlands: Springer International Publishing. https://doi.org/10.1007/978-3-319-25855-3.

Clemente, Filipe M., Hugo Sarmento, Gibson M. Praça, Pantelis T. Nikolaidis, Thomas Rosemann, and Beat Knechtle. 2019. "Variations of Network Centralities Between Playing Positions in Favorable and Unfavorable Close and Unbalanced Scores During the 2018 FIFA World Cup." *Frontiers in Psychology* 10. https://doi.org/10.3389/fpsyg.2019.01802.

Costa, Bruno R. S., Rodrigo F. Almeida, and Israel T. Costa. 2015. "Comparative study of tactical behavior performed by under-13 and under-15 players" *Revista Da Educação Física* 26: 557–66. https://doi.org/10.4025/reveducfis.
v26i4.26830.

Costa, Israel T., Julio Garganta, Pablo J. Greco, Isabel Mesquita, and Ezequiel Muller. 2011. "Relationship between pitch size and tactical behavior of soccer player" *Rev. Bras. Educ. Fís. Esporte* 25: 79–96.

Costa, Israel T., Julio Garganta, Pablo J. Greco, Isabel Mesquita, and Jana Maia. 2011. "System of Tactical Assessment in Soccer (FUT-SAT): Development and Preliminary Validation." *Motricidade* 7: 69–84.

Cummings, Jonathon N., and Rob Cross. 2003. "Structural Properties of Work Groups and Their Consequences for Performance." *Social Networks* 25: 197–210. https://doi.org/10.1016/S0378-8733(02)00049-7.

Duarte, Ricardo, Duarte Araújo, Vanda Correia, and Keith Davids. 2012. "Sports Teams as Superorganisms: Implications of Sociobiological Models of Behaviour for Research and Practice in Team Sports Performance Analysis." *Sports Medicine* 42: 633–42.

Duarte, Ricardo, Duarte Araújo, Hugo Folgado, Pedro Esteves, Pedro Marques, and Keith Davids. 2013. "Capturing Complex, Non-Linear

Team Behaviours during Competitive Football Performance." *Journal of Systems Science and Complexity* 26: 62–72.

Duch, Jordi, Joshua S. Waitzman, and Luis A. Amaral. 2010. "Quantifying the Performance of Individual Players in a Team Activity." *PloS One* 5: e10937.

Egaña, Guillermo-Gorospe, Antonio Hernández-Mendo, Maria T. Anguera, and Raul Martínez-Santos. 2005. "Desarrollo y Optimización de Una Herramienta Observacional En El Tenis de Individuales." ["Development and Optimization of an Observational Tool in Singles Tennis."] *Psicothema* 17: 123–27.

Folgado, Hugo, Ricardo Duarte, Orlando Fernandes, and Jaime Sampaio. 2014. "Competing with Lower Level Opponents Decreases Intra-Team Movement Synchronization and Time-Motion Demands during Pre-Season Soccer Matches." Edited by Jeffrey M. Haddad. *Plos One* 9: e97145. https://doi.org/10.1371/journal.pone.0097145.

Folgado, Hugo, Koen P M Lemmink, Wouter Frencken, and Jaime Sampaio. 2014. "Length, Width and Centroid Distance as Measures of Teams Tactical Performance in Youth Football." *European Journal of Sport Science* 14: S487-92. https://doi.org/10.1080/17461391.2012.730060.

Fradua, Luis, Asier Zubillaga, Oscar Caro, Angel Iván Fernández-García, Carlos Ruiz-Ruiz, and Albin Tenga. 2013. "Designing Small-Sided Games for Training Tactical Aspects in Soccer: Extrapolating Pitch Sizes from Full-Size Professional Matches." *Journal of Sports Sciences* 31: 573–81. https://doi.org/10.1080/02640414.2012.746722.

Frencken, W, K Lemmink, N Delleman, and C Visscher. 2011. "Oscillations of Centroid Position and Surface Area of Football Teams in Small-Sided Games." *European Journal of Sport Science* 11: 215–23.

Frencken, Wouter, Harjo De Poel, Chris Visscher, and Koen Lemmink. 2012. "Variability of Inter-Team Distances Associated with Match Events in Elite-Standard Soccer." *Journal of Sports Sciences* 30: 1207–13. https://doi.org/10.1080/02640414.2012.703783.

Garganta, Julio, and Joao Pinto. 1994. "O Ensino Do Futebol. [Teacing soccer]" In *O Ensino Dos Jogos Desportivos* [*Teaching team sports*], edited by A Graça and J Oliveira, 95–136. Faculdade de Ciências do Desporto e de Educação Física da Universidade do Porto: Rainho & Neves Lda.

Gréhaigne, Jean F., and Paul Godbout. 1997. "Performance Assessment in Team Sports." *Journal of Teaching in Physical Education* 16: 500–516.

Grund, Thomas. 2012. "Network Structure and Team Performance: The Case of English Premier League Soccer Teams." *Social Networks* 34: 682–90.

Horvath, Shaun. 2011. *Weighted Network Analysis: Applications in Genomics and Systems Biology*. New York: Springer.

James, Nic. 2006. "Notational Analysis in Soccer: Past, Present and Future." *International Journal of Performance Analysis in Sport* 6: 67–81. https://doi.org/10.1080/24748668.2006.11868373.

Jonsson, Gudberg K., Maria T. Anguera, Ángel Blanco-Villaseñor, José L. Losada, Antonio Hernández-Mendo, Toni Ardá, Oleguer Camerino, and Julen Castellano. 2006. "Hidden Patterns of Play Interaction in Soccer Using SOF-CODER." *Behavior Research Methods* 38: 372–81. https://doi.org/10.3758/BF03192790.

Li, A., and S. Horvath. 2007. "Network Neighborhood Analysis with the Multi-Node Topological Overlap Measure." *Bioinformatics* 23: 222–31. https://doi.org/10.1093/bioinformatics/btl581.

Lopes, Jose 2007. "*Análise Diacrónica Heterocontingente Dos Métodos de Jogo Ofensivo No Futebol.* [*Heterocontingent Diachronic Analysis Of Offensive Game Methods In Football*]" Universidade do Porto.

Lusher, Dean, Garry Robins, and Peter Kremer. 2010. "The Application of Social Network Analysis to Team Sports." *Measurement in Physical Education and Exercise Science* 14: 211–24. https://doi.org/10.1080/1091367X.2010.495559.

Magnusson, Magnus. 2000. "Discovering Hidden Time Patterns in Behavior: T-Patterns and Their Detection." *Behavior Research Methods, Instruments, & Computers* 32: 93–110.

Malta, Pedro, and Bruno Travassos. 2014. "Characterization of the Defense-Attack Transition of a Soccer Team." *Motricidade* 10: 27–37.

Mason, Oliver, and Mark Verwoerd. 2007. "Graph Theory and Networks in Biology." *IET Systems Biology* 1: 89–119. http://www.ncbi.nlm.nih.gov/pubmed/17441552.

McHale, Ian G., and Samuel D. Relton. 2018. "Identifying Key Players in Soccer Teams Using Network Analysis and Pass Difficulty." *European Journal of Operational Research* 268 : 339–47. https://doi.org/10.1016/j.ejor.2018.01.018.

Memmert, Daniel, and Stephen Harvey. 2008. "The Game Performance Assessment Instrument (GPAI): Somce Concerns and Solutions for Further Development." *Journal of Teaching in Physical Education* 27: 220–40.

Memmert, Daniel, Koen Lemmink, and Jaime Sampaio. 2017. "Current Approaches to Tactical Performance Analyses in Soccer Using Position Data." *Sports Medicine* 47: 1–10. https://doi.org/10.1007/s40279-016-0562-5.

Nieminen, Jurgen. 1974. "On the Centrality in a Graph." *Scandinavian Journal of Psychology* 15: 332–36.

Oslin, Judith L., Stephen A. Mitchell, and Linda L. Griffin. 1998. "The Game Performance Assesment Instrument (GPAI): Development and Preliminary Validation." *Journal of Teaching in Physical Education* 17: 231–43.

Padilha, Maickel B., José C. Moraes, and Israel T. Costa. 2013. "O Estatuto Posicional Pode Influenciar o Desempenho Tático Ente Jogadores Da Categoria Sub-13?" ["Positional Status Can Influence Tactical Performance Among Under-13 Players."] *Revista Brasileira de Ciência e Movimento* 21: 73–79.

Peña, Javier L., and Hugo Touchette. 2012. "A Network Theory Analysis of Football Strategies." In *Sports Physics: Proc. 2012 Euromech Physics of Sports Conference*, edited by C. Clanet, 517–28. Palaiseau, France: 'Editions de l'\'Ecole Polytechnique, Palaiseau.

Praça, Gibson M., Juan C. Pérez-Morales, Pedro E. D. Moreira, Gustavo H. C. Peixoto, Sarah T. Bredt, Mauro H. Chagas, Israel T. Costa, and

Pablo J. Greco. 2017a. "Tactical Behavior in Soccer Small-Sided Games: Inluence of Team Composition Criteria." *Brazilian Journal of Kinanthropometry and Human Performance* 19. https://doi.org/10.5007/1980-0037.2017v19n3p354.

Praça, Gibson M., Juan C. Pérez-Morales, Pedro E. D. Moreira, Gustavo Henrique Cunha Peixoto, Sarah Teles Bredt, Mauro Heleno Chagas, Israel T., and Pablo J. Greco. 2017b. "Tactical Behavior in Soccer Small-Sided Games: Influence of Team Composition Criteria." *Revista Brasileira de Cineantropometria & Desempenho Humano* 19: 354–63. https://doi.org/10.5007/1980-0037.2017v19n3p354.

Praça, Gibson M., Juan C. Pérez-Morales, and Pablo J. Greco. 2016. "Influência Do Estatuto Posicional No Comportamento Tático Durante Jogos Reduzidos No Futebol: Um Estudo de Caso Em Atletas Sub-17 de Elite. [Influence of Positional Status on Tactical Behavior During small-sided soccer games: A Case Study in Elite Under-17 Athletes]" *Revista Portuguesa de Ciências Do Desporto* 16 : 194–206.

Praça, Gibson M., Gustavo Fernandes Barbosa, Cristiano da Conceição Ferreira Murta, Sarah Teles Bredt, Daniel Barreira, Mauro Heleno Chagas, and Pablo J. Greco. 2019. "Influence of Floaters and Positional Status on Players' Tactical, Physical, and Physiological Responses in Soccer Small-Sided Games." *Human Movement* In press.

Praça, Gibson M., and Pablo J. Greco. 2019. "Pequenos Jogos No Futebol: Princípios Táticos Fundamentais Em Situações de Superioridade Numérica." ["Small Games in Soccer: Fundamental Tactical Principles in Situations of Numerical Superiority."] *Revista Brasileira de Educação Física e Esporte* 33.

Praça, Gibson M., Juan C. Pérez Morales, Sarah da Glória Teles Bredt, Raphael Brito e Sousa, André Gustavo Pereira de Andrade, and Pablo J. Greco. 2017. "The Development of Tactical Skills in U-14 and U-15 Soccer Players throughout a Season: A Comparative Analysis." *Human Movement* 18: 39–47. https://doi.org/10.1515/humo-2017-0046.

Praça, Gibson M., Raphael B. Sousa, Sarah G. T. Bredt, Filipe M. Clemente, Israel T. Costa, Henrique Oliveira, Gustavo Conti, et al.

2018. "Defensive Interactions in Soccer Small-Sided Games: An Integrated Approach between the Fundamental Tactical Principles and the Social Network Analysis." *Brazilian Journal of Kinanthropometry and Human Performance* 20: 422–31. https://doi.org/10.5007/1980-0037.2018v20n5p422.

Práxedes, Alba, Fernando Del Villar Álvarez, Alberto Moreno, Alexander Gil-Arias, and Keith Davids. 2019. "Effects of a Nonlinear Pedagogy Intervention Programme on the Emergent Tactical Behaviours of Youth Footballers." *Physical Education and Sport Pedagogy*, 1–12. https://doi.org/10.1080/17408989.2019.1580689.

Ramos, João, Rui J. Lopes, Pedro Marques, and Duarte Araújo. 2017. "Hypernetworks Reveal Compound Variables That Capture Cooperative and Competitive Interactions in a Soccer Match." *Frontiers in Psychology* 8. https://doi.org/10.3389/fpsyg.2017.01379.

Sarmento, Hugo. 2012. "*Análise Do Jogo de Futebol - Padrões de Jogo Ofensivo Em Equipas de Alto Rendimento: Uma Abordagem Qualitativa*." ["*Football Match Analysis - Patterns of Offensive Play in High-Performance Teams: A Qualitative Approach*."] Universidade de Trás os Montes e Alto Douro.

Sarmento, Hugo, Maria T. Anguera, J. Camapaniço, and Jose C. Leitão. 2013. "A Metodologia Observacional Como Método Para Análise Do Jogo de Futebol - Uma Prespetiva Teórica. [Observational Methodology as a Method for Analyzing the Football Game - A Theoretical Perspective.]" *Boletim Da Sociedade Portuguesa de Educação Física* 37: 9–20.

Sarmento, Hugo, A. Barbosa, M. T. Anguera, Jorge Campaniço, and Jose C. Leitão. 2014. "Regular Patterns of Play in the Counter-Attack of the FC Barcelona and Manchester United Football Teams." In *Performance Analysis of Sport IX*, edited by D. M. Peters and P. O'Donoghue, 57–64. Routledge.

Sarmento, Hugo, Pedro Roma, Adilson Marques, and Jose C. Leitão. 2016. "Tactical Analysis of Barcelona, Inter Milan and Manchester United – A Mixed Method Approach." In *International Research in Science &*

Soccer II, edited by T. Favero, B. Drust, and B. Dawson. London, UK: Routledge.

Sarmento, Hugo, Filipe M. Clemente, Duarte Araújo, Keith Davids, Allistair McRobert, and António Figueiredo. 2018. "What Performance Analysts Need to Know About Research Trends in Association Football (2012–2016): A Systematic Review." *Sports Medicine* 48: 799–836. https://doi.org/10.1007/s40279-017-0836-6.

Sarmento, Hugo, Rui Marcelino, Maria T. Anguera, Jorge Campaniço, Nuno Matos, and Jose C. Leitão. 2014. "Match Analysis in Football: A Systematic Review." *Journal of Sports Sciences* 32: 1831–43. https://doi.org/10.1080/02640414.2014.898852.

Serra-Olivares, Jaime, Sixto Gonzalez-Villora, Luis M. Garcia-Lopez, and Duarte Araujo. 2015. "Game-Based Approaches' Pedagogical Principles: Exploring Task Constraints in Youth Soccer." *Journal of Human Kinetics* 46: 251–61. https://doi.org/10.1515/hukin-2015-0053.

Silva, Pedro, Luís Vilar, Keith Davids, Duarte Araújo, and Julio Garganta. 2016. "*Sports Teams as Complex Adaptive Systems: Manipulating Player Numbers Shapes Behaviours during Football Small-Sided Games*." SpringerPlus 5: 191. https://doi.org/10.1186/s40064-016-1813-5.

Sousa, Raphael Brito, Sarah T. Bredt, Pablo J. Greco, Filipe M. Clemente, and Gibson M. Praça. 2019. "Influence of Limiting the Number of Ball Touches on Players' Tactical Behaviour and Network Properties during Football Small-Sided Games." *International Journal of Performance Analysis in Sport* 19.

Squartini, Tiziano, Francesco Picciolo, Franco Ruzzenenti, and Diego Garlaschelli. 2013. "Reciprocity of Weighted Networks." *Scientific Reports* 3: 2729. https://doi.org/10.1038/srep02729.

Taki, Tsuyoshi, and Jun-ichi Hasegawa. 2000. "Visualization of Dominant Region in Team Games and Its Application to Teamwork Analysis." In *Proceedings Computer Graphics International 2000*, 227–35. IEEE Comput. Soc. https://doi.org/10.1109/CGI.2000.852338.

Tenga, Albin, Anders Mortensholm, and Peter O'Donoghue. 2017. "Opposition Interaction in Creating Penetration during Match Play in

Elite Soccer: Evidence from UEFA Champions League Matches." *International Journal of Performance Analysis in Sport* 17: 802–12. https://doi.org/10.1080/24748668.2017.1399326.

Travassos, Bruno, Keith Davids, Duarte Araújo, and Pedro T. Esteves. 2013. "Performance Analysis in Team Sports : Advances from an Ecological Dynamics Approach." *International Journal of Performance Analysis in Sport* 13: 83–95.

Wäsche, Hagen. 2015. "Interorganizational Cooperation in Sport Tourism: A Social Network Analysis." *Sport Management Review* 18: 542–54. https://doi.org/10.1016/j.smr.2015.01.003.

Wasserman, Stan, and Katherine Faust. 1994. *Social Network Analysis: Methods and Applications*. New York, USA: Cambridge University Press.

Yue, Zengyan, Holger Broich, Florian Seifriz, and Joachim Mester. 2008. "Mathematical Analysis of a Football Game. Part I: Individual and Collective Behaviors." *Studies in Applied Mathematics* 121: 223–43.

In: An Essential Guide to Sports Performance ISBN: 978-1-53617-608-7
Editors: Daniel Castillo Alvira et al.

Chapter 2

The Influence of Situational Variables on Technical Performance in Elite Spanish Goalkeepers during Official Competition

*Daniel Castillo**, PhD, Miguel Escalona,*
Ángel Lago-Rodríguez, PhD, María Soto, PhD,
Silvia Sánchez-Díaz and Javier Raya-González, PhD
Faculty of Health Sciences, Universidad Isabel I, Burgos, Spain

Abstract

The knowledge of the technical demands encountered by goalkeepers during match-play is crucial to design specific soccer training tasks. The aim of this investigation was to examine the influence of situational factors (i.e., game location, quality of the opponent, and match outcome) on technical performance indicators of elite goalkeepers competing at the

---

* Corresponding Author's Email: danicasti5@gmail.com.

First Spanish Division (*La Liga*). Twenty goalkeepers, who completed a total of 344 matches during the 2018-19 season in the First Spanish Division, participated in this investigation. Technical performance measures, such as goals conceded, goal attempts, saves, clear-outs, successful short passes, successful long passes, and game restarts were registered during official matches using an observational tool (Wyscout, Chiavari, Genova, Italy). The situational variables introduced for the analysis were: game location (home and away), quality of the opponent (Champions League, UEFA, intermediate, and low-level) and match outcome (winner, drawer, and loser). Results show that goalkeepers conceded higher goal attempts ($P < 0.01$; ES = -0.49, small), performed greater saves ($P < 0.01$; ES = -0.48, small) and made larger game restarts ($P < 0.01$; ES = -0.54, moderate) when playing away, in comparison to playing at home. In addition, in general no significant differences ($P > 0.05$) in goalkeepers' technical performance were found attending to the quality of the opponent. Finally, loser goalkeepers conceded higher goals ($P < 0.01$; ES = -1.21/-1.21, large) and goal attempts ($P < 0.01$; ES = -0.52/-0.66, moderate) compared to drawer and winner goalkeepers, and winner goalkeppers performed significantly more clear-outs ($P < 0.01$; ES = 0.43, small) and less short successful passes ($P < 0.05$; ES = -0.39, small) in comparison to loser and drawer goalkeepers, respectively. These results provide a more thorough understanding of goalkeeper's performance profiles, what allows to design novel approaches for the goalkeepers' training and development process.

Keywords: *La Liga*, technical measures, game location, quality of the opponent, match outcome

INTRODUCTION

Goalkeeper's primary role in soccer is to protect his/her goal, whilst a secondary purpose lies in ball distribution during the initiation of an attack (White et al. 2018). In addition, the rules of the game provide goalkeepers a special role during the development of the game in comparison to other outfield playing positions, since they are allowed to handle the ball inside the penalty area (Almeida, Volossovitch, and Duarte 2016). Given that the ultimate objective of soccer is to out-score the opponent team to win matches, it stands to reason that the specific-actions upon goalkeepers have the potential to directly influence the final outcome of match-play (Seaton and Campos 2011). Thus, gathering knowledge of the game demands encountered by goalkeepers during match-play is crucial in order to design goalkeeper-specific training tasks, not only the additional training apart from the team but also the in-group participation. Considering these game demands, the periodization of the training contents could be optimized within the microcycle, maximizing their soccer competence.

In the last two decades, the number of studies focused on soccer has increased substantially (Mujika 2018), especially those related to the technical demands encountered by outfield players during match-play (Liu et al. 2016). However, few studies have analyzed goalkeepers' technical performance during match-play (Sainz-de Baranda, Ortega, and Palao 2008; Park et al. 2016). In this line, goalkeepers usually participate in 15% of the total match time, both directly and indirectly, during the development of the game. Focusing on goalkeeper's defensive role, Sainz de Baranda, Ortega and Palao (2008) reported that saves were the most frequent technical action, observing ~10 saving actions per match during the 2002 World Cup in Korea and Japan, whereas other studies reported ~2-5 saves per match during Spanish *La Liga* (Serrano et al. 2018; Liu, Gomez, and Lago-Peñas 2015). In addition, it has been shown that elite goalkeepers perform several other technical defensive actions, such as ~2 clearances and ~2 open palm actions per match (Sainz de Baranda, Ortega, and Palao 2008; Liu, Gomez, and Lago-Peñas 2015). As for their offensive role, goalkeepers perform ~20 successful passes per match, which represent 60-70% of the total passes (Serrano et al. 2018; Liu, Gomez, and Lago-Peñas 2015). However, more studies are needed in order to increase the knowledge regarding goalkeepers' performance during official competitions, especially those studies based on short and long successful passes and game restarts.

Soccer is a team sport influenced by technical-tactical and strategic factors (Ric et al. 2016), so it is reasonable to suggest that situational variables may somehow influence both teams' and players' behaviors, which are crucial in order to achieve the game outcome. Regarding this, situational variables such as match location, quality of the opponent and match outcome have been suggested as the most important factors for soccer performance, so its evaluation would help coaches to understand the game and to design specific training strategies (Taylor et al. 2017). Therefore, research regarding the influence of situational variables on technical-tactical performance in outfield soccer players and goalkeepers would be relevant to understand game demands. Considering that most previous studies were focused on the evaluation of outfield players, further research is needed on the influence of situational factors over goalkeepers' performance.

Regarding to match location, Pollard (1986) found an advantage in favour to home teams, which obtained about 64% of all points gained in the English Football League. Similarly, Thomas, Reeves and Davies (2004) observed that 61% of total matches played in the English Premier League were won by the home team. It seems that various factors such as crowd support, travel fatigue and/or playing field could contribute to understand this phenomenon (Lago-Peñas and Lago-Ballesteros 2011). Analyzing technical performance during two British domestic league seasons, some authors showed that soccer teams playing at home performed higher number of shots, passes, dribbles and crosses, compared to teams playing away (Taylor et al. 2008), while other authors observed higher possession time for teams playing at home during the First Division Spanish League (Acero and Peñas 2005). Results showed that home teams had significant higher means for goal scored, total shots, shots on goal, attacking moves, box moves, crosses, offsides committed, assists, passes made, successful passes, dribbles made, successful dribbles, ball possession, and gains of possession, while visiting teams presented higher means for losses of possession and yellow cards in Spanish professional men's league.

Other situational factor which influences players' performance is the quality of the opponent, by means of the final team's position on the table at the end of the competitive season (Castillo et al. 2018). For technical performance, teams in the top-ranked group exhibited significantly greater amount of possession in opponent's field half, number of entry passes in the final third of the field and the penalty area, and 50-50 challenges, compared to lower-ranked teams (Yang et al. 2018). In addition, Lago-

Peñas and Lago-Ballesteros (2011) showed that playing against strong opposition was associated with a decreased possession time in Spanish professional soccer teams. The fact that better-ranked teams present greater technical performance in offensive role denote that goalkeeper's behavior could be influenced by higher technical actions in its defensive role. Thus, it may be interesting to analyze goalkeepers' technical performance during match-play according to the quality of the opponent.

Individual and collective performance of soccer players have been also associated with match outcome (Lago-Peñas, Lago-Ballesteros, and Rey 2011). In this respect, higher shots' success has been reported for professional British football winning teams, in comparison with losing or drawing teams (Taylor et al. 2008). In addition, it has been shown that Spanish professional teams performed higher amount of shots and crosses at won matches, in comparison to drew or lost matches (Lago-Peñas et al. 2010). Other authors showed that the percentage of ball possession was greater when losing than when winning or drawing (Lago-Peñas, Lago-Ballesteros, and Rey 2011). However, Yang et al. (2018) observed that larger possession time increased the probability of winning. Again, it would reasonable to expect that the greater technical performance showed by winner teams during the development of the game would increase the number of defensive technical actions encountered by the opponent goalkeepers. Therefore, it would be relevant to analyze the influence of match outcome in goalkeepers' technical profiles.

The majority of the studies have analyzed the effect of situational variables on technical performance in outfield soccer players, but only one study has been focused on professional goalkeepers (Liu, Gomez, and Lago-Peñas 2015). Therefore, the aim of this investigation was to examine the influence of situational factors (i.e., game location, quality of the opponent and match outcome) on the technical performance indicators of elite goalkeepers during Spanish *La Liga* competition.

METHODS

Participants

Twenty goalkeepers, belonged to the soccer teams of the First Spanish Division (*La Liga*) across the 2018-19 season, participated in this study. All participants trained at least five times a week, and were involved in an official match at weekends. One goalkeeper from each team was chosen to be part in this investigation, selecting those who played more time for each team during the first round of the competitive season. The criteria for allocating the goalkeepers technical actions during official matches was based on three situational variables: game location (home vs. away), quality of the opponent (matches playing against teams whose final position in the classification table was Champions League [1st - 4th position], UEFA [5th - 7th position], intermediate [8th - 17th position] or low-level [18th – 20th position]), and match outcome (those matches in which goalkeepers' team won, drew or lost). All clubs authorized researchers to use the technical data collection. This investigation was performed in accordance to the Declaration of Helsinki (2013) and met the ethical standards in Sport and Exercise Science Research (Harriss & Atkinson. 2013).

Experimental Design

The design used in this study was descriptive and based on an observational methodology applied to the acquired data, which was obtained across a total of 344 official matches through a computerized semi-automatic video match-analysis system (Wyscout. Chiavari. Genova. Italia) in order to analyze the technical-tactical actions of soccer goalkeepers who competed in Spanish *La Liga* competition. This system does not use different cameras distributed throughout the stadium, but it makes the recording through a fixed tactical camera. The dependent variables in terms of technical measures such as goals conceded, goal attempts, saves, clear-outs, successful short passes, successful long passes and restarts were registered during the official matches. The independent variables were the situational variables: game location (home and away), quality of the opponent (Champions League, UEFA, intermediate and low-level) and match outcome (winner, drawer and loser).

Procedures

Technical performance. The technical actions selected to be registered during the data acquisition process were based on previous studies (Sainz de Baranda, Ortega, & Palao. 2008; Serrano et al. 2018) and performed by the goalkeepers during official matches: goals conceded, goal attempts (shots on goal and outside performed by the opponent team), saves (catching or blocking a shot, which prevents the opponent from scoring a goal), clear-outs (technique adopted to clear a crossed ball that cannot be caught; either by punching the ball over the goalkeepers' head, or guiding the ball over the crossbar); successful short passes (those short pass that end with an outfield player managing the ball), successful long passes (those long pass that end with an outfield player managing the ball) and restarts (goalkeeper starts the game as goal kicks or direct/indirect free kicks).

Statistical Analysis

Results are presented as means ± standard deviations (SD). Normality distribution of the considered variables was tested using the Kolmogorov-Smirnov test and statistical parametric techniques were conducted. A *t*-test for independent samples was used to compare the results of technical performances between those matches in which goalkeepers played at home and away. A one-way analysis of variance (ANOVA), with the Bonferroni correction test for post hoc analysis, was used to determine the differences in the goalkeepers' technical performance attending to the quality of the opponent and match outcome, respectively. Practical significance was assessed by calculating Cohen's effect size (ES). ES were classified as trivial (<0.2), small (0.2–0.5), moderate (0.5–0.8) and large (>0.8) (Cohen, 1988). In addition, mean differences between/among groups were expressed as percentage using the formula: $\Delta\% = ([\text{mean } 2 - \text{mean } 1] / \text{mean } 1) * 100$. Data analysis was carried out using the Statistical Package for Social Sciences (SPSS 21.0. SPSS™ Inc. Chicago. IL. USA). Statistical significance was set at $P < 0.05$.

RESULTS

Elite goalkeepers, who competed in a Spanish First Division (*La Liga*), conceded 1.75 ± 0.99 goals and 4.59 ± 2.37 goal attempts per match. In addition, goalkeepers performed 3.41 ± 1.99 saves, 2.02 ± 1.29 clear-outs, 8.96 ± 6.45 successful short passes, 7.76 ± 4.84 successful long passes and 7.03 ± 3.71 restarts of game per match.

Table 1 shows differences of the technical actions performed by goalkeepers between matches played at home and away. Goalkeepers conceded greater goal attempts ($P < 0.01$; ES = -0.49, small), performed greater saves ($P < 0.01$; ES = -0.48, small) and made larger restarts ($P < 0.01$; ES = -0.54, moderate) when playing away, in comparison to playing at home.

Figure 1 represents differences on the technical actions performed by goalkeepers according to the quality of the opponent (i.e., Champions League, UEFA, intermediate level and low-level teams). In general, no significant differences ($P > 0.05$) were found in technical actions encountered by goalkeepers during Spanish First Division competition based on the quality of the opponent (i.e., Champions League, UEFA, intermediate and low-level). However, goalkeepers performed higher clear-outs ($P < 0.05$; ES = -0.62, moderate) against Champions League teams than when played against low-level teams. In addition, higher successful long passes were performed by goalkeepers when played against UEFA teams in respect to low-level teams ($P < 0.05$; ES = 0.53, moderate).

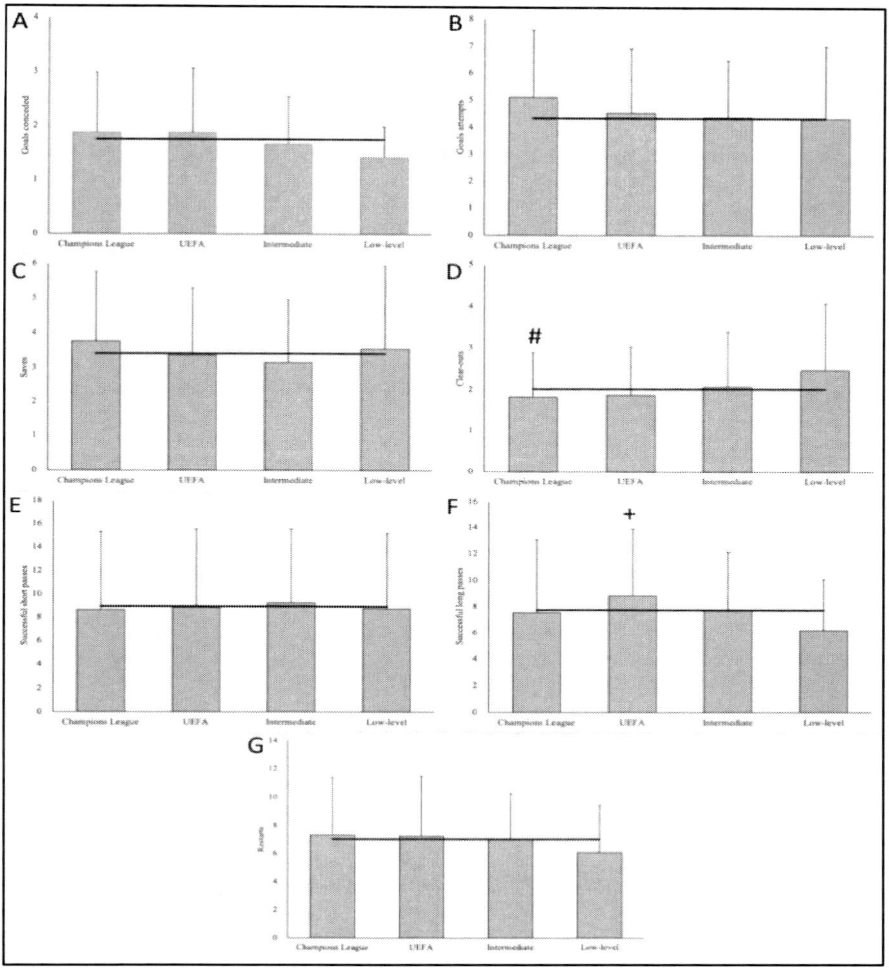

Differences in technical actions when goalkeepers played against Champions League and low-level teams; + Differences in technical actions when goalkeepers played against UEFA and low-level teams.

Figure 1. Comparisons of the technical actions performed by goalkeepers when played against opponents of different quality (in bars) and total mean results (in line).

Table 2 shows the differences on the technical actions performed by goalkeepers among matches won, drew and lost. Goalkeepers conceded higher goals ($P < 0.01$; ES = -1.21/-1.21, large) and goal attempts ($P < 0.01$; ES = -0.52/-0.66, moderate) during lost matches, in comparison to drew and won matches. In addition, goalkeepers performed higher clear-outs during won matches, in comparison to lost matches ($P < 0.01$; ES = 0.43, small). Moreover, goalkeepers made higher successful short passes during lost matches versus won matches ($P < 0.01$; ES = -0.39, small).

Table 1. Comparison of the technical actions performed by goalkeepers between matches played at home and away

Variable	Home	Away	Mean difference (%)	ES
Goals conceded	1.75 ± 1.08	1.74 ± 0.93	-0.57	0.01
Goal attempts	4.08 ± 2.06	5.08 ± 2.54	24.51	-0.49**
Saves	3.03 ± 1.58	3.78 ± 2.26	24.75	-0.48**
Clear-out	1.91 ± 1.23	2.13 ± 1.33	11.52	-0.18
Successful short passes	9.36 ± 6.58	8.56 ± 6.30	-8.55	0.12
Successful long passes	7.59 ± 4.94	7.92 ± 4.73	4.35	-0.07
Restarts of game	6.23 ± 2.99	7.84 ± 4.17	25.84	-0.54**

ES = effect size. **Significance level set at $P < 0.01$.

Table 2. Differences on the technical actions performed by goalkeepers among matches won, drew and lost

Variable	Won	Drew	Lost	ES Won-Drew	ES Won-Lost	ES Drew-Lost
Goals conceded	1.35 ± 0.67	1.38 ± 0.69	2.21 ± 1.13	-0.04	-1.29**	-1.21**
Goal attempts	4.04 ± 2.21	4.26 ± 2.39	5.50 ± 2.23	-0.10	-0.66**	-0.52**
Saves	3.53 ± 1.94	3.33 ± 2.18	3.38 ± 1.83	0.10	0.08	-0.02
Clear-out	2.37 ± 1.59	1.94 ± 1.07	1.68 ± 0.94	0.27	0.43**	0.24
Successful long passes	7.55 ± 4.56	8.35 ± 5.37	7.35 ± 4.48	-0.18	0.04	0.19
Successful short passes	7.77 ± 5.95	9.11 ± 6.45	10.08 ± 6.79	0.21	-0.39*	-0.15
Restarts	7.39 ± 3.87	6.88 ± 3.63	6.81 ± 3.61	0.13	0.15	0.02

ES = effect size; **Significance level set at $P < 0.01$; *Significance level set at $P < 0.05$.

Discussion

The main aim of this investigation was to examine the influence of situational factors (i.e., game location, quality of the opponent and match outcome) on the technical performance indicators of elite goalkeepers during Spanish *La Liga* competition. Up to date, no previous literature has addressed the success of short and long passes encountered by goalkeepers attending to situational variables during official competition. The results of our study revealed differences in goalkeepers' technical performance attending to match location, quality of the opponent and match outcome. Specifically, goalkeepers playing away conceded higher goal attempts, performed greater saves and made larger game restarts in comparison to playing at home. In addition, minor significant differences in goalkeepers' technical performance were found attending to the quality of the opponent. Finally, loser goalkeepers conceded higher goals and goal attempts versus the drawer and winner ones, and winner goalkeepers performed higher clear-outs and lower short successful passes versus the loser ones. These results provide a more thorough understanding of goalkeeper's performance profiles, what allows to design novel approaches for the goalkeepers' training and development process.

The majority of the studies quantifying the technical actions during match-play have been focused on outfield players (Bradley et al. 2013; Rampinini et al. 2009; Clemente et al. 2016). However, few studies have analyzed the technical performance profiles of soccer goalkeepers (Sainz-de Baranda, Ortega, and Palao 2008; Liu, Gomez, and Lago-Peñas 2015; Serrano et al. 2018). In line with evidence reported in previous studies (Serrano et al. 2018; Liu, Gomez, and Lago-Peñas 2015), elite goalkeepers in our study performed ~3 saves per match. In addition, similar to results reported by Sainz-de Baranda et al. (2008), we observed that goalkeepers performed ~2 clear-outs per match. Some studies reported a total of ~20 successful passes per match for goalkeepers, which represents 60-70% of the total passes completed by these players (Serrano et al. 2018; Liu, Gomez, and Lago-Peñas 2015), whereas a total of ~15 successful passes have been observed in our study. These differences could be explained by the different observational tool used (MediaCoach vs. Wyscout) or the goalkeepers' competitive level. Moreover, this is the first study which differentiates the effectivity on short and long passes, and the first one analyzing game restarts perform by goalkeepers, which represents an important finding for understanding the game technical demands in soccer and for optimizing the training process of goalkeepers.

The home advantage in team sports has a crucial role on the final match score (Pollard & Gómez, 2009). In addition, previous studies showed higher offensive indicators such as shots, goals, off-sides, successful passes, possessions for teams playing at home, compared to teams playing away during official competitions (Acero & Lago-Peñas, 2005; Lago-Peñas & Lago-Ballesteros, 2011; Taylor et al. 2008). However, there is a lack of literature reporting specific data regarding goalkeepers. Results from our study point out that match location influences goalkeepers' technical performance. In this sense, we observed that goalkeepers conceded lower goal attempts, performed lower saves and made lower game restarts when playing at home, in comparison to playing away. Some explanations for these aforementioned results may be the operational strategy chosen by the coaches, the attempt to take the initiative of the game, the knowledge of their own field or the crowd support taking place when teams play at home (Pollard and Gómez 2009; Thomas, Reeves, and Davies 2004). On the contrary, teams playing away could be more conservative, giving up the initiative through possession and taking a defensive positioning in a medium-low block.

Attending to the quality of the opponent, our results showed no significant differences in technical actions encountered by goalkeepers during Spanish First Division competition when played against Champions League, UEFA, intermediate and low-level teams. Nevertheless, two unique differences were observed. On one hand, higher clear-outs were performed by goalkeepers against Champions League teams versus low-level teams, possibly explained by the higher number of interventions shown by goalkeepers from low-level teams; and on the other hand, higher successful long passes were performed by goalkeepers when playing against UEFA teams in respect to low-level teams, due to a high-level team try to press in the opponent area and the goalkeeper try to pass the ball to the distant player. In contrast, Liu et al. (2015) showed higher percentage of successful passes encountered by goalkeepers when played against low-level teams in Spanish *La Liga*. In addition, Serrano et al. (2018) found higher successful passes in goalkeepers from high-level versus low-level teams over six consecutive seasons in the Spanish First Division. These differences could not be explained by the postulate of Serrano et al. (2018), who support the idea of better teams controlling matches with longer and more precise possessions, in which goalkeepers are actively involved. Moreover, despite we did not find differences on the number of saves encountered by goalkeepers depending on the quality of the opponent team, other studies showed contradictory results. While Liu et al. (2015) observed that high-level ranked goalkeepers performed higher saves when playing against a low-level team than when playing against a high-level team, Serrano et al. (2018) observed higher saves in those goalkeepers from lower competitive-level. So, further research is needed to understand the number of saves according to the quality of the opponent.

Match outcome has been considered as a fundamental factor which influences game demands in soccer players. Previous investigations demonstrated that players who won the matches performed higher shots on goal, successful passes, crosses and possession times in respect to the draw or lost ones throughout the Champions League or Spanish First Division (Lago-Peñas, Lago-Ballesteros, and Rey 2011; Lago-Peñas et al. 2010). In this respect, our results showed that goalkeepers conceded higher goals and goal attempts during lost matches, in comparison with drew and won ones. Obviously, these results are explained because goalkeepers who conceded less goals and goal attempts are likely to win the matches. Moreover, we observed that winner goalkeepers made lower successful short passes versus the loser ones. These results are in contrast with previous data reported by Grant, Williams and Reilly (1999), who observed that winner teams registered higher effectivity in passes. It might be reasonable to suggest this discrepancy results from the type of pressing strategy adopted by losing teams, which would be initiated closer to the opponent's penalty area, thus influencing the number of successful passes performed by the winning team.

This investigation is not exempt of limitations, being the main one that only one competitive season has been analyzed, although it should be noted that a total of 344 official matches were examined through a computerized semi-automatic video match-analysis system. For further research, it would be interesting to analyze the evolution of goalkeepers' technical indicators over several seasons. Another limitation was the analysis of goalkeepers' technical actions throughout only one competition, although elite level (i.e., *La Liga*) was considered. Thus, it may be relevant to compare the technical performance among goalkeepers from different soccer elite-level leagues. Finally, this study examined the technical indicators encountered by goalkeepers according to situational variables separately, although the study of a combination of different situational factors would be convenient for a deeper understanding of goalkeepers' technical performance.

CONCLUSION

In Spanish *La Liga* competition, goalkeeper's technical performance is partially influenced by match location, the quality of the opponent, and the final match outcome. Data from this study may help coaches with the training process and development process of their goalkeepers, allowing them to adapt the planning of training sessions to match requirements. These results suggest a practical approach to the goalkeepers' training and development process in order to design the specific training attending to the pre-week and post-week match-play aimed to optimize their soccer competence.

References

Acero, Rafael M., and Carlos Lago Peñas. 2005. "Análisis de Variables Determinantes en el Fútbol de Alto Rendimiento: El Tiempo de Posesión del Balón (Abriendo la Caja Negra del Fútbol). [Analysis of Determinants Variables in Elite Soccer Perfomance: The Ball Possession Period (Opening the Black Box of Soccer]" *Revista de Entrenamiento Deportivo* 19:13–9.

Almeida, Carlos H., Anna Volossovitch, and Ricardo Duarte. 2016. "Penalty Kick Outcomes in UEFA Club Competitions (2010-2015): The Roles of Situational, Individual and Performance Factors." *International Journal of Performance Analysis in Sport* 16: 508–22. doi:10.1080/24748668.2016.11868905.

Bradley, Paul S., Christopher Carling, Antonio Gomez-Diaz, Peter Hood, Chris Barnes, Jack Ade, Mark Boddy, Peter Krustrup, and Magni Mohr. 2013. "Match Performance and Physical Capacity of Players in the Top Three Competitive Standards of English Professional Soccer." *Human Movement Science* 32: 808–21. doi:10.1016/j.humov.2013.06.002.

Castillo, Daniel, Carlo Castagna, Jesús Cámara, Aitor Iturricastillo, and Javier Yanci. 2018. "Influence of Team's Rank on Soccer Referees' External and Internal Match Loads during Official Matches." *Journal of Strength and Conditioning Research* 32 (6): 1715–22. doi:10.1519/JSC.0000000000002040.

Clemente, Filipe M., Antonio J. Figueiredo, Fernando M. Lourenco-Martins, Rui Sousa-Mendes, and Del P. Wong. 2016. "Physical and Technical Performances are not Associated with Tactical Prominence in U14 Soccer Matches." *Research in Sports Medicine* 24: 352–62. doi:10.1080/15438627.2016.1222277.

Cohen, Jacob. 1988. *Statistical Power Analysis for the Behavioral Sciences*. Hillsdale: Lawrence Erlbaum Associates.

Grant, Abt G., Andrew M. Williams, and Thomas Reilly. 1999. "Analysis of the Goals Scored in the 1998 World Cup." *Journal of Sports Sciences* 17: 826–27.

Harriss, Dave, and Greg Atkinson. 2013. "Ethical Standards in Sport and Exercise Science Research: 2014 Update." *International Journal of Sports Medicine* 34: 1025–28. doi:10.1055/s-0033-1358756.

Lago-Peñas, Carlos, and Joaquin Lago-Ballesteros. 2011. "Game Location and Team Quality Effects on Performance Profiles in Professional Soccer." *Journal of Sports Science & Medicine* 10: 465–71.

Lago-Peñas, Carlos, Joaquin Lago-Ballesteros, Alexandre Dellal, and Maite Gomez. 2010. "Game-Related Statistics that Discriminated Winning, Drawing and Losing Teams from the Spanish Soccer League." *Journal of Sports Science & Medicine* 9: 288–93.

Lago-Peñas, Carlos, Joaquín Lago-Ballesteros, and Ezequiel Rey. 2011. "Differences in Performance Indicators between Winning and Losing Teams in the UEFA Champions League." *Journal of Human Kinetics* 27: 135–46. doi:10.2478/v10078-011-0011-3.

Liu, Hongyou, Miguel A. Gomez, Bruno Goncalves, and Jaime Sampaio. 2016. "Technical Performance and Match-to-Match Variation in Elite Football Teams." *Journal of Sports Sciences* 34: 509–18. doi:10.1080/02640414.2015.1117121.

Liu, Hongyou, Miguel A. Gomez, and Carlos Lago-Peñas. 2015. "Match Performance Profiles of Goalkeepers of Elite Football Teams." *International Journal of Sports Science & Coaching* 10: 669–82. doi:10.1260/1747-9541.10.4.669.

Mujika, I. 2018. "The Biggest Event of The Beautiful Game Is Back!" *International Journal of Sports Physiology and Performance* 13:537. doi:10.1111/1467-937X.00249.

Park, Young-Shoo, Man-Sik Choi, Sang-Yeol Bang, and Jeong-Keun Park. 2016. "Analysis of Shots on Target and Goals Scored in Soccer Matches: Implications for Coaching and Training Goalkeepers." *South African Journal for Research in Sport, Physical Education and Recreation* 38: 123–37.

Pollard, Richard. 1986. "Home Advantage in Soccer: A Retrospective Analysis." *Journal of Sports Sciences* 4: 237–48. doi:10.1080/02640418608732122.

Pollard, Richard, and Miguel A. Gómez. 2009. "Home Advantage in Football in South-West Europe: Long-Term Trends, Regional Variation, and Team Differences." *European Journal of Sport Science* 9: 341–52. doi:10.1080/17461390903009133.

Rampinini, Ermanno, Franco M. Impellizzeri, Carlo Castagna, Aaron J. Coutts, and Ulrik Wisløff. 2009. "Technical Performance during Soccer Matches of the Italian Serie A League: Effect of Fatigue and Competitive Level." *Journal of Science and Medicine in Sport* 12: 227–33. doi:10.1016/j.jsams.2007.10.002.

Ric, Angel, Carlota Torrents, Bruno Goncalves, Jaime Sampaio, and Robert Hristovski. 2016. "Soft-Assembled Multilevel Dynamics of Tactical Behaviors in Soccer.' *Frontiers in Psychology* 7:1513. doi:10.3389/fpsyg.2016.01513.

Sainz de Baranda, Pilar, Enrique Ortega, and José M. Palao. 2008. "Analysis of Goalkeepers' Defence in the World Cup in Korea and Japan in 2002." *European Journal of Sport Science* 8: 127–34. doi:10.1080/17461390801919045.

Seaton, Marcus, and Jose Campos. 2011. "Distribution Competence of a Football Clubs Goalkeepers." *International Journal of Performance Analysis in Sport* 11:314–24. doi:10.1080/24748668.2011.11868551.

Serrano, Carlos, Victor Paredes-Hernandez, Javier Sanchez-Sanchez, Jana Gallardo-Perez, Ricardo Da Silva, David Porcel, Enrique Colino, Jorge Garcia-Unanue, and Leonor Gallardo. 2018. "The Team's Influence on Physical and Technical Demands of Elite Goalkeepers in LaLiga: A Longitudinal Study in Professional Soccer." *Research in Sports Medicine*, 16:1–15. doi:10.1080/15438627.2018.1555755.

Taylor, Jeffrey B., Alexis A. Wright, Steven L. Dischiavi, Allison Townsend, and Adam R. Marmon. 2017. "Activity Demands during Multi-Directional Team Sports: A Systematic Review." *Sports Medicine* 47:2533–51. doi:10.1007/s40279-017-0772-5.

Taylor, Joseph B, Stephen D. Mellalieu, Nic James, and David A. Shearer. 2008. "The Influence of Match Location, Quality of Opposition, and Match Status on Technical Performance in Professional Association

Football." *Journal of Sports Sciences* 26: 885–95. doi:10.1080/02640410701836887.

Thomas, Sion, Colin Reeves, and Simon Davies. 2004. "An Analysis of Home Advantage in the English Football Premiership." *Perceptual and Motor Skills* 99:1212–16. doi:10.2466/pms.99.3f.1212-1216.

White, Anthony, Samuel P. Hills, Carlton B. Cooke, Trevor Batten, Liam P. Kilduff, Christian J. Cook, Craig Roberts, and Mark Russell. 2018. "Match-Play and Performance Test Responses of Soccer Goalkeepers: A Review of Current Literature." *Sports Medicine* 48: 2497–2516. doi:10.1007/s40279-018-0977-2.

Yang, Gai, Anthony S. Leicht, Carlos Lago-Peñas, and Miguel A. Gomez. 2018. "Key Team Physical and Technical Performance Indicators Indicative of Team Quality in the Soccer Chinese Super League." *Research in Sports Medicine* 26: 158–67. doi:10.1080/15438627.2018.1431539.

In: An Essential Guide to Sports Performance ISBN: 978-1-53617-608-7
Editors: Daniel Castillo Alvira et al. © 2020 Nova Science Publishers, Inc.

Chapter 3

ANTHROPOMETRIC CHARACTERISTICS AND PHYSICAL PERFORMANCE OF SENIOR SOCCER PLAYERS: EFFECT OF COMPETITIVE LEVEL AND FIELD POSITION

Javier Yanci[1*], Julio Calleja-González[1], Jurdan Mendigutxia[2], Alexandre Dellal[3], Aitor Iturricastillo[1] and Asier Los Arcos[1]

[1]Department of Physical Education and Sport,
Faculty of Education and Sport, University of the Baque Country,
UPV/EHU, Vitoria-Gasteiz, Spain
[2]Zentrum Rehabilitation and Performance Centre,
Department of Physical Therapy, Pamplona, Spain
[3]FIFA Medical Excellence Centre, Santy Orthopedicae Clinical,
Sport Science and Research Department, Lyon, France

---

[*] Corresponding Author's Email: Javier.yanci@ehu.eus.

Abstract

The aims of this investigation were to determine the differences in anthropometric, acceleration, vertical jump and change of direction ability among amateur and professional senior soccer players, and describe differences in the anthropometric characteristics and physical performance among playing positions. 46 male soccer players were divided into 2 groups according to their level: a) amateur players (n = 32) competed in third division and b) professional players (n = 14) competed in second division B of Spanish league or into 6 groups according to their playing position goalkeepers (n = 6), central defenders (n = 8), lateral defenders (n = 9), central midfields (n = 9), lateral midfields (n = 7) and forwards (n = 7). The evaluation sessions consisted of anthropometric measurements, vertical jump (squat jump, countermovement jump and arm swim countermovement jump), acceleration (5, 10 and 15 m) and change of direction ability tests (modified agility test, 505 and 20 yards test). No statistically significant differences were observed between groups in anthropometrics characteristics in means parameters, vertical jump height and change of direction ability. The professional group showed significant better results than the amateur group in 5 m (3%, $p < 0.05$, $d = 0.81$), 10 m (5%, $p < 0.05$, $d = 0.69$), and 15 m (5%, $p < 0.05$, $d = 0.75$) and in CMJ-SJ ($p < 0.05$, $d = 0.68$). According to position, significant differences were found in both groups with goalkeepers in 10 m ($p < 0.05$), 15 m ($p < 0.01$) and 20 yards tests ($p < 0.05$). The acceleration capacity appeared to distinguish professional and amateur players, reflecting as a discriminate reason according to the competition level and the acceleration capacity (10 and 15 m) and 20 yards change of direction ability test appeared to distinguish among goalkeepers and others playing positions.

Keywords: soccer, sprint, change of direction, vertical jump, performance

Introduction

Soccer performance is dependent on a multitude of factors (Little and Williams 2006) and is a multifaceted sport, in which success depends on several: physical, technical, and tactical factors (Stølen et al. 2005). The physical performance characteristics required to play soccer have been extensively reported (Barker et al. 1993) and follow-up investigations explored the relationship between these parameters and soccer playing ability (Arnold et al. 1980). Reilly et al. (2000) indicated that a number of physical and anthropometric prerequisites are necessary to compete in soccer. However, the contribution of physique and body composition in soccer performance was recognized, and the parameters of physical fitness were not well studied in professional players (Nikolaidis and Karydis 2011).

In the last years, it has been found that during adolescence, soccer players presented significant differences in terms of body composition and physical capacity (Nikolaidis and Karydis 2011) and elite players differ from their non-elite counterparts in terms of anthropometrical features, while explosive strength and kicking speed are not sensitive enough to distinguish between levels. On the other hand, the findings indicated few positional variations, and only goalkeepers tend to have a specific anthropometric and fitness profile. Anthropometric variables, explosive strength and experience have an influence on kicking speed (Sedano et al. 2009).

Apart from body composition, sprint performance was described as an essential factor in anaerobic performance (Ozkan et al. 2012) and may also indicates that short-term anaerobic production training is effective for improving acceleration and intermittent exercise performance (Ingebrigtsen et al. 2013). To our knowledge, few studies have compared within the same research design the specific fitness characteristics between professional and amateur players (Bekris et al. 2018; Rampinini et al. 2009). Information in this context would be of particular interest to coaches and sport scientists for the development of talent selection procedures (Dellal et al. 2011) and specific training protocols (Reilly et al. 2000).

Thus, the main aim of the present investigation was to determine the differences in anthropometric characteristics, acceleration capacity, vertical jump (VJ) and change of direction ability (CODA) between amateur and professional soccer players. A secondary purpose was to describe the differences in the anthropometric characteristics and physical performance among field position in two soccer groups: professionals vs. amateurs. For this purpose, a heterogeneous group of 46 soccer players was required to attend the exercise-testing laboratory on 2 separate occasions to do several physical tests, hypothesizing that neuromuscular characteristics is a discriminate factor according to the competitive level (professional vs. amateur).

METHODS

Participants

The sample consisted of forty-six male soccer players (age: 23.07 ± 2.42 years, height: 179.96 ± 5.76 cm, body mass: 76.87 ± 7.95 kg, BMI: 23.72 ± 1.95 kg.m^{-2}). Participants were volunteered to take part in this investigation and were divided into 2 different groups according to their soccer level: a) amateur soccer players (AM: n = 32, age: 23.53 ± 2.63 years, height: 180.19 ± 5.75 cm, body mass: 77.47 ± 8.02 kg, BMI: 23.85 ± 2.04 kg.m^{-2}) competed in third division of Spanish soccer league (training experience = 15.56 ± 2.86 years) and b) professional soccer players (PROF: n = 14, age: 22.01 ± 1.41 years, height: 179.43 ± 5.96 cm, body mass: 75.51 ± 7.90 kg, BMI: 23.42 ± 1.77 kg.m^{-2}) competed in second division B of Spanish soccer league (training experience = 14.50 ± 1.65 years). The inclusion criteria for the participants in the study were: belong to a second or third soccer division, to have played usually of the official games in the season and not be previous injured during 6 months before starting the time of research. The selection of highly trained and motivated soccer players for this study was based on our experience that competitive players are generally willing and able to withstand considerable discomfort and to exercise until the development of physiological test. They performed regular physical conditioning training: endurance, strength, acceleration and specific soccer practice from 3-6 days per week, for more than 6 years. Written informed consent was obtained from each of the participants after a detailed written and oral explanation of the potential risks and benefits resulting from their participation and that they had the option to voluntarily withdraw from the study at any time. Also, the study was conducted with the consent of the club to which they belonged and according to the Declaration of Helsinki and was approved beforehand by the local Ethics Committee.

Procedure

The tests were performed on a synthetic indoor court during the in-season period (may). The air temperature ranged from 21 to 27°C and all test sessions were conducted between 18:00 h and 21:00 h in order to present the same circadian variations. In the prior sessions, specific exercises were performed to familiarize participants with the correct execution of the tests, and explanations and concrete corrections were also given to the players. The players were instructed to perform all tests at maximum intensity. No strenuous exercises were performed during the 48 h immediately prior to the tests and the researches supervised the study all time. Participants were required to attend the exercise-testing laboratory on 2 separate occasions. The first visit served as a players returned to the laboratory after 7 days for second testing sessions (sprint and CODA). Before each testing session a 10 min standardized warm-up consisting in 6 min self paced low-intensity running, 4 min skipping exercises, strides and two 15 m sprints and VJs were performed.

The first evaluation session consisted of anthropometric measurements and VJ tests with a randomized controlled trial: squat jump (SJ), countermovement jump (CMJ) and arm swim countermovement jump (CMJAS) were tested. The second evaluation session consisted of an acceleration test (5, 10 and 15 m) and CODA tests measured by modified agility test (MAT), 505 agility test (505) and 20 yards agility test (20Y).

Measures

Anthropometric Characteristics

The anthropometric variables of height (cm), body mass (kg) were measured in each player. Height was measured to the nearest 0.1 cm using a stadiometer (Holtain Ltd®, Crymych, United Kingdom) with a precision ±2 mm and a range 130-210 cm. Body mass was obtained to the nearest 0.1 kg using an electronic scale (Seca Instruments Ltd®, Hamburg, Germany). The BMI was calculated: BMI = body mass (kg) x height (m^{-2}). Bio-impedance (BIA) was measured, after lying for 10 min in a horizontal position on a clinical bed, using a Tanita BC-418 analyser (Tanita®, Tokyo, Japan).

Physical Capacities

VJ test: Soccer players' 3 x SJ, 3 x CMJ, and 3 x CMJAS were tested using the Opto Jump Next® (Microgate, Italy), according to the procedures proposed by Bosco et al. (1983). In both jumps (except CMJAS), the hands were placed on the hips during the take-off, flight, and landing phases. The maximal flexion of the knees during the take-off phase was required to be about 90°. During both jumps, a minimal flexion of the trunk during take-off was permitted. Any jump that did not meet the considered requirements was excluded from calculations and repeated. Flight time was used to calculate the change in the height of the body's centre of gravity (Bosco and Komi, 1979). The calculation of jump height assumed that the take-off and landing positions of the body's centre of gravity (Ostojic, Mazic, and Dikic, 2006). To assess limb stretch-shortening cycle efficiency, difference between CMJ and SJ jumping height (CMJ-SJ) was assessed (Castagna and Castellini 2013; McGuigan et al. 2006).

Acceleration

The participants undertook a sprint test consisting of three maximal acceleration of 5, 10 and 15 m, with a 120 s rest period among each sprint, enough time to walk back to the start and wait for turn, previously described by Los Arcos et al. (2014). The participants were placed at 0.5 m from the starting point, and began when they felt (Los Arcos et al. 2014). Time was recorded using photocell gates (Microgate® Polifemo, Bolzano, Italy) placed 0.4 m above the ground (Los Arcos et al. 2014) with an accuracy of ±0.001 s. The timer was activated automatically as the volunteers passed the first gate at the 0.0 m mark and split times were then recorded at 5, 10 and 15 m.

Change of Direction Ability Tests (CODA)

Modified agility test (MAT): The participants began with both feet together at 0.5 m from cone A, and complete the circuit (Figure 1A), using the protocol by Sassi et al. (2009). The players performed the test using the same directives but the displacements are free, it is not required move laterally and facing forward (Yanci et al. 2015). A-B displacement (5 m): At his own discretion, each subject sprinted forward to cone B and touched the top with the right hand. B-C displacement (2.5 m): Facing forward they shuffled to the left to cone C and touched the top with the left hand. C-D displacement (5 m): The participants then shuffled to the right to cone D and touched the top. D-B displacement (2.5 m): They shuffled back to the left to cone B and touched the top. B-A displacement (5 m): Finally, the participants moved as quickly as possible and returned to start line. All participants performed the test 3 times with at least 3 min of rest among trials. The total distance covered was 20 m and the height of the cones was 0.3 m. Seven days after, the retest was performed under the same conditions. A photocell (Powertimer, Newtest® Oy, Oulu, Finland) located over cone A was used to record the time. Time measurement started and finished when the player crossed the line between both tripods. The calculated margin of error was ± 0.001 s and the sensors were set approximately 0.40 m above the floor. 505 test: The players sprinted forward to a line 5 m ahead and pivoted 180° before returning to the start position (Figure 1B). A photocell (Powertimer, Newtest® Oy, Oulu, Finland) located over start/finish line was used to record the time. Time measurement started and finished when the subject crossed the line between the tripods. The calculated margin of error was ± 0.001 s, and the sensors were set approximately 0.40 m above the floor. 20Y test: 20Y required an ability to accelerate, decelerate, and change the direction by rotating the body for 180º. On an indoor surface, a 2-ft piece of tape was placed to mark the centerline. From the centerline, 5 m was measured in both directions, and these spots were also marked with tape. Each participant was instructed to straddle the centerline with his feet on the line. On the given command, the player ran toward the line of his choice and touched it with his foot, changed the direction and ran past the centerline to the opposite line and touched it with his foot. After, the subject changed the direction and ran through the centerline (Figure 1C). The drill was over when the subject crossed the centerline with his body (Salaj and Markovic, 2011). A photocell (Powertimer, Newtest® Oy, Oulu, Finland) was used to record the final time.

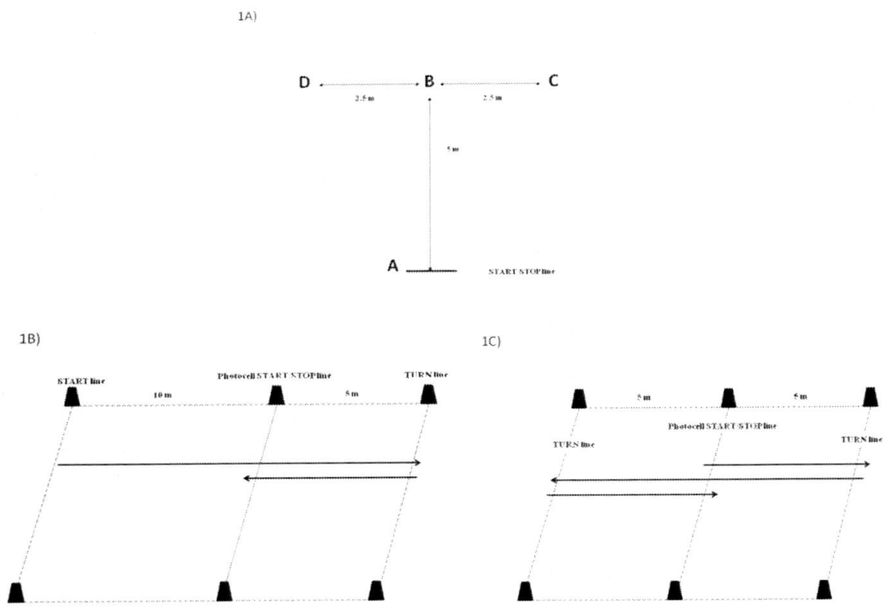

Figure 1. Change of direction ability (CODA) tests design. 1A) Modified agility T-test (MAT). 1B) 505 agility test (505); 1C) 20 yards agility test (20Y).

Data Analysis

The results are presented as mean ± standard deviation from the mean (SD). All the variables were normal and satisfied the equality of variances according to the Shapiro-Wilk test for $n \leq 50$ and Levene tests respectively. Only the maximum score of each test was included in the data analysis and the parametric analysis techniques were used. Coefficient of variation (CV) was calculated for all test variables to determine the stability of measurement among trials (CV = [SD/mean] x 100). Independent parametric Student t-tests were used to compare general descriptive characteristics between two groups and different tests. Practical differences were assessed by calculating Cohen's d effect size. Effect sizes (ES) of >0.8, 0.8-0.5, 0.5-0.2 and <0.2 were considered as large, moderate, small, and trivial, respectively (Cohen, 1988). A one-way analysis of variance (ANOVA) was used for playing position comparisons, and Bonferroni post-hoc analysis was applied to any set of hypothesis tests. Statistical significance was set at $p < 0.05$. Data analysis was performed using the Statistical Package for Social Sciences (version 23.0 for Windows, SPSS® Inc, Chicago, IL, USA) for Windows.

RESULTS

Descriptive statistics for anthropometric characteristics and training experience of players by competitive level and field position are presented in Table 1. No statistically significant difference was observed between AM and PROF groups in height, body mass, BMI, body fat, body water and training experience. However, the AM group showed significant higher values in age ($p < 0.05$, ES = 0.58, moderate) than the PROF group. According to the playing position, significant differences in body water and body fat were observed among various groups (Table 1). FW group was the group that presented the lowest fat percentage (9.96 ± 2.42%). However, LM group described more fat percentage (18.19 ± 4.55%).

Table 1. Soccer players' anthropometric characteristics by competitive level and field position. Values are mean (standard deviation) and effect size (ES)

	Sample (n = 46)	Professional (n = 14)	Amateur (n = 32)	ES	GK (n = 6)	CD (n = 8)	LD (n = 9)	CM (n = 9)	LM (n = 7)	FW (n = 7)
Age (yr)	23.07 ± 2.42	22.00 ± 1.41	23.53 ± 2.63*	0.58	23.67 ± 2.42	23.75 ± 1.75	22.44 ± 2.35	22.56 ± 2.35	24.29 ± 3.35	22.00 ± 2.08
Training experience (yr)	15.24 ± 2.58	14.50 ± 1.65	15.56 ± 2.86	0.37	14.83 ± 2.14	15.88 ± 1.13	14.56 ± 2.35	15.00 ± 2.74	16.86 ± 3.89	14.43 ± 2.64
Height (cm)	179.96 ± 5.76	179.43 ± 5.96	180.19 ± 5.75	0,13	180.50 ± 3.27	183.75 ± 4.27	179.22 ± 6.78	178.00 ± 3.77	175.71 ± 6.18	182.86 ± 6.57
Body mass (kg)	76.87 ± 7.95	75.51 ± 7.90	77.47 ± 8.02	0.24	80.60 ± 3.59	82.75 ± 6.11	71.90 ± 6.10	77.32 ± 4.69	75.44 ± 12.46	74.21 ± 8.80
BMI ($kg.m^{-2}$)	23.72 ± 1.95	23.42 ± 1.77	23.85 ± 2.04	0,21	24.75 ± 0.88	24.51 ± 1.58	22.39 ± 1.50	24.41 ± 1.56	24.31 ± 2.78	22.14 ± 1.57
Muscular mass (%)	38.98 ± 8.57	37.46 ± 4.73	39.65 ± 9.78	0.22	41.32 ± 2.10	41.04 ± 2.00	34.97 ± 2.42	37.82 ± 1.96	34.96 ± 5.22	45.30 ± 19.98
Body water (%)	48.52 ± 4.85	48.11 ± 5.71	48.70 ± 4.50	0.13	52.57 ± 2.52	52.28 ± 2.62	45.20 ± 2.98#*f*	48.33 ± 2.49	44.89 ± 6.37#*f*	48.93 ± 5.90
Body fat (%)	13.51 ± 4.42	12.90 ± 3.04	13.78 ± 4.93	0.18	10.78 ± 2.29	13.30 ± 4.70	13.87 ± 3.83	14.28 ± 4.04	18.19 ± 4.55#	9.96 ± 2.42‡

Legend: BMI = body mass index; GK = goalkeepers; CD = central defenders; LD = lateral defenders; CM = central midfields; LM = lateral midfields; FW = forwards. Significant differences between elite and amateur soccer players * $p < 0.05$. Significant differences with goalkeeper's # $p < 0.05$. Significant differences with central defenders *f* $p < 0.05$. Significant differences between lateral midfields and forwards † $p < 0.05$, ‡ $p < 0.01$.

The differences between PROF and AM groups of the acceleration's tests are presented in Figure 2. The PROF soccer group showed significant better results than the AM group in 5 m (3%, $p < 0.05$, ES = 0.81, large), 10 m (5%, $p < 0.05$, ES = 0.69, moderate), and 15 m (5%, $p < 0.05$, ES = 0.75, moderate). The CV obtained for 5, 10 and 15 m was 2.4%, 1.6% and 1.1%, respectively.

The CV obtained for SJ, CMJ and CMJAS was 4.6%, 2.7% and 2.7%, respectively. No significant differences were observed between AM and PROF groups in SJ, CMJ, CMJAS and CMJAS-CMJ. However, the PROF group showed significant higher values in CMJ-SJ ($p < 0.05$, ES = 0.68, moderate) than the AM group. These results were presented in Figure 3 and 4.

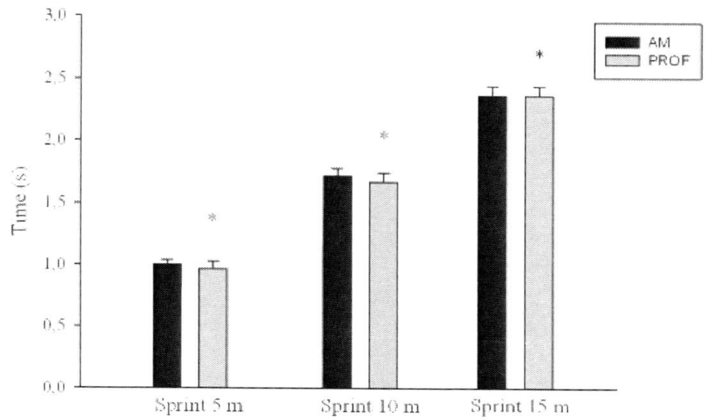

Figure 2. Differences between professional (PROF) and amateur (AM) soccer players in sprint 5, 10 y 15 m test. Legend: Significant differences between competitive levels * $p < 0.05$.

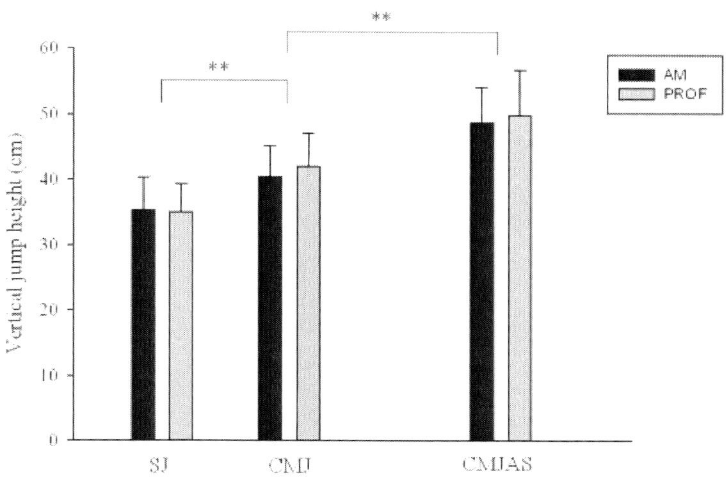

Legend: SJ = squat jump; CMJ = countermovement jump; CMJAS = arm swing countermovement jump. Significant differences between types of test results ** $p < 0.01$.

Figure 3. Differences between professional (PROF) and amateur (AM) soccer players in vertical jump (VJ) tests and differences between types of test.

Table 2. Performance of soccer players in sprint, vertical jump and change of direction ability (CODA) tests by field position. Values are mean (standard deviation)

	Sample (n = 46)	GK (n = 6)	CD (n = 8)	LD (n = 9)	CM (n = 9)	LM (n = 7)	FW (n = 7)
Sprint (s)							
5 m	0.99 ± 0.06	1.04 ± 0.05	0.98 ± 0.04	0.99 ± 0.05	0.99 ± 0.05	1.00 ± 0.03	0.96 ± 0.05
10 m	1.71 ± 0.06	1.79 ± 0.07	1.68 ± 0.05#	1.68 ± 0.05#	1.71 ± 0.07	1.70 ± 0.03	1.66 ± 0.08##
15 m	2.34 ± 0.06	2.45 ± 0.08	2.33 ± 0.06	2.33 ± 0.07	2.35 ± 0.08	2.33 ± 0.03	2.30 ± 0.10##
Vertical jump (cm)							
SJ	35.34 ± 4.71	34.35 ± 3.90	36.53 ± 2.91	34.60 ± 4.89	36.81 ± 4.38	35.17 ± 7.47	34.07 ± 5.32
CMJ	40.97 ± 4.87	39.20 ± 3.13	41.35 ± 3.12	39.03 ± 5.03	43.30 ± 4.88	41.33 ± 6.25	41.67 ± 6.57
CMJ-SJ	5.63 ± 3.06	4.85 ± 1.94	4.83 ± 4.33	4.43 ± 1.71	6.49 ± 3.35	6.17 ± 2.63	7.60 ± 3.31
CMJAS	49.15 ± 5,86	48.67 ± 3.50	50.76 ± 5.73	46.97 ± 6.58	50.15 ± 5.16	50.27 ± 5.83	48.32 ± 8.53
CMJAS-CMJ	8.18 ± 2.87	9.47 ± 1.00	9.41 ± 4.33	7.93 ± 3.06	6.85 ± 1.43	8.93 ± 2.97	6.65 ± 2.15
Change of direction ability (s)							
MAT	4.91 ± 0.16	5.01 ± 0.14	4.81 ± 0.11	4.94 ± 0.20	4.87 ± 0.12	4.92 ± 0.14	4.92 ± 0.18
505	2.51 ± 0.09	2.56 ± 0.07	2.48 ± 0.05	2.52 ± 0.08	2.51 ± 0.13	2.49 ± 0.09	2.49 ± 0.06
Y20	4.84 ± 0.17	5.00 ± 0.22	4.72 ± 0.13#	4.89 ± 0.12	4.84 ± 0.20	4.81 ± 0.10	4.81 ± 0.17

Legend: SJ = squat jump; CMJ = countermovement jump; CMJAS = arm swing countermovement jump; MAT = modified agility test; 505 = 505 agility test; Y20 = 20 yards agility test; GK = goalkeepers; CD = central defenders; LD = lateral defenders; CM = central midfields; LM = lateral midfields; FW = forwards. Significant differences between elite and amateur soccer players * $p < 0.05$. Significant differences with goalkeepers # $p < 0.05$, ## $p < 0.01$.

The CV obtained in MAT, 505 and 20Y test was 2.2%, 2.9% and 1.8%, respectively. No significant differences among PROF and AM groups were found in CODA tests (MAT = 4.90 ± 0.15 s vs. 4.91 ± 0.16 s, ES = 0.06, trivial; 505 = 2.52 ± 0.09 s vs. 2.50 ± 0.08 s, ES = 0.16, trivial;

20Y = 4.85 ± 0.16 s vs. 4.84 ± 0.18 s, ES = 0.01, trivial). The differences among players based on field position are presented in Table 2. Only significant differences were found in some groups with goalkeepers' group in 10 m ($p < 0.05$), 15 m ($p < 0.01$) and 20Y tests ($p < 0.05$).

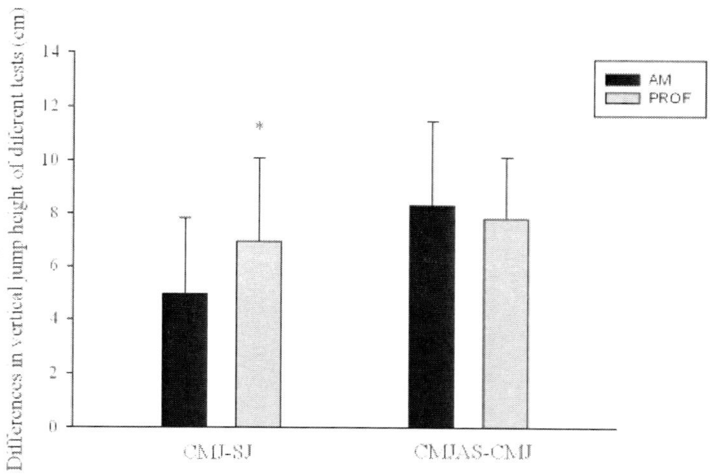

Legend: SJ = squat jump; CMJ = countermovement jump; CMJAS = arm swing countermovement jump. Significant differences between competitive levels * $p < 0.05$.

Figure 4. Differences between professional (PROF) and amateur (AM) soccer players in CMJ-SJ and CMJAS-CMJ values.

DISCUSSION

For our knowledge, this is the first study to examine selected fitness profile of male Spanish soccer players based on different competitive level and field position in a single research design. The main aim of this research was to determine the differences in acceleration, VJ and CODA between amateur and professional soccer players. A secondary purpose was to describe the differences in the physical characteristics and performance among playing position in two soccer groups. The main finding of the present study was that the PROF soccer group showed significant better results than the AM group in 5, 10, and 15 m test. According to the player position, significant differences were found in some groups with goalkeepers' group in 10 m, 15 m and 20Y tests.

Acceleration capacity during short distances has been certified to be a conditioning prerequisite for professional soccer players (Reilly et al. 2000). Besides, Cometti et al. (2001) showed that professional soccer players were faster over 10 m than amateur players. In the same line, Rampinini et al. (2009) observed that the repeat sprint ability performance differentiates between professional and amateur standard soccer players. In the present study, we did confirm these conclusions. Sprint abilities were found to discriminate between professional and amateur players presenting higher values 3% (ES = 0.81, large), 5% (ES = 0.69, moderate), 5% (ES = 0.75, moderate) in 5, 10, and 15 m, respectively. The higher values were in 10 and 15 m test. Therefore, it seems that sprint performance can be a differentiating capacity between players of different competitive levels.

The assessment of high-intensity activities during a match is a valid measure of physical performance in elite soccer, although the present study only showed the difference between PROF and AM. In the past years, sprinting activities have been analyzed in more depth (Di Salvo et al. 2010). It should also be emphasized that about 90% of sprints performed by professional soccer players were shorter than 5 s (Andrzejewski et al. 2013). Moreover, sprinting characteristics (Deprez et al. 2015; Di Salvo et al. 2010) and anaerobic power (Deprez et al. 2015) are influenced by playing position. This study was conducted to analyze the differences between groups in sprints 5, 10, and 15 m and we observed significant differences ($p < 0.05$) among central defenders, lateral defenders and forwards vs. goalkeepers in 10 m sprint. Specially, this difference was significant ($p > 0.01$) in 10 and 15 m between forwards and goalkeepers. Previous studies with elite players described those goalkeepers also are the slowest players in the team when sprinting ability over 10 and 20 m is required (Sporis et al. 2009). Significant differences were found between forwards and goalkeepers in 15 m test ($p > 0.01$), as previous studies had demonstrated when attackers were the quickest players in the team when looking at sprint values over 5, 10, and 20 m (Sporis et al. 2009), given that the speed dribbling ability test is not used much for goalkeepers. Correspondingly, speed-dribbling ability is not a specific indicator for goalkeepers, and this test should not be used for the choice of goalkeepers (Taskin 2008), and therefore future studies should utilize a similar adapted testing protocol for goalkeepers.

The VJ test has been reported a discriminant performance parameter in men's soccer (Bekris et al. 2018). Additionally, Arnason et al. (2004) showed that VJ performance could be considered as a discriminating variable in male soccer players of different competitive standard. In our investigation there are no differences between both groups in jump capacities, except CMJ-SJ values. Recently, the interest over performance potentiation in stretch-shortening movements has grown in sport performance analysis (Bobbert and Casius 2005). The ability to use the stretch-shortening cycle efficiently is critical in team sports (McGuigan et al. 2006). This is commonly measured comparing CMJ with SJ and expressing jumping height as difference (McGuigan et al. 2006). In this study, PROF players presented higher values in CMJ-SJ (28.2%, $p < 0.05$, $ES = 0.68$) compared with AM group. These results provide evidence for a less developed eccentric utilization ability of AM soccer players. Castagna and Castellini (2013) did no found significant competitive level differences for the absolute (CMJ-SJ) measurements in male players.. However, the U17 team CMJ-SJ was moderately different ($ES = 0.67$) from U21 and U20 teams (Castagna and Castellini 2013). This is of great interest for the strength and conditioning professional coaches given that the magnitude of the eccentric utilization ratio was reported to be useful in designing specific training interventions (McGuigan et al. 2006). Specifically, soccer players with greater gain over SJ performance through CMJ should supposedly possess the ability to develop force slowly (Bobbert and Casius 2005; Castagna and Castellini 2013). This conclusion suggests that strength and coaches should consider stretch-shortening cycle efficiently when dealing with prospective male soccer players. The use of either absolute expression of stretch-shortening cycle efficiently should be considered in parallel with CMJ and SJ heights (Castagna and Castellini 2013).

On the other hand, CODA is considered determinant for successful performance in soccer (Chaouachi et al. 2012) and the response to different and rapid movements is essential in soccer players. For this reason, CODA has been tested in order to asses soccer players conditioning (Chaouachi et al. 2012; Magal et al. 2009). A previous study showed that Portuguese soccer players, agility appeared to distinguish elite from non-elite in various field positions (Rebelo et al. 2013). However, in the present study, no significant differences by competitive level among PROF and AM groups were found in CODA tests (MAT, ES = 0.06, trivial; 505, ES = 0.16, trivial; 20Y, ES = 0.01, trivial). Only significant differences were found in central defenders with goalkeepers' group in 20Y tests ($p < 0.05$). A study conducted by Orendurff et al. (2010), demonstrated that central defenders attenuated the intensity of the work and recovery bouts late in the match staying closer to a more moderate work rate with fewer high- or low-intensity bouts, verifying the specificity of the position. In our study we observed that central defenders presented significant difference than goalkeepers in 20Y test ($p > 0.01$). This could be due as a result the used CODA test may possess a different degree of association with game activities and to the test specificity spectrum according to their relevance to soccer (Brughelli et al. 2008), although futures studies aiming to develop soccer specific tests are warranted (Chaouachi et al. 2012), for each position. The results obtained in this study should be taken with caution. The low number of players in each playing position group to have influenced the results. It would be interesting future studies with a larger players sample in each group.

Conclusion

According to our results the professional group showed significant better results than the amateur group in 5, 10, and 15 m. Based on the player position, significant differences were found in some groups with goalkeepers' group in 10 m, 15 m and 20Y tests. Acceleration is considered as a discriminate factor according to the competition level.

Based in our results, this conclusion suggests that the stretch-shortening cycle efficiently when dealing with prospective male soccer players. Therefore, training prescriptions in soccer should also be based on the specific requirements of the playing positions thereby ensuring players are better able to fulfill their tactical responsibilities during the game. Future studies should examine these differences among players on different training situations and at different times of the season.

REFERENCES

Andrzejewski, Marcin, Jan Chmura, Beata Pluta, Ryszard Strzelczyk, and Andrzej Kasprzak. 2013. "Analysis of Sprinting Activities of Professional Soccer Players." *Journal of Strength and Conditioning Research* 27: 2134–40. https://doi.org/10.1519/JSC.0b013e318279423e.

Arnason, Arni, Stefan B Sigurdsson, Arni Gudmundsson, Ingrad Holme, Lars Engebretsen, and Bahr Roald. 2004. "Physical fitness, injuries, and team performance in soccer." *Medicine and Science in Sports and Exercise* 36:278–285.

Arnold, James A, Barry Brown, Ralph Perry Micheli, and Tom P Coker. 1980. "Anatomical and Physiological Characteristics to Predict Football Ability." *American Journal of Sports Medicine* 8: 119–22.

Barker, Michael, Toni J Wyatt, Rober L Johnson, Michael H Stone, Harold S. O´Bryant, Carl Poe, and Michael Kent. 1993. "Performance Factors, Psychological Assessment, Physical Characteristics, and Football Playing Ability." *Journal of Strength and Conditioning Research* 7: 224–33.

Bekris, Evangelos, Georgios Pidoulas, Pantelis Pidoulas, Ioannis Gissis, Athanasios Katis, and Stergios Komsis. 2018. "Examination of Physical Fitness Parameters Between Professional and Amateur Greek Soccer Players During the Transition Period." *Journal of Strength and Conditioning Research*, October, 1. https://doi.org/10.1519/jsc.0000000000002770.

Bobbert, Maarten F, and LJ Richard Casius. 2005. "Is the Effect of a Countermovement on Jump Height Due to Active State Development?" *Medicine and Science in Sports and Exercise* 37: 440–46. https://doi.org/10.1249/01.MSS.0000155389.34538.97.

Bosco, Carmelo, and Paavo V Komi. 1979. "Mechanical Characteristics and Fiber Composition of Human Leg Extensor Muscles." *European Journal of Applied Physiology and Occupational Physiology* 41: 275–84. https://doi.org/10.1007/BF00429744.

Bosco, Carmelo, Paavo V Komi, Joszef Tihanyi, G Fekete, and Peter Apor. 1983. "Mechanical power test and fiber composition of human leg extensor muscles." *European Journal of Applied Physiology and Occupational Physyology* 51:129-135.

Brughelli, Matt, John Cronin, Greg Levin, and Chaouachi, Anis. 2008. "Understanding Change of Direction Ability in Sport: A Review of Resistance Training Studies." *Sports Medicine*. Adis International Ltd. https://doi.org/10.2165/00007256-200838120-00007.

Castagna, Carlo, and Elena Castellini. 2013. "Vertical Jump Performance in Italian Male and Female National Team Soccer Players." *Journal of Strength and Conditioning Research* 27: 1156–61. https://doi.org/10.1519/JSC.0b013e3182610999.

Chaouachi, Anis, Vincenzo Manzi, Anis Chaalali, Del P Wong, Karim Chamari, and Carlo Castagna. 2012. "Determinants Analysis of Change-of-Direction Ability in Elite Soccer Players." *Journal of Strength and Conditioning Research* 26: 2667–76. https://doi.org/10.1519/JSC.0b013e318242f97a.

Cohen, Jacob. 1988. *Statistical Power Analysis for the Behavioral Sciences*. Neew York: Routledge. https://doi.org/https://doi.org/10.4324/9780203771587.

Cometti, Gilles, Nicola Maffiuletti, Michel Pousson, Jean-Claud Chatard, and Nicola Maffulli. 2001. "Isokinetic strength and anaerobic power of elite, subelite and amateur French soccer players." *International Journal of Sports Medicine*, *22*: 45–51. https://doi.org/10.1055/s-2001-11331.

Dellal, Alexandre, R Jannault, Manuel Lopez-Segovia, Vincent Pialoux. 2011. "Influence of the Numbers of Players in the Heart Rate Responses of Youth Soccer Players Within 2 vs. 2, 3 vs. 3 and 4 vs. 4 Small-Sided Games." *Journal of Human Kinetics* 28: 107–14. https://doi.org/10.2478/v10078-011-0027-8.

Deprez, Dieter, Job Fransen, Jan Boone, Matthieu Lenoir, Renaat Philippaerts, and Roel Vaeyens. 2015. "Characteristics of High-Level Youth Soccer Players: Variation by Playing Position." *Journal of Sports Sciences* 33: 243–54. https://doi.org/10.1080/02640414.2014.934707.

Di Salvo, Valter, Ramon Baron, Carlos González-Haro, Christian Gormasz, Fabio Pigozzi, and Norbert Bachl. 2010. "Sprinting Analysis of Elite Soccer Players during European Champions League and UEFA Cup Matches." *Journal of Sports Sciences* 28: 1489–94. https://doi.org/10.1080/02640414.2010.521166.

Ingebrigtsen, Jørgen, Shaher A I Shalfawi, Espen Tønnessen, Peter Krustrup, and Andreas Holtermann. 2013. "Performance Effects of 6 Weeks of Aerobic Production Training in Junior Elite Soccer Players." *Journal of Strength and Conditioning Research* 27: 1861–67. https://doi.org/10.1519/JSC.0b013e31827647bd.

Little, Thomas, and Alun G Williams. 2006. "Suitability of Soccer Training Drills for Endurance Training." *Journal of Strength and Conditioning Research* 20: 316–19. https://doi.org/10.1519/R-17094.1.

Los Arcos, Asier, Javier Yanci, Jurdan Mendiguchia, Juan J. Salinero, Matt Brughelli, and Carlo Castagna. 2014. "Short-Term Training Effects of Vertically and Horizontally Oriented Exercises on Neuromuscular Performance in Professional Soccer Players." *International Journal of Sports Physiology and Performance* 9: 480–88. https://doi.org/10.1123/IJSPP.2013-0063.

Magal, Meir, Ron T Smith, Jon J Dyer, and Jay R Hoffman. 2009. "Seasonal Variation in Physical Performance-Related Variables in Male NCAA Division III Soccer Players." *Journal of Strength and Conditioning Research* 23: 2555–59. https://doi.org/10.1519/JSC.0b013e3181b3ddbf.

McGuigan, Michael R, Timothy L A Doyle, Michael Newton, Dylan J Edwards, Sophia Nimphius, and Robert U Newton. 2006. "Eccentric Utilization Ratio: Effect of Sport and Phase of Training." *Journal of Strength and Conditioning Research* 20: 992–95. https://doi.org/10.1519/R-19165.1.

Nikolaidis, Pantelis Theodoros, and Nikos Vassilios Karydis. 2011. "Physique and Body Composition in Soccer Players across Adolescence." *Asian Journal of Sports Medicine* 2: 75–82. https://doi.org/10.5812/asjsm.34782.

Orendurff, Micael S, Jason D. Walker, Mladen Jovanovic, Kirsten L. Tulchin, Morris Levy, and David K. Hoffmann. 2010. "Intensity and duration of intermittent exercise and recovery during a soccer match" *Journal of Strength and Conditioning Research* 24: 2683–2692. https://doi.org/10.1519/JSC.0b013e3181bac463.

Ostojic, Sergej M, Sanja Mazic, and Nenad Dikic. 2006. "Profiling in basketball: Physical and physiological characteristics of elite players." *Journal of Strength and Conditioning Research* 24: 740–744. https://doi.org/10.1519/R-15944.1.

Ozkan, Ali, Gürhan Kayıhan, Yusuf Köklü, Nevin Ergun, Mitat Koz, Gülfem Ersöz, and Alexandre Dellal. 2012. "The Relationship between Body Composition, Anaerobic Performance and Sprint Ability of Amputee Soccer Players." *Journal of Human Kinetics* 35: 141–46. https://doi.org/10.2478/v10078-012-0088-3.

Rampinini, Ermanno, Aldo Sassi, Andrea Morelli, Stefano Mazzoni, Maurizio Fanchini, and Aaron J Coutts. 2009. "Repeated-Sprint Ability in Professional and Amateur Soccer Players." *Applied Physiology, Nutrition and Metabolism* 34: 1048–54. https://doi.org/10.1139/H09-111.

Rebelo, Antonio, Joao Brito, José Maia, Manuel J. Coelho-e-Silva, Antonio J Figueiredo, Jens Bangsbo, Robert Malina, and André Seabra. 2013. "Anthropometric Characteristics, Physical Fitness and Technical Performance of under-19 Soccer Players by Competitive Level and Field Position." *International Journal of Sports Medicine* 34: 312–17. https://doi.org/10.1055/s-0032-1323729.

Reilly, Thomas, Andrew Mark Williams, Alan Michael Nevill, and A Franks. 2000. "A Multidisciplinary Approach to Talent Identification in Soccer." *Journal of Sports Sciences* 18: 695–702. https://doi.org/10.1080/02640410050120078.

Salaj, Sanja, and Goran Markovic. 2011. "Specificity of Jumping, Sprinting, and Quick Change-of-Direction Motor Abilities." *Journal of Strength and Conditioning Research* 25: 1249–55. https://doi.org/10.1519/JSC.0b013e3181da77df.

Sassi, Radhouane Haj, Wajdi Dardouri, Mohamed Haj Yahmed, Nabil Gmada, Mohamed Elhedi Mahfoudhi, and Zied Gharbi. 2009. "Relative and absolute reliability of a Modified Agility T-Test and its relationship with vertical jump and straight sprint." *Journal of Strength and Conditioning Research* 23: 1644-1651.

Sedano, Silvia, Roel Vaeyens, Renaat Philippaerts, Juan Carlos Redondo, and Gonzalo Cuadrado. 2009. "Anthropometric and Anaerobic Fitness Profile of Elite and Non-Elite Female Soccer Players." *Journal of Sports Medicine and Physical Fitness* 49: 387-394.

Sheppard Jeremy, and Warren B. Young. 2006. "Agility literature review: classifications, training and testing." *Journal of Sports Sciences* 24: 919-932.

Sporis, Goran, Igor Jukic, Sergej M Ostojic, and Dragan Milanovic. 2009. "Fitness Profiling in Soccer: Physical and Physiologic Characteristics of Elite Players." *Journal of Strength and Conditioning Research* 23: 1947–53. https://doi.org/10.1519/JSC.0b013e3181b3e141.

Stølen, Tomas, Karim Chamari, Carlo Castagna, and Ulrik Wisløff. 2005. "Physiology of Soccer: An Update." *Sports Medicine*. https://doi.org/10.2165/00007256-200535060-00004.

Taskin, Halil. 2008. "Evaluating Sprinting Ability, Density of Acceleration, and Speed Dribbling Ability of Professional Soccer Players with Respect to Their Positions." *Journal of Strength and Conditioning Research* 22: 1481–86. https://doi.org/10.1519/JSC.0b013e318181fd90.

Yanci, Javier, Asier Los Arcos, Jurdan Mendiguchia, and Matt Brughelli. 2015. "Relationships between Sprinting, Agility, One- and Two-Leg Vertical and Horizontal Jump in Soccer Players" *Kinesiology* 46: 194–201.

In: An Essential Guide to Sports Performance ISBN: 978-1-53617-608-7
Editors: Daniel Castillo Alvira et al.

Chapter 4

DIFFERENCES IN POWER PERFORMANCE ATTENDING TO SPRINT CAPACITY AND ASYMMETRY LEVEL IN YOUNG ELITE SOCCER PLAYERS

Javier Raya-González*[1,*]*, PhD, Marco Beato*[2]*, PhD and Daniel Castillo*[1]*, PhD

[1]Faculty of Health Sciences,
Universidad Isabel I, Burgos, Spain
[2]School of Health and Sports Sciences,
University of Suffolk, Ipswich, UK

ABSTRACT

The aim of this study was to analyze the differences in power performance attending to sprint capacity and asymmetry level in young

* Corresponding Author's Email: rayagonzalezjavier@gmail.com.

elite soccer players, using a median split analysis to separate faster and slower athletes and players with higher and lower asymmetry scores. Thirty-one young elite male soccer players participated in this study and completed the following physical tests: countermovement jump (CMJ), Abalakov jump (ABK), 30-m linear sprint test, and change of direction sprint test. The differences between faster and slower and between lower and higher asymmetry score groups (LAS and HAS, respectively) were calculated using the magnitude-based inferences method. Faster soccer players performed better in all the speed-power tests, without differences in change of direction deficit (CODd) in comparison to slower players. Nevertheless, no differences were found in the proposed tests when soccer players were discriminated by their asymmetry score, except in CODd, demonstrating a greater deficit in those players with greater asymmetry values. These findings show the importance of separating young soccer players by their speed performance to identify its specific training needs, as well as to reduce the inter-limb asymmetries to improve the capacity to efficiently change direction.

Keywords: sprint capacity, change of direction, agility, change of direction deficit, team sports

INTRODUCTION

Soccer is considered as an intermittent team-sport characterized by the combination of low-intensity (e.g., walking or jogging) and high-intensity actions (e.g., jumping, sprinting and changes of direction [COD]) (Ade, Fitzpatrick, and Bradley 2016). These latter actions occur mainly during decisive moments of the match-play, pointing out the key role of high-intensity activities to achieve a great on-field performance (Faude et al. 2014). Specifically, soccer players are required to perform a great number of successive accelerations, decelerations, and re-accelerations, as well as quick and decisive changes in movement direction (Chaouachi et al. 2012). Such actions are dependent on external stimuli (e.g., ball trajectory, opponents' and team-mates' movements) (Born et al. 2016). Thus, COD capacity is considered a key factor in soccer players' on-field performance, although a more comprehensive analysis of this capacity, not only based on COD velocity (CODv), is required. In this sense, the COD deficit (CODd) has emerged as an indicator of the athlete's efficiency to change direction, and it refers to the additional time that a COD requires when compared to a linear straight sprint test (LSST) over the same distance (Nimphius et al. 2016) or the difference in velocity between the LSST and a COD task of equal distance (Pereira et al. 2018). The CODd is definitely a practical tool to better isolate and identify a young soccer player's ability to change direction.

Traditionally, the study of the physical conditioning of soccer players, in terms on physical performance analysis attending to different capacities (e.g., acceleration, velocity, COD, etc.), has been developed for the whole team (Beato et al. 2019, 2017) or based on the age-category (Loturco et al. 2019b) or competitive level (Ayarra et al. 2018). However, given the existing associations between the decisive neuromuscular capacities in soccer (e.g., jumping, sprinting and COD) (Pereira et al. 2018; Cronin and Hansen 2005), it would be interesting to investigate the selective influence of the initial physical fitness level on performance (e.g., differentiating the players their performance in some physical test), in order to design the training strategies towards the specific players' profile. Regarding this, Loturco, et al. (2019a) used a median split analysis based on the player's acceleration capacity (e.g., 5-m performance) to classify the soccer players into faster and slower. These authors observed that those players able to accelerate faster over short distances (e.g., 5-m) performed better in jumping, sprinting and COD capacities, although they showed lower COD efficiency (e.g., CODd) in comparison to slower professional players. Also, Freitas et al. (2018) reported greater values in jumping, sprinting and COD test by those rugby players with a greater capacity to reach high velocities in a 40-m LSST, in addition to a higher CODd. Due to the contradictory results on the influence of the individual players sprint performance for the different physical capacities, it is deemed appropriate to deepen this analysis.

Several studies have analyzed the magnitude and direction of asymmetries in soccer players (Bishop et al. 2018; Bishop et al. 2019c; Bishop et al. 2019d). This interest is justified by the fact that thresholds of >10% are to be accepted as cutoffs where reduced physical performance

(Bishop, Turner, and Read 2018b) and increased risk of injury are present (Rohman et al. 2015). Despite this, a controversy exists when analyzing the influence of the asymmetries on the physical performance. On the one hand, Bishop et al. (2019d) showed that drop jump height asymmetry was associated with reduced 30-m sprint ($r = 0.58$) and 505 test performance on both limbs ($r = 0.52$-0.66) in female soccer players. Additionally, Bishop et al. (2019b) showed that countermovement jump (CMJ) height asymmetry was associated with slower 5-m ($r = 0.60$-0.86), 10-m ($r = 0.54$-0.87), 20-m ($r = 0.56$-0.79), and 505 test performance on both limbs ($r = 0.61$-0.85) in elite soccer players ranging from under-16 to under-23. On the other hand, several authors observed no significant relationship between CMJ height asymmetry and COD (Bishop et al. 2019b; Bishop et al. 2019c). To further gather knowledge about this topic, it would be relevant to analyze whether young soccer players with greater asymmetry scores (HAS) exhibit equal or different physical performances in comparison to lower asymmetry scores (LAS).

Since no previous studies had analyzed the selective influence of the sprint capacity and the asymmetry level on power performances in young soccer players, the aim of this study was to analyze the differences on power performances attending to sprint capacity and asymmetry level in elite young soccer players, using a median split analysis to separate faster and slower athletes and players with higher and lower asymmetry scores. Based on previous studies (Bishop et al. 2019c; Loturco et al. 2019a) we hypothesized that faster players would be able to perform better physically than their slower counterparts as well as the most symmetric players in comparison to the asymmetric players.

METHODS

Participants

Thirty-one young elite male soccer players (age: 15.7 ± 1.1 years, height: 172 ± 5 cm, body mass: 64.3 ± 7.7 kg, and body mass index (BMI):

20.7 ± 1.0 kg m^{-2}) of the same elite soccer academy participated in this study. Participants played in the highest division corresponding to their age-category level in Spain. Goalkeepers were excluded from the study sample, due to their specific role in the game. Prior to the study beginning, each player completed a questionnaire about their medical and injury history, and we excluded those participants who suffered an injury in the two months before the assessment. Additionally, players who did not complete all tests were omitted in the subsequent statistical analysis. Players trained three days per week and were involved in an official match at the weekends. All the participants were informed of the objectives of the research, participated voluntarily and had the possibility to withdraw at any time from the investigation without any penalty. A written informed consent was filled out by participants′ parents as they were under the age of 18. The study followed the guidelines set out in the Declaration of Helsinki (2013) and was conducted under the established ethical standards for sport science and exercise research (Harriss and Atkinson 2015).

Experimental Design

A cross-sectional comparative study design was used to the differentiate power performances attending to sprint capacity and asymmetry level in young elite soccer players. All the participants undertook similar soccer training routines and were familiarized with the testing procedures following the assessment routines carried out in the clubs. The tests were completed during the in-season period, in an only testing session, and following the next order: vertical jump tests (i.e., CMJ and ABK), 30-m LSST and COD test. Five minutes for recovery were given to participants between each test. All tests were performed on an artificial grass field where the team had their usual training sessions and players wore their normal soccer boots. In addition, all tests were supervised by accredited strength and conditioning coaches, who gave verbal encouragement to each participant to ensure both parties were satisfied with requirements before data collection (Bishop Berney, et al.

2019). Before the data collection, a standardized 15-min warm-up was performed, consisting of seven minutes of slow jogging and strolling locomotion, followed by eight minutes of jump and progressive acceleration and sprint actions over 10 and 30-m distances.

Procedures

Vertical Jump Tests

Players performed three bilateral CMJ and three bilateral Abalakov (ABK) jumps on a platform with infrared rays (Optojump Next, Microgate ®, Bolzano, Italy) separated by 45 s of passive recovery (Núñez et al. 2018). During the CMJ, players were instructed to perform a downward movement followed by a complete, explosive extension of the lower limbs, maintaining their hands on the hip (Sáez de Villarreal et al. 2015). For the ABK, the same movement pattern was performed but swinging of the arms was allowed (Maulder and Cronin 2005). For the subsequent statistical analysis, the best performance of each test was selected. The intraclass correlation coefficients (ICCs) and the coefficients of variation (CVs) for the jump tests were 0.96 (0.92–0.98) and 3.1% for CMJ and 0.96 (0.92–0.98) and 3% for ABK, respectively.

30-m Linear Straight Sprint Test (30-LSST)

Participants were assessed over a 30-LSST with split times on 10-m, 20-m and 30-m. Four pairs of photoelectric cells (Polifermo Light Radio, Microgate®, Bolzano, Italy) were used to record the sprint times. The starting position was placed 0.5-m before the first timing gate, and players started when ready eliminating reaction time. Two trials with a rest of two min between each sprint were completed, and the fastest time was considered for the subsequent statistical analysis. The sprint velocity ($m \cdot s^{-1}$) was calculated as the distance traveled over a measured time interval and sprint momentum ($kg \cdot m \cdot s^{-1}$) was obtained by multiplying the athlete's body mass by the respective velocity during the linear sprint (Freitas et al. 2019). The ICC for the 30-LSST ranged from 0.77 to 0.90 while the CV ranged from 1.0 to 3.3.

Change of Direction (COD) Sprint Test

Participants were evaluated over a 20-m COD sprint test using two pairs of photoelectric cells (Polifermo Light Radio, Microgate®, Bolzano, Italy). The same starting position as in LSST was adopted. Four maximum 10+10-m sprints with a COD turn of 90° (i.e., two trials with the right leg on the outside during the turn and two trials with the left leg on the outside) were performed, and two minutes of passive recovery were allowed between trials. The best time obtained with each leg was identified, and the mean between both best trials was calculated and selected for the subsequent analysis. CODv was calculated as the distance traveled over a measured time interval. To evaluate de COD maneuverability, an adapted CODd calculation was used as in previous studies (Freitas et al. 2018; Loturco et al. 2019a), which was calculated as follows: 20-m LSST – CODv. For this test, the ICC was 0.96 (0.91–0.98) and the CV 2%.

Statistical Analysis

Results are presented as mean ± standard deviations (SD). Median split analysis was used to divide the soccer players into two groups according to their linear sprint velocity (faster and slower players) and attending to their asymmetry level (LAS and HAS groups). All data were log-transformed for analysis to reduce bias arising from non-uniformity error and then analyzed for practical significance using magnitude-based inferences (Hopkins et al. 2009). Effect sizes (ES) with the uncertainty of the estimates shown as 90% confidence limits (CL) were used to quantify the magnitude of the difference between groups in all variables analyzed. Threshold values for assessing magnitudes of the ES were: trivial (<0.2), small (0.2–0.6), moderate (0.6–1.2), large (1.2–2.0), very large (2.0–4.0) and extremely large (>4.0) (Hopkins et al. 2009). Quantitative chances of higher or lower differences were evaluated qualitatively as follows: possibly (25–75%), likely (75–95%), very likely (95–99.5%), and most likely (>99.5%) (Hopkins et al. 2009). Inference was classified as unclear if the 90% CL overlapped the thresholds for the smallest worthwhile positive and negative effects (Hopkins et al. 2009). A dedicated spreadsheet, available at http://www.sportsci.org, was used to perform all the statistical analyses (Hopkins 2006).

RESULTS

Figure 1 depicts the comparison of the vertical jump tests between faster and slower players and between LAS and HAS groups. Vertical jump performance was substantially higher in the faster group when compared to slower players (likely moderate for CMJ and Abalakov), while no substantial differences were observed between LAS and HAS groups (unclear) in these vertical tests.

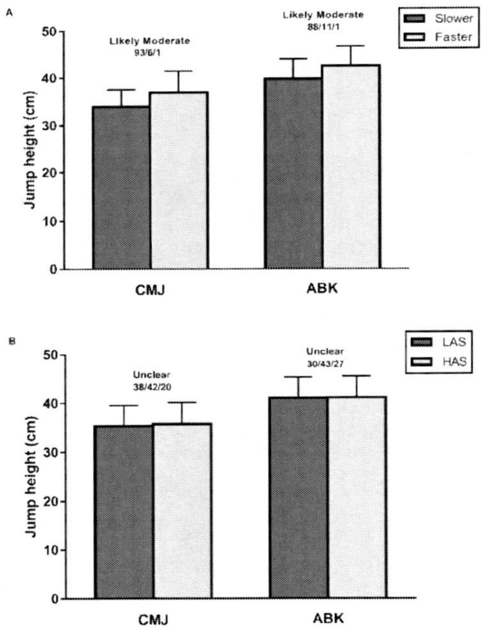

CMJ = countermovement jump; ABK = Abalakov jump.

Figure 1. Practical differences in the vertical jumps between faster and slower (A) and between lower (LAS) and higher (HAS) asymmetry score (B) groups.

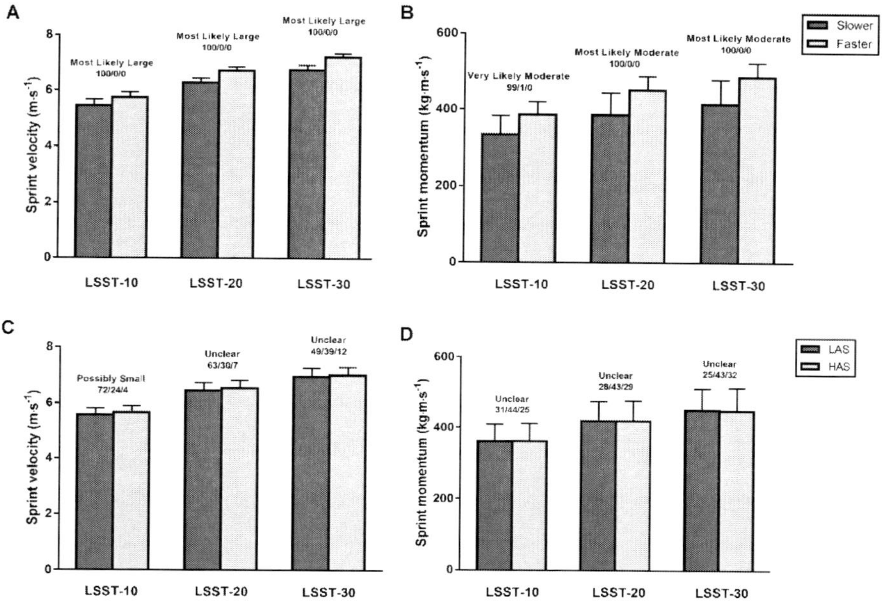

LSST-10 = 10-m linear straight sprint test; LSST-20 = 20-m linear straight sprint test; LSST-30 = 30-m linear straight sprint test.

Figure 2. Practical differences in the sprint velocity and momentum between faster and slower (A, B) and between lower (LAS) and higher (HAS) asymmetry score (C, D) groups.

The differences in the sprint velocity and sprint momentum between faster and slower players and between LAS and HAS groups are shown in Figure 2. Very likely moderate to most likely large differences in sprint velocity and sprint momentum was found between the faster group and the slower one. Regarding to the LAS and HAS groups, no substantial (unclear and possibly small) differences were reported in sprint variables.

Figure 3 shows the comparisons of the CODv and CODd between faster and slower players and between LAS and HAS groups. Faster players showed higher CODv compared with slower players (likely moderate), without meaningful differences (unclear) in CODd comparing faster and slower players. LAS and HAS groups showed no substantial differences in CODv (unclear), while a greater CODd value was observed in the HAS group in comparison with the LAS group (likely small).

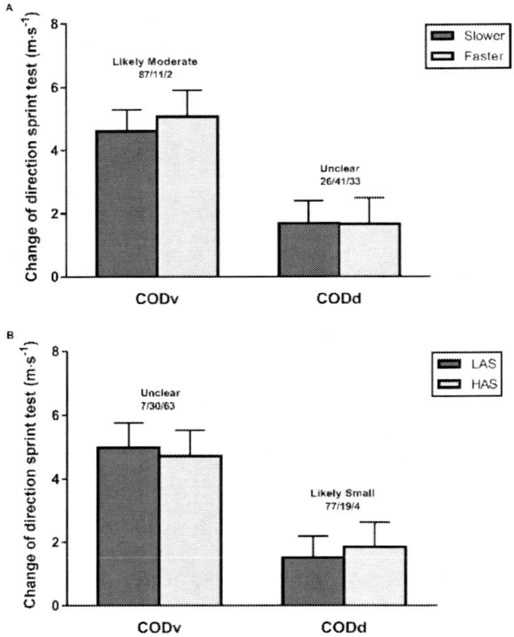

CODv = change of direction velocity; CODd = change of direction deficit.

Figure 3. Practical differences in the change of direction sprint test between faster and slower (A) and between lower (LAS) and higher (HAS) asymmetry score (B) groups.

DISCUSSION

The main aim of the current study was to analyze the differences on power performance attending to sprint capacity and asymmetry level in young elite soccer players, using a median split analysis to separate faster and slower athletes and players with higher and lower asymmetry scores. This is the first study that examined the influence of the initial physical level performance on physical conditioning in elite young players. The main results of the study were that soccer players able to perform better sprint results obtained better results in all the physical conditioning tests analyzed, showing a similar maneuverability efficiency (e.g., CODd) in comparison to slower players. However, no differences were found in power performance tests when soccer players were discriminated by their asymmetry score, except in CODd, checking a greater deficit in those players with greater asymmetry values.

Regarding the vertical jump capacity, faster players showed greater performance in both tests (e.g., CMJ and ABK) in comparison to the slower ones, similar to the results obtained by Freitas et al. (2018) with professional rugby players. This is due to the demonstrated relationship among several tests in which the rapid power application is a key factor (Yanci et al. 2014), especially in team-sports like soccer. In this sense, Köklü et al. (2015) observed a moderate correlation (r = -0.59; $P = 0.02$) between 30-m LSST performance and CMJ height when assessing young soccer players. Similarly, Yanci et al. (2014) found a significant correlation (r = -0.54; $P < 0.05$) between 15-m LSST and CMJ performance in semiprofessional soccer players. Additionally, McFarland et al. (2016) examined the relationship among different power performance tests in male and female soccer players, showing moderate correlation between 30-m LSST and CMJ tests in both genders (r = -0.57 and -0.67 for males and females respectively; $P < 0.05$). Nevertheless, our results suggest that there is no relationship between the asymmetry level, measured by a COD test, and vertical jump capacity. Conversely, the only previous study that analyzed the COD asymmetry effects on jump capacity showed that the most symmetrical athletes had a better performance in CMJ tests (Madruga-Parera et al. 2019). These differences could be due to the sample assessed in the Madruga-Parera's study (e.g., male and female tennis players), since the locomotor pattern and physical demands of tennis players are different in comparison to soccer players (Fernandez-Fernandez, Sanz-Rivas, and Mendez-Villanueva 2009) mainly related to jump capacity, with soccer players performing vertical jumps with only one leg. These findings suggest the necessity to apply specific fitness test which are sensitive to detect the asymmetries' influence on performance in soccer players (e.g., jumping test) (Bishop et al. 2019a; Bishop et al. 2019d).

As expected, better sprint performances in the 30-m distance test were obtained by faster players in comparison to slower ones. In addition, the faster group also showed better sprint performances on short distances (e.g., 10 and 20-m) due to the necessity to effectively accelerate over short distances to achieve greater performances in linear sprints above 20-m distance (Loturco et al. 2019a). These results are supported by previous studies such as Freitas et al. (2018), who observed that faster rugby players in a 40-m LSST achieved greater velocities at 10, 20, 30 and 40-m distances. Also, Loturco et al. (2019a) showed that players with a better acceleration capacity (e.g., 5-m) were able to reach greater performances in LSST over several distances (e.g., 10 and 20-m). Sprint momentum ($kg \cdot ms^{-1}$) is an interesting variable to take into account in collision sports such as soccer (Baker and Newton 2008). Some authors (Freitas et al. 2018) have shown no differences in sprint momentum when dividing the participants between faster and slower players, mainly due to the fact that slower players had 15% higher body mass than faster players. In this sense, it has been suggested the need to achieve an "ideal relationship" between velocity and body mass to maximize sprint momentum (Barr et al. 2014). In contrast to the aforementioned study, current results showed that faster players generated a greater sprint momentum than lower players, due to the higher velocity and body mass (e.g., 67.1 kg vs. 61.2 kg) in the first group. These results raise the importance of focusing the training not only on the body mass increase through strength training, but towards speed development over short distances (e.g., below to 20-m). Considering the differentiation by asymmetry scores, no differences between groups were observed for speed velocity and sprint momentum here. The fact that the nature of LSST, in which a constant force application is required, differs widely from the COD test, which is characterized by the presence of a braking action with an immediate requirement to transition into high propulsive forces, could be the reason why there were no differences between groups.

Similar to previous studies (Loturco et al. 2019a; Freitas et al. 2018; Freitas et al. 2019), faster players in LSST reached higher velocities during the COD test, despite the fact that in this activity other factors (e.g., the capacity to turn), in addition to the speed, influence the physical performance (Hader, Palazzi, and Buchheit 2015). In this sense, the relatively high linear running distance (e.g., 10+10-m) demanded in the

COD test could have influenced these results in favour of the faster group. Attending to the CODd, it seems logical to expect that faster and more powerful soccer players presented a lower capacity to effectively change direction (Loturco et al. 2018). This is justified by the fact that those players able to generating greater momentum sprint, and therefore, greater inertia, need to apply higher braking forces through longer ground contact times (Dos'Santos et al. 2018a), besides increasing the demands of eccentric contractions in the muscles involved (Dos'Santos et al. 2018b). Nevertheless, in the current study no differences between velocity groups were observed, since the COD test used only required performing a single COD maneuver. Conversely, previous studies that used multi-COD maneuvers tests (Freitas et al. 2018; Loturco et al. 2016) showed that faster players presented a lower capacity to change direction (e.g., greater COD deficits). According to this, to include tasks in training sessions based on actions that enhance the players' capacity to tolerate higher approaching velocities (e.g., sequentially accelerate, decelerate, and re-accelerate) would be an interesting strategy to improve COD efficiency (and reduce CODd). Notably, when discriminating players based on their asymmetry scores, no differences were found in CODv, while the HAS group generated a greater CODd in comparison with LAS, showing that HAS players are not capable to perform the COD maneuver efficiently. In this regard, to apply regular and multifaceted training strategies (i.e., strength training programs and tasks based on COD movement pattern) seems to be essential in order to reduce asymmetries (and COD deficit) in players with greater asymmetry values (Bishop, Turner, and Read 2018a).

This study presents several limitations that must be considered. Firstly, only a single COD test was used to assess COD performance. Secondly, asymmetry scores were calculated based on only one test. In this sense, a fitness test battery should be applied to provide a holistic picture of the asymmetries in the soccer players. Thirdly, due to the particular characteristics of the participants studied herein, the results obtained are difficult to generalize to other competitive levels. Finally, future research should study the influence of eccentric strength (dividing players according to their level) on COD performances.

Conclusion

Elite young soccer players that had a better performance during sprint tests obtained better results for all the physical conditioning variables (jump height, sprint velocity, sprint momentum, and CODv), showing a similar maneuverability efficiency (e.g., CODd) in comparison to slower players. On the other hand, no differences were found in the power performance tests when soccer players were discriminated by their asymmetry score, except in CODd, demonstrating a greater deficit in those players with greater asymmetry values. The finding obtained in this study suggests the importance of applying a median split analysis based on the individual sprint capacities to identify the specific training needs for each soccer player, as well as to reduce the inter-limb asymmetries to improve the capacity to efficiently change direction.

References

Ade, Jack, John Fitzpatrick, and Paul S. Bradley. 2016. "High-Intensity Efforts in Elite Soccer Matches and Associated Movement Patterns, Technical Skills and Tactical Actions. Information for Position-Specific Training Drills." *Journal of Sports Sciences* 34: 2205–14. doi:10.1080/02640414.2016.1217343.

Ayarra, Rubén, Fabio Y. Nakamura, Aitor Iturricastillo, Daniel Castillo, and Javier Yanci. 2018. "Differences in Physical Performance According to the Competitive Level in Futsal Players." *Journal of Human Kinetics* 64: 275–85. doi:10.1515/hukin-2017-0201.

Baker, Daniel G., and Robert U. Newton. 2008. "Comparison of Lower Body Strength, Power, Acceleration, Speed, Agility, and Sprint Momentum to Describe and Compare Playing Rank among Professional Rugby League Players." *Journal of Strength and Conditioning Research* 22: 153–58. doi:10.1519/JSC.0b013e318 15f9519.

Barr, Matthew J., Jeremy M. Sheppard, Tim J. Gabbett, and Robert U. Newton. 2014. "Long-Term Training-Induced Changes in Sprinting Speed and Sprint Momentum in Elite Rugby Union Players." *Journal of Strength and Conditioning Research* 28: 2724–31. doi:10.1519/JSC.0000000000000364.

Beato, Marco, Mattia Bianchi, Giuseppe Coratella, Michele Merlini, and Barry Drust. 2018. "Effects of Plyometric and Directional Training on Speed and Jump Performance in Elite Youth Soccer Players." *Journal of Strength and Conditioning Research* 32: 289-96. doi:10.1519/JSC.0000000000002371.

Beato, Marco, Mattia Bianchi, Giuseppe Coratella, Michele Merlini, and Barry Drust. 2019. "A Single Session of Straight Line and Change-of-Direction Sprinting per Week Does Not Lead to Different Fitness Improvements in Elite Young Soccer Players." *Journal of Strength and Conditioning Research*. doi:10.1519/JSC.0000000000003369.

Bishop, Chris, Jake Berney, Jason Lake, Irineu Loturco, Richard Blagrove, Anthony Turner, and Paul Read. 2019a. "Bilateral Deficit During Jumping Tasks: Relationship With Speed and Change of Direction Speed Performance." *Journal of Strength and Conditioning Research*. doi:10.1519/JSC.0000000000003075.

Bishop, Chris, Calum Brashill, Will Abbott, Paul Read, Jason Lake, and Anthony Turner. 2019b. "Jumping Asymmetries Are Associated With Speed, Change of Direction Speed, and Jump Performance in Elite Academy Soccer Players." *Journal of Strength and Conditioning Research*. doi:10.1519/JSC.0000000000003058.

Bishop, Chris, Jason Lake, Irineu Loturco, Kostas Papadopoulos, Anthony Turner, and Paul Read. 2018. "Interlimb Asymmetries: The Need for an Individual Approach to Data Analysis." *Journal of Strength and Conditioning Research*. doi:10.1519/JSC.0000000000002729.

Bishop, Chris, Paul Read, Jon Brazier, Paul Jarvis, Shyam Chavda, Tom Bromley, and Anthony N Turner. 2019c. "Effects of Inter-Limb Asymmetries on Acceleration and Change of Direction Speed: A Between-Sport Comparison of Professional Soccer and Cricket

Athletes." *Journal of Strenght and Conditioning Research*. doi:10. 1519/JSC.0000000000003135.

Bishop, Chris, Anthony Turner, Sean Maloney, Jason Lake, Irineu Loturco, Tom Bromley, and Paul Read. 2019d. "Drop Jump Asymmetry Is Associated with Reduced Sprint and Change-of-Direction Speed Performance in Adult Female Soccer Players." *Sports* 7: 29. doi:10.3390/sports7010029.

Bishop, Chris, Anthony Turner, and Paul Read. 2018a. "Training Methods and Considerations for Practitioners to Reduce Interlimb Asymmetries." *Strength and Conditioning Journal* 40: 40–46. doi:10.1519/SSC.0000000000000354.

Bishop, Chris, Anthony Turner, and Paul Read. 2018b. "Effects of Inter-Limb Asymmetries on Physical and Sports Performance: A Systematic Review." *Journal of Sports Sciences* 36: 1135–44. doi:10.1080/ 02640414.2017.1361894.

Born, Dennis-Peter, Christoph Zinner, Peter Düking, and Billy Sperlich. 2016. "Multi-Directional Sprint Training Improves Change-Of-Direction Speed and Reactive Agility in Young Highly Trained Soccer Players." *Journal of Sports Science & Medicine* 15: 314–19.

Chaouachi, Anis, Vincenzo Manzi, Anis Chaalali, Del P. Wong, Karim Chamari, and Carlo Castagna. 2012. "Determinants Analysis of Change-of-Direction Ability in Elite Soccer Players." *Journal of Strength and Conditioning Research* 26: 2667–76. doi:10.1519/JSC. 0b013e318242f97a.

Cronin, John B., and Keir T. Hansen. 2005. "Strength and Power Predictors of Sports Speed." *The Journal of Strength and Conditioning Research* 19: 349-57. doi:10.1519/14323.1.

Dos'Santos, Thomas, Christopher Thomas, Paul Comfort, and Paul A. Jones. 2018a. "The Effect of Angle and Velocity on Change of Direction Biomechanics: An Angle-Velocity Trade-Off." *Sports Medicine* 48: 2235–53. doi:10.1007/s40279-018-0968-3.

Dos'Santos, Thomas, Christopher Thomas, Paul A Jones, and Paul Comfort. 2018b. "Assessing Asymmetries in Change of Direction Speed Performance; Application of Change of Direction Deficit."

Journal of Strength and Conditioning Research. doi:10.1519/JSC.0000000000002438.

Faude, Oliver, Anke Steffen, Michael Kellmann, and Tim Meyer. 2014. "The Effect of Short-Term Interval Training during the Competitive Season on Physical Fitness and Signs of Fatigue: A Crossover Trial in High-Level Youth Football Players." *International Journal of Sports Physiology and Performance* 9: 936–44. doi:10.1123/ijspp.2013-0429.

Fernandez-Fernandez, Jaime, David Sanz-Rivas, and Alberto Mendez-Villanueva. 2009. "A Review of the Activity Profile and Physiological Demands of Tennis Match Play." *Strength and Conditioning Journal* 31: 15–26. doi:10.1519/SSC.0b013e3181ada1cb.

Freitas, Tomás, Pedro Alcaraz, Chris Bishop, Julio Calleja-González, Ademir Arruda, Aristide Guerriero, Valter Reis, Lucas Pereira, and Irineu Loturco. 2018. "Change of Direction Deficit in National Team Rugby Union Players: Is There an Influence of Playing Position?" *Sports* 7: 2. doi:10.3390/sports7010002.

Freitas, Tomás, Pedro Alcaraz, Julio Calleja-González, Ademir Arruda, Aristide Guerriero, Ronaldo Kobal, Valter Reis, Lucas Pereira, and Irineu Loturco. 2019. "Differences in Change of Direction Speed and Deficit Between Male and Female National Rugby Sevens Players." *Journal of Strength and Conditioning Research*. doi:10.1519/JSC.0000000000003195.

Hader, Karim, Dino Palazzi, and Martin Buchheit. 2015. "Change of Direction Speed in Soccer: How Much Braking Is Enough?" *Kinesiology* 47: 67–74.

Harriss, Dave, and Greg Atkinson. 2015. "Ethical Standards in Sport and Exercise Science Research: 2016 Update." *International Journal of Sports Medicine* 36: 1121–24. doi:10.1055/s-0035-1565186.

Hopkins, William G. 2006. "Spreadsheets for Analysis of Controlled Trials, with Adjustment for a Subject Characteristic." *Sportscience* 10: 46–50.

Hopkins, William G., Stephen W. Marshall, Aalan M. Batterham, and Juri Hanin. 2009. "Progressive Statistics for Studies in Sports Medicine and

Exercise Science." *Medicine & Science in Sports & Exercise* 41: 3–13. doi:10.1249/MSS.0b013e31818cb278.

Köklü, Yusuf, Utku Alemdaroğlu, Ali Özkan, Mitat Koz, and Gülfem Ersöz. 2015. "The Relationship between Sprint Ability, Agility and Vertical Jump Performance in Young Soccer Players." *Science & Sports* 30: 1–5. doi:10.1016/J.SCISPO.2013.04.006.

Loturco, Irineu, Lucas Pereira, Tomás Freitas, Pedro Alcaraz, Vinicius Zanetti, Chris Bishop, and Ian Jeffreys. 2019a. "Maximum Acceleration Performance of Professional Soccer Players in Linear Sprints: Is There a Direct Connection with Change-of-Direction Ability?" *PloS One* 14: e0216806. doi:10.1371/journal.pone.0216806.

Loturco, Irineu, Ian Jeffreys, César C. Cal Abad, Ronaldo Kobal, Vinicius Zanetti, Lucas Pereira, and Sophia Nimphius. 2019b. "Change-of-Direction, Speed and Jump Performance in Soccer Players: A Comparison across Different Age-Categories." *Journal of Sports Sciences* 6: 1–7. doi:10.1080/02640414.2019.1574276.

Loturco, Irineu, Sophia Nimphius, Ronaldo Kobal, Altamiro Bottino, Vinicius Zanetti, Lucas Pereira, and Ian Jeffreys. 2018. "Change-of Direction Deficit in Elite Young Soccer Players." *German Journal of Exercise and Sport Research* 48: 228–34. doi:10.1007/s12662-018-0502-7.

Loturco, Irineu, Lucas Pereira, Ronaldo Kobal, Thiago Maldonado, Alessandro Piazzi, Altamiro Bottino, Katia Kitamura, Cesar Cal Abad, Miguel de Arruda, and Fabio Y. Nakamura. 2016. "Improving Sprint Performance in Soccer: Effectiveness of Jump Squat and Olympic Push Press Exercises." Edited by Stephen E Alway. *PloS One* 11: e0153958. doi:10.1371/journal.pone.0153958.

Madruga-Parera, Marc, Chris Bishop, Azahara Fort-Vanmeerhaeghe, Maria R. Beltran-Valls, Oliver G. Skok, and Daniel Romero-Rodríguez. 2019. "Interlimb Asymmetries in Youth Tennis Players." *Journal of Strength and Conditioning Research*. doi:10.1519/JSC.0000000000003152.

Maulder, Peter, and John B. Cronin. 2005. "Horizontal and Vertical Jump Assessment: Reliability, Symmetry, Discriminative and Predictive

Ability." *Physical Therapy in Sport* 6: 74–82. doi:10.1016/J.PTSP. 2005.01.001.

McFarland, Isaiah, Jay Dawes, Craig Elder, and Robert G. Lockie. 2016. "Relationship of Two Vertical Jumping Tests to Sprint and Change of Direction Speed among Male and Female Collegiate Soccer Players." *Sports* 4: 1–7. doi:10.3390/sports4010011.

Nimphius, Sophia, Samuel J. Callaghan, Tania Spiteri, and Robert G. Lockie. 2016. "Change of Direction Deficit: A More Isolated Measure of Change of Direction Performance than Total 505 Time." *Journal of Strength and Conditioning Research* 30: 3024–32. doi:10.1519/JSC. 0000000000001421.

Núñez, Francisco Javier, Alfredo Santalla, Irene Carrasquila, Jose Antonio Asian, Jose I. Reina, and Luis Suarez-Arrones. 2018. "The Effects of Unilateral and Bilateral Eccentric Overload Training on Hypertrophy, Muscle Power and COD Performance, and Its Determinants, in Team Sport Players." *PloS One* 13: e0193841. doi:10.1371/journal. pone.0193841.

Pereira, Lucas, Sophia Nimphius, Ronaldo Kobal, Katia Kitamura, Luiz A.L. Turisco, Rita C. Orsi, César Cal Abad, and Irineu Loturco. 2018. "Relationship Between Change of Direction, Speed, and Power in Male and Female National Olympic Team Handball Athletes." *Journal of Strength and Conditioning Research* 32: 2987–94. doi:10.1519/JSC. 0000000000002494.

Rohman, Eric, Tyler Steubs, and Marc Tompkins. 2015. "Changes in Involved and Uninvolved Limb Function during Rehabilitation after Anterior Cruciate Ligament Reconstruction: Implications for Limb Symmetry Index Measures." *The American Journal of Sports Medicine* 43: 1391–98. doi:10.1177/0363546515576127.

Sáez de Villarreal, Eduardo, Luis Suarez-Arrones, Bernardo Requena, Gregory G. Haff, and Carlos Ferrete. 2015. "Effects of Plyometric and Sprint Training on Physical and Technical Skill Performance in Adolescent Soccer Players." *Journal of Strength and Conditioning Research* 29: 1894–1903. doi: 10.1519/JSC.0000000000000838.

Yanci, Javier, Asier Los Arcos, Jurdan Mendiguchia, and Matt Brughelli. 2014. "Relationships Between Sprinting, Agility, One-and Two-Leg Vertical and Horizontal Jump in Soccer Players." *Kinesiology* 46: 194–201.

In: An Essential Guide to Sports Performance ISBN: 978-1-53617-608-7
Editors: Daniel Castillo Alvira et al. © 2020 Nova Science Publishers, Inc.

Chapter 5

ROLE OF AEROBIC FITNESS IN RECOVERY CAPACITY ASSESSMENT THROUGH HEART RATE RECOVERY IN YOUNG SOCCER PLAYERS

Alejandro Rodríguez Fernández[1,*], José Antonio Rodríguez-Marroyo[2], Javier Sánchez Sánchez[3] and José Gerardo Villa Vicente[2]

[1]Faculty of Health Sciences, University Isabel I, Burgos, Spain
[2]Department of Physical Education and Sport, University of León, León, Spain
[3]Faculty of Education, Pontifical University of Salamanca, Salamanca, Spain

---

[*] Corresponding Author's Email: alejandro.rodriguez.fernandez@ui1.es; Faculty of Sport Sciences, University Isabel I, Burgos, Spain.

ABSTRACT

Aerobic fitness is a decisive performance factor in soccer players. Previous studies have correlated the distance travelled in an intervallic test (Yo-Yo IR test) with the distance covered in competition, demonstrating that a high aerobic capacity contributes to better recovery in high intensity intermittent exercises typical of training and soccer matches. In addition, an increase in the capacity of the oxygen transport mechanism leads to greater energy spent through the aerobic metabolism and consequently reduces fatigue through glycogen savings and the prevention of decreased muscle pH. Heart rate recovery (HRR) is the rate at which the heart rate (HR) decreases (i.e., the time taken for HR to recover) following a moderate-to-heavy exercise in response to a combination of parasympathetic activation and sympathetic withdrawal. Based on this background, the aim of this study was to check if soccer players with better aerobic fitness have better recovery (both after maximum efforts in laboratory and field tests, and after submaximal efforts at progressive intensities in a field test). Eighty (n=80) young soccer players (mean ± SD, age 16.7 ± 0.8 yr; body mass 67.5 ± 7.6 kg; height 175.1 ± 6.9 cm; fat mass 13.6 ± 3.3%; and VO_2max 3.7 ± 0.6 L/min and 55.5 ± 5.1 ml/kg/min) took part in this study. All players performed a laboratory ergoespirometric maximal test on a treadmill (LabTest) and an incremental intervallic intermittent field test (TIVRE-Soccer© test). Soccer players with better aerobic capacity ($VO_2max \geq 60$ ml/kg/min) present significantly (p = 0.039) better HRR after the 30 s laboratory test and significantly (p = 0.028) better HRR in recovery stages after the anaerobic threshold in the TIVRE-Soccer© test. It is possible that soccer players with better aerobic fitness could better adapt to maximal or submaximal efforts and, therefore, present a better HRR.

Keywords: football, performance, specific endurance, intermittent endurance

INTRODUCTION

Soccer is the most popular sport with more than 270 million people actively involved in the sport worldwide (Turner and Stewart 2014). Different studies have analysed performance factors in this sport and have concluded that this sport is characterised by maximal and submaximal short-term actions (Ade, Fitzpatrick, and Bradley 2016). The players run 110–120 m/min, with a distance per match of 9–14 km (Palucci Vieira et al. 2019), for which the energy provision of the aerobic system during a match is between 70% and 80% (Bangsbo 1994). Although aerobic training is traditionally an important component of physical training in soccer, because some studies show a relationship between maximal oxygen uptake (VO_2max) and level of the team or distance covered during the match (Krustrup et al. 2003), the implementation of new technologies (GPS and time-motion analysis) have shown that other variables (i.e., distance covered at high intensities) are more valid to measure physical performance in soccer players (Bradley et al. 2010). Thus, in recent years, the assessment of VO_2max has diminished in the interests of researchers. However, high aerobic fitness appears to improve recovery during high-intensity intermittent exercise, which is typical of soccer performance and training (Tomlin and Wenger 2001); therefore, we cannot neglect training and assessment of this capacity.

Heart rate recovery (HRR) is the assessment of the rate at which heart rate (HR) decreases and reflects the coordinated interaction between parasympathetic re-activation and sympathetic withdrawal (Borresen and Lambert 2007). HRR is one of the measures of the autonomic HR regulation method (Bellenger et al. 2016) and because changes in training load (Pichot et al. 2000), aerobic (Buchheit et al. 2010; Darr et al. 1988; Du et al. 2005; Lamberts et al. 2009) and strength fitness (Otsuki et al. 2007) and body composition (Esco, Williford, and Olson 2011; Nagashima et al. 2010) are reflected in the balance of parasympathetic and sympathetic modulation of the autonomic nervous system, interest in the study of this subject has increased among researchers.

Previous studies have shown that subjects with greater VO_2max have faster HRR after maximal exercise (Darr et al. 1988; Du et al. 2005; Ostojic et al. 2010; Rodríguez-Fernández et al. 2017), suggesting that aerobic fitness, along with autonomic modulation, might play a role in HRR; this reflects a positive adaptation to exercise training and, possibly, a superior capacity in endurance events (Bosquet, Gamelin, and Berthoin 2008). This high HRR may be due to the restoration of parasympathetic tone, changes in plasma volume, or accumulation of metabolic factors (Javorka et al. 2002). However, HRR is improved after heavy overreaching training with lower performance (Thomson et al. 2016), while previous studies have shown a faster HRR associated with performance improvements (Buchheit et al. 2010). These discrepancies indicate that we have to interpret the changes in HRR, because it is conditioned not only by the level of aerobic fitness, but by the intensity and type of previous exercises.

The studies that have analysed the relationship between HRR and VO_2max always analysed HRR after continuous, incremental, and maximum efforts (after laboratory ergoespirometric tests) that meet maximality criteria; however, in team sports those types of efforts are not reproduced by match demands because, in the match, distances run at maximal or submaximal intensity ($>$ 24 km/h) represent only $\approx$ 2% of effort in soccer (Asian Clemente et al. 2019) or $\approx$ 6% (18 to 36 km/h) for rugby elite players (Glassbrook et al. 2019) and this effort is not incremental or continuous. This may be due to the fact that, to our knowledge, there is only one test that specifically assesses endurance and is also able to determine the HRR between the different stages that make up the test (TIVRE-Soccer© test;(Garcia-Lopez et al. 2003). To our knowledge, only one study has analysed the relationship between aerobic fitness and HRR after incremental maximal and submaximal intensities that characterise team sport match play (Rodríguez-Fernández et al. 2017). This study concluded that soccer players with high aerobic fitness have better HRR after maximal ($\approx$ 2%) and total HRR in intervallic tests ($\approx$ 3%); however, this study did not analyse the relationship between VO_2max and HRR.

The aim of the present study is to determine if soccer players with high aerobic fitness have better HRR both after continuous incremental maximal effort and between recovery phases in incremental intervallic specific tests, and to analyse the correlation between VO_2max and HRR. We hypothesize that HRR recovery will be faster in soccer players with better aerobic fitness.

METHODS

Participants

Eighty young male soccer players (age 16.7 ± 0.8 yr; body mass 67.5 ± 7.6 kg; height 175.1 ± 6.9 cm; fat mass 13.6 ± 3.3%; and VO_2max 3.7 ± 0.6 L/min and 55.5 ± 5.1 ml/kg/min) that compete in the same league performed a maximal laboratory test (LabTest) and a specific endurance intermittent test, TIVRE-Soccer© test (TST). Over the course of three months players trained for three sessions per week and played one official match at the weekend. The inclusion criteria were as follows: not to have been injured during the last month before the test, to have taken part in at least 80% of training sessions in the last three months, to have reached the maximum criteria in the LabTest (Midgley et al. 2007), and for their HR to have reached a maximum in the TST (Midgley, McNaughton, and Carroll 2006). All players possessed at least six years of experience in soccer training and competition. The soccer players were classified according to their VO_2max in high VO_2max (HVO_2max: ≥ 60 ml/kg/min) and low VO_2max (LVO_2max: < 60 ml/kg/min). All players (and their parents if they were minors) and coaches were informed about the aims, methods, benefits, and risks of the study and signed their informed consent. The study was performed in accordance with the Declaration of Helsinki.

Experimental Design

All players undertook the test on two different days. On the first day, anthropometric measures and the LabTest were performed. Forty-eight to seventy-two hours later, a TST was performed. All tests of all players were performed in a three-week period. Players were instructed before each test to produce maximal effort, follow their normal diet, and to refrain from any form of intense physical activity for the 24 h period prior to the test. The LabTest was always performed at the same time of day and the TST was performed in the usual training surface for each team (all natural grass). During all testing sessions, the HR and the HRR were assessed by Polar Team (PolarTeam®, Polar Electro Oy, Kempele, Finland) which has been previously validated (Engström et al. 2012).

Procedures

Aerobic Power and Capacity

Soccer players were tested in a maximal incremental ergoespiromtric laboratory test (LabTest) using a treadmill (Cosmos Pulsar 4.0®, Cosmos Sports & Medical, Nussdorf-Traunstein, Germany) and a calibrated computer system (Ergo Card®, Medisoft, Sorinnes, Belgium). The test began at 8 km/h and at each minute the speed was increased by 1 km/h until the player stopped due to volitional exhaustion. If the last stage was not fully completed, the peak treadmill speed was calculated using the following formula: $S + (t/60 \times 1)$, where S was the last completed speed (km/h) and t the time (s) of the uncompleted stage, with a previously established high reliability (ICC = 0.91) (Kuipers et al. 1985). Maximal oxygen uptake (VO_2max), and aerobic (VT1) and anaerobic (VT2) thresholds were determined by Medisoft software (Medisoft®, Sorinnes, Belgium). VO_2max was determined when soccer players attained a VO_2 plateau ($\leq$ 150 mL/min), RER $\geq$ 1.15, and HR was $\pm$ 10 beats from the theoretical maximal heart rate (Midgley et al. 2009). VT1 was determined when an increase in the ventilatory equivalent for oxygen (VE/VO_2) was produced with no increase in the ventilatory equivalent for carbon dioxide (VE/VCO_2) and a first exponential increase of ventilation (VE) and VT2 was determined when an increase in VE/VO_2 and VE/VCO_2 and a second exponential increase of VE were produced (Lucia et al. 1999). Maximal heart rate (HR_{max}) and heart rate recovery of 30 (HRR_{30}), 60 (HRR_{60}), and 120 (HRR_{120}) seconds were recorded using continuous twelve-channel electrocardiography (CardioDetect® med card, Rennesens GmbH, Berlin, Germany). Fifteen minutes before the test, anthropometric measures were registered to determine fat mass (body mass, height, and six skinfolds; (Carter 1982).

Specific Endurance and Recovery Capacity

The TIVRE-Soccer© test (TST) was conducted in the centre of a standard soccer pitch (Garcia-Lopez et al. 2003). The soccer players ran around the specific circuit (Figure 1) delimited by fourteen cones (9.15 m between cones) at a speed indicated by the software (TIVRE-Soccer© test, DSD Inc.®, León, Spain) and reproduced on a laptop (Acer Aspire 6530G, Acer, Taipei, Taiwan). Players had to adapt their speed to that indicated by the audio signals. Each of the stages is made up of two laps (2 x 128 m). The test began at 9 km/h, increasing by 0.6 km/h at each stage. The next stage started after 30 s of recovery and the participants completed that stage in the opposite direction. The test ended when the subject did not reach three consecutive cones at the indicated speed or reached exhaustion. Throughout the test, players carried a heart rate monitor (PolarTeam®, Polar Electro Oy, Kempele, Finland). The intervallic anaerobic threshold was determined by the HR deflexion point (Vucetic et al. 2014) by two experienced exercise physiologists using specific software (Polar Pro Trainer 5®, Polar Electro Oy, Kempele, Finland). Total distance completed (disTST), end speed (vTST), speed at intervallic anaerobic threshold (vIAT), mean HRR in stages before IAT (%Rec-PreIAT) and in stages after IAT (%Rec-PostIAT) and total stages (%Rec-T) were determined.

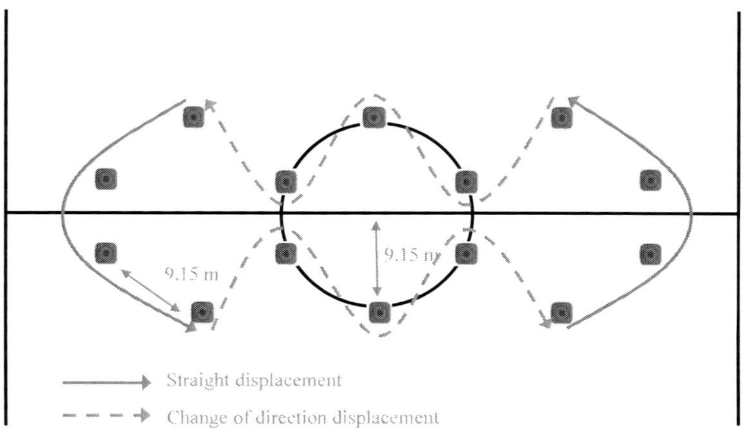

Figure 1. Schematic representation of TIVRE-Soccer© test (Rodríguez-Fernández et al. 2017).

Statistical Analyses

Results are presented as means ± standard deviations (SD). Before conducting the parametric test, the condition of normal variation was verified using the Kolmogorov–Smirnov test. The difference in recovery capacity between soccer players with high aerobic capacity and soccer players with low aerobic capacity were compared through paired *t* student tests and a one-way ANOVA adjusted using the Bonferroni method. To investigate the correlation between aerobic performance and recovery capacity, descriptive correlations were used by using Pearson's product-moment correlation coefficient (r). Magnitude of correlation coefficients were considered as trivial ($r < 0.1$), small ($r \geq 0.1$ and < 0.3), moderate ($r \geq 0.3$ and < 0.5), large ($r \geq 0.5$ and < 0.7), very large ($r \geq 0.7$ and < 0.9), nearly perfect ($r \geq 0.9$), and perfect ($r = 1.0$) (Hopkins 2000). The level of significance was set at $p < 0.05$. The data were analysed using the statistical package SPSS, version 20.0 (SPSS Inc., Chicago, IL, USA).

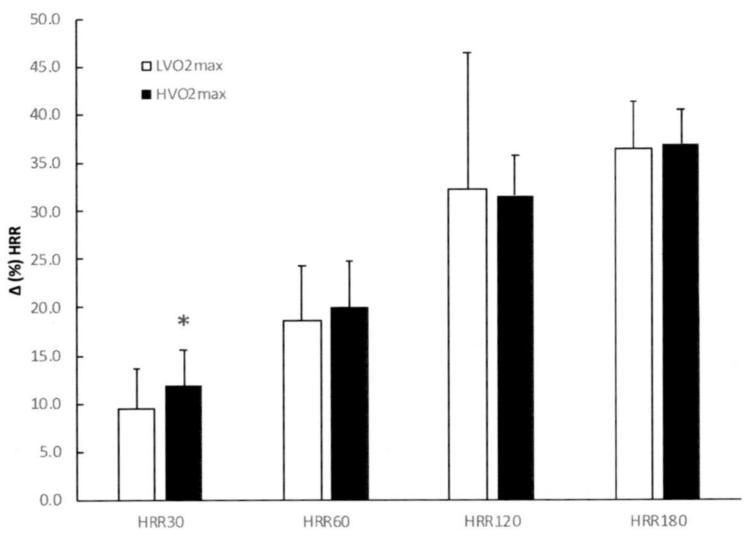

* denotes significant differences. $p < 0.05$

Figure 2. Heart Rate Recovery 30 (HRR30), 60 (HRR60), 120 (HRR120), and 180 (HRR180) seconds after LabTest in soccer players with low $VO_2max < 60$ ml/kg/min (LVO_2max) and high $VO_2max \geq 60$ ml/kg/min (HVO_2max).

RESULTS

There are significant differences ($p = 0.000$) in VO_2max between soccer players with high VO_2max (HVO_2max, n = 20, 61.6 ± 1.7 ml/kg/min) and soccer players with low VO_2max (LVO_2max, n = 60, 53.6 ± 4.3 ml/kg/min). In addition, HVO_2max players covered significantly ($p = 0.024$) more distance (3152.9 ± 343.8 vs. 2898.1 ± 492.4) and reached significantly ($p = 0.005$) greater maximal speeds (16.4 ± 0.9 vs 15.5 ± 1.3) than soccer players with LVO_2max in TST.

HVO_2max players have a significantly ($p = 0.039$) better percentage of HRR than LVO_2max players at 30 s after the end of the LabTest (Figure 2).

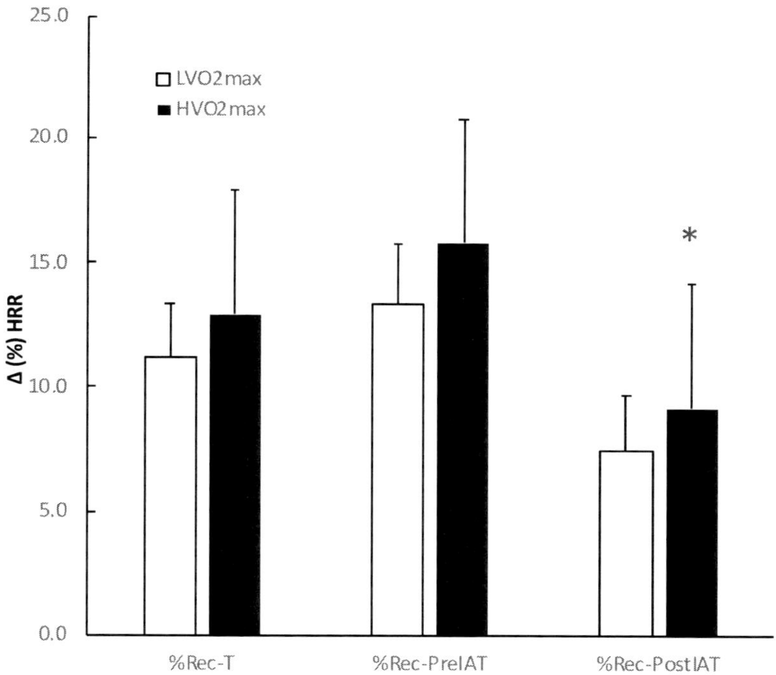

* denotes significant differences. $p < 0.05$.

Figure 3. Heart Rate Recovery (HRR) in all stages (%Rec-T), stages before vIAT (%Rec-PreIAT) and stages after vIAT (%Rec-PostIAT) in soccer players with low $VO_2max < 60$ ml/kg/min (LVO_2max) and high $VO_2max \geq 60$ ml/kg/min (HVO_2max).

Table 1. Pearson correlation between maximal values in LabTest and TST, and HRR in LabTest and TST

		HRR_{30}	HRR_{60}	HRR_{120}	HRR_{180}	%Rec-PreIAT	%Rec-PostIAT	%Rec-T
VO_2max	LVO_2max	- 0.179 ($p = 0.178$)	- 0.216 ($p = 0.92$)	0.026 ($p = 0.842$)	0.086 ($p = 0.519$)	- 0.199 ($p = 0.195$)	- 0.408 ($p = 0.006$)*	- 0.290 ($p = 0.039$)*
	HVO_2max	- 0.112 ($p = 0.669$)	- 0.210 ($p = 0.338$)	- 0.154 ($p = 0.529$)	- 0.133 ($p = 0.587$)	- 0.173 ($p = 0.572$)	- 0.126 ($p = 0.681$)	- 0.166 ($p = 0.554$)
	Total	- 0.042 ($p = 0.719$)	- 0.153 ($p = 0.173$)	- 0.005 ($p = 0.962$)	- 0.050 ($p = 0.667$)	0.133 ($p = 0.326$)	- 0.026 ($p = 0.848$)	0.129 ($p = 0.301$)
vVO_2max	LVO_2max	- 0.181 ($p = 0.174$)	- 0.164 ($p = 0.203$)	- 0.239 ($p = 0.061$)	- 0.040 ($p = 0.714$)	- 0.416 ($p = 0.005$)*	- 0.446 ($p = 0.002$)*	- 0.362 ($p = 0.009$)*
	HVO_2max	0.298 ($p = 0.245$)	0.338 ($p = 0.156$)	0.456 ($p = 0.050$)*	0.380 ($p = 0.108$)	0.481 ($p = 0.096$)	0.320 ($p = 0.286$)	0.584 ($p = 0.022$)
	Total	- 0.019 ($p = 0.874$)	- 0.057 ($p = 0.611$)	- 0.201 ($p = 0.072$)	- 0.090 ($p = 0.433$)	- 0.061 ($p = 0.652$)	- 0.193 ($p = 0.150$)	- 0.047 ($p = 0.705$)
disTST	LVO_2max	- 0.233 ($p = 0.100$)	- 0.307 ($p = 0.024$)*	- 0.116 ($p = 0.403$)	0.000 ($p = 0.999$)	- 0.388 ($p = 0.009$)*	- 0.317 ($p = 0.036$)*	- 0.308 ($p = 0.028$)*
	HVO_2max	- 0.044 ($p = 0.886$)	- 0.593 ($p = 0.020$)*	- 0.586 ($p = 0.022$)*	- 0.528 ($p = 0.043$)*	- 0.077 ($p = 0.802$)	- 0.119 ($p = 0.698$)	0.031 ($p = 0.912$)
	Total	- 0.116 ($p = 0.359$)	- 0.138 ($p = 0.259$)	- 0.084 ($p = 0.492$)	- 0.073 ($p = 0.559$)	- 0.185 ($p = 0.168$)	- 0.197 ($p = 0.143$)	- 0.138 ($p = 0.269$)
vTST	LVO_2max	- 0.191 ($p = 0.180$)	- 0.319 ($p = 0.019$)	- 0.116 ($p = 0.403$)	0.000 ($p = 0.999$)	- 0.401 ($p = 0.007$)*	- 0.274 ($p = 0.072$)	- 0.279 ($p = 0.047$)*
	HVO_2max	- 0.157 ($p = 0.607$)	0.266 ($p = 0.338$)	0.385 ($p = 0.157$)	0.476 ($p = 0.073$)	0.326 ($p = 0.278$)	0.090 ($p = 0.771$)	0.414 (pv0.125)
	Total	- 0.107 ($p = 0.399$)	- 0.183 ($p = 0.132$)	- 0.116 ($p = 0.343$)	- 0.072 ($p = 0.566$)	- 0.055 ($p = 0.686$)	- 0.093 ($p = 0.492$)	- 0.003 ($p = 0.980$)

Note: LVO_2max = players with $VO_2max < 60$ ml/kg/min; $HVO_2max = VO_2max \geq 60$ ml/kg/min; HRR_{30} = heart rate recovery 30 s after end of laboratory test; HRR_{60} = heart rate recovery 60 s after end of laboratory test; HRR_{120} = heart rate recovery 120 s after end of laboratory test; HRR_{180} = heart rate recovery 180 s after end of laboratory test; %Rec-PreIAT = percentage of recovery in all recovery stages before anaerobic threshold in TIVRE-Soccer© test; %Rec-PostIAT = percentage of recovery in all recovery stages after anaerobic threshold in TIVRE-Soccer© test; %Rec-T = percentage of recovery in all recovery stages in TIVRE-Soccer© test; vVO_2max = end speed in laboratory test; disTST = total distance in TIVRE-Soccer© test; vTST = end speed in TIVRE-Soccer© test. *denotes significant correlation $p < 0.05$.

HVO_2max players showed a significantly (p = 0.000) higher VT2 speed determined in the LabTest than the LVO_2max players (14.9 ± 0.9 km/h vs. 13.3 ± 1.5 km/h, respectively). Although the trend is similar in the results of the TST speed at vIAT, the differences obtained are not significant (13.6 ± 0.9 km/h vs. 13.0 ± 1.2 km/h, respectively). The HRR determined in all stages of recovery after the vIAT (%REC-PostIAT) is significantly (p = 0.028) better in HVO_2max players than in LVO_2max players. There were no differences in %Rec-PreIAT and %REC-T according to aerobic fitness level (Figure 3).

The correlation between the aerobic fitness in different tests and HRR is shown in Table 1.

DISCUSSION

To our knowledge, this study is original because it reveals the influence of aerobic fitness in HRR after continuous incremental maximal effort and in submaximal efforts (recovery stages in an incremental intervallic specific test). The main findings of this study were that soccer players with high aerobic fitness levels (≥ 60 ml/kg/min) have significantly better HRR in the first 30 s after the maximal test and these soccer players have better HRR in recovery stages after the anaerobic intervallic threshold in a specific soccer test (TIVRE-Soccer© test). The results suggest that aerobic fitness (VO_2max) might play a role in HRR after maximal and submaximal efforts.

Previous studies have analysed HRR in relation to endurance (Haraldsdottir et al. 2018; Lamberts et al. 2010; Mourot et al. 2015) and team sport (Harry and Booysen 2019;Ostojic et al. 2010; Ostojic, Stojanovic, and Calleja-Gonzalez 2011; Suzic Lazic et al. 2017) athletes after maximal effort; and their relationship with aerobic fitness (Buchheit and Gindre 2006; Darr et al. 1988; Du et al. 2005; Haraldsdottir et al. 2018; Ostojic, Stojanovic, and Calleja-Gonzalez 2011), previous training load (Lamberts et al. 2009; Thomson et al. 2016), and changes in physical performance (Buchheit et al. 2010, 2012; Lamberts et al. 2010). Studies with team sport athletes show a ≈ 8% (Ostojic, Stojanovic, and Calleja-Gonzalez 2011) and 15% (Suzic Lazic et al. 2017) in HRR_{30} and HRR_{60} after incremental maximal tests, respectively. Similarly, in our study, HVO_2max players have 11.8 ± 3.8% and 19.9 ± 4.8% and LVO_2max players have 9.4 ± 4.1% and 18.6 ± 5.6% for HRR_{30} and HRR_{60} after incremental maximal tests, respectively, establishing significant ($p < 0.05$) differences between groups only in HRR_{30}. This may be due to a better aerobic capacity, because VO_2max has been related to HRR (Darr et al. 1988). However, previous studies have not demonstrated a relationship between VO_2max and HRR in rowers (Haraldsdottir et al. 2018), middle-aged individuals (Buchheit and Gindre 2006), and girls and boys (Mahon et al. 2003). This difference may be because in addition to considering HRR_{60}, HRR was evaluated for a shorter time (HRR_{30}) for which significant differences existed when compared with HRR_{60} and when compared with previous studies. It could be postulated that HRR in the first thirty seconds may represent a better adaptation to high intensity exercise (Bosquet, Gamelin, and Berthoin 2008) and possible mechanisms such as the restoration of parasympathetic tone, changes in plasma volume, or accumulation of metabolic factors (Javorka et al. 2002) can explain that adaptation. Another possible explanation is that our athletes practice intermittent sports, and previous studies have shown a better HRR in athletes of these disciplines which require similar aerobic fitness (Ostojic, Stojanovic, and Calleja-Gonzalez 2011).

Age is a key factor in HRR, because the ageing process induces a decline in HRR (Antelmi et al. 2008; Carnethon et al. 2005; Trevizani, Benchimol-Barbosa, and Nadal 2012). This aspect may be due to a decrease in HRmax and a decrease in maximal cardiac output, produced by the reduction in intrinsic HR, such as, for example, attenuated chronotropic response to beta-adrenergic stimulation (Christou and Seals 2008). In our study, the ages of the soccer players were lower (16.7 ± 0.8 vs. ≈55 and ≈20 age) than in studies which did not obtain a relationship between VO_2max and HRR (Buchheit and Gindre 2006; Haraldsdottir et al. 2018) and this age difference can condition the results obtained. In addition, this may explain why higher HRR was obtained than in previous studies (Ostojic, Stojanovic, and Calleja-Gonzalez 2011; Suzic Lazic et al. 2017).

In team sport (Casamichana et al. 2018; Glassbrook et al. 2019; Narazaki et al. 2009) and specifically in soccer (Ade, Fitzpatrick, and Bradley 2016; Bradley et al. 2013; Carling, Le Gall, and Dupont 2012; Suarez-Arrones et al. 2014; Whitehead et al. 2018), efforts are characterized by being carried out at submaximal or maximum intensity intermittently and with brief recovery periods. Therefore, it is interesting to assess the HRR not only after continuous progressive and maximal effort, but after the realization of intermittent efforts of different intensity that better represent match demands. To our knowledge, only TST is able to assess HRR at different intensities (Rodríguez-Fernández et al. 2017). In addition, because the anaerobic threshold can be determined by deflection of the HR (Buchheit, Solano, and Millet 2007; Mikulic, Vucetic, and Sentija 2011; Vucetic et al. 2014) this allows us to determine the HRR pre- and post-anaerobic threshold in TST (Garcia-Lopez et al. 2004; Villa-Vicente et al. 2000). The distance run by our players in TST is higher (23% and 17% for LVO_2max and LVO_2max respectively) than that reported by other studies with similar tests, such as the Yo-Yo IR test ($\approx$ 2400 m) (Deprez et al. 2015), in soccer players with similar ages. If we compare the maximum speed reached in TST (16.4 $\pm$ 0.9 and 15.5 $\pm$ 1.3 for HVO_2max and LVO_2max, respectively), this is lower than that shown by a test with similar characteristics, such as 30-15 IFT ($\approx$ 19 km/h) (Rabbani and Buchheit 2015) and Yo-Yo IRT ($\approx$ 17 km/h) (Deprez et al. 2015; Bangsbo, Iaia, and Krustrup 2008), in soccer players of a similar age.

To our knowledge, only three studies have analysed inter-effort recovery in a specific intervallic test (Haydar et al. 2011; Rodríguez-Fernández et al. 2017; Vaquera Jiménez et al. 2007), but one of these estimated recovery by comparing the performance between the protocol with recovery stages and simulated the same protocol without recovery stages (Haydar et al. 2011). In our results, HVO_2max players have significantly better (p = 0.028) %REC-PostIAT than LVO_2max players. These efforts, despite being carried out at an intensity higher than the anaerobic threshold, have a duration greater than 60 s and there is a predominance of oxidative phosphorylation (Chamari and Padulo 2015); therefore, players with a higher VO_2max will have a greater aerobic contribution to these efforts (Bentley, Newell, and Bishop 2007), and recovery periods will be optimized. On the other hand, there are no significant differences in %Rec-PreIAT between HVO_2max and LVO_2max players. These intensities can represent a low intensity effort, so no significant differences were obtained in speed at vIAT between HVO_2max and LVO_2max players, and these efforts represent intensities of less than 85% of maximal speed in TST in both HVO_2max and LVO_2max players.

Previous studies have not obtained a significant relationship ($p > 0.05$) between any of the post-exercise HRR responses and VO_2max (Buchheit and Gindre 2006; Mahon et al. 2003). These studies assume that any effect of fitness on HRR should be attributed to training adaptations (Saltin and Rowell 1980), that these two variables are independent of one another, and that this confirms that VO_2max is of limited value in tracking or predicting athletic ability (Noakes 2008). However, a longitudinal study reported a correlation ($r = 0.15$, $n = 3.446$) between HRR_{120} and performance on a treadmill test (Carnethon et al. 2005). In the same line, in a study of well-trained cyclists, a positive correlation between changes in HRR and performance was observed (Lamberts et al. 2009); however, the exercise protocol preceding the HRR measurement was a 40 km time trial, and comparisons with an incremental maximal exercise test should be drawn with caution (Haraldsdottir et al. 2018). In our results, only LVO2max players had a significant relationship between any of the post-exercise HRR responses and aerobic fitness variables, and this relationship was always negative. Previous studies have already shown a negative relationship between VO_2max and HRR_{60} (Suzic Lazic et al. 2017). The authors argue that HRR_{60} is a parasympathetic phenomenon and VO_2max may be highly influenced by the sympathetic drive. To assess VO_2max, maximal exercise tests have been used, and parasympathetic activity is shown to be negligible in the level of peak exercise (Robinson et al. 1953).

This study has several limitations. Modern soccer players are experiencing an increase in match-play physical demands, in part due to a greater number of high-intensity running actions (Silva et al. 2018).

Therefore, the recovery time of 30 s may not be the most appropriate. In addition, the type of recovery assessment (passive) is not always performed by the players, because this is characterized by being static, walking, or jogging (Carling, Le Gall, and Dupont 2012; Casamichana and Castellano 2010); it would be interesting to evaluate this type of recovery while it affects the HRR after maximal exercise (Haraldsdottir et al. 2018). Previous studies have shown the effects of the previous microcycle training load on the HRR (Aubry et al. 2015; Thomson et al. 2016); thus, it would have been interesting to quantify the training load in the previous microcycle.

This study provides novel information about HRR values after different intensities of effort by soccer players with respect to aerobic fitness. In conclusion, the soccer players with high aerobic fitness show better HRR_{30} and better HRR in recovery stages after the anaerobic threshold in an incremental intermittent specific test. It is possible that these soccer players could better adapt to maximal or submaximal efforts.

REFERENCES

Ade, J., John, Fitzpatrick. & Paul, S. Bradley. (2016). "High-Intensity Efforts in Elite Soccer Matches and Associated Movement Patterns, Technical Skills and Tactical Actions. Information for Position-Specific Training Drills." *Journal of Sports Sciences*, *33*, 2205–14.

Antelmi, Ivana., Eliseu, Y. Chuang., Cesar, J. Grupi., Maria, R. Dias de Oliveira. & Alfredo, J. Mansur. (2008). "Heart Rate Recovery after Treadmill Electrocardiographic Exercise Stress Test and 24-Hour Heart Rate Variability in Healthy Individuals." *Arquivos Brasileiros de Cardiologia*, *90*, 380–85. doi: 10.1590/s0066-782x2008000600005.

Asian, Clemente., Jose, A., Bernardo, Requena., Igor, Jukic., Jack, Nayler., Alfredo, Santalla. & Christopher, Carling. (2019). "Is Physical Performance a Differentiating Element between More or Less Successful Football Teams?" *Sports*, *7*. doi: 10.3390/sports7100216.

Aubry, Anael., Christophe, Hausswirth., Julien, Louis., Aaron, J. Coutts., Martin, Buchheit. & Yann, Le Meur. (2015). "The Development of Functional Overreaching Is Associated with a Faster Heart Rate Recovery in Endurance Athletes." *PloS One*, *10*, e0139754. doi: 10.1371/journal.pone.0139754.

Bangsbo, J. (1994). "The Physiology of Soccer--with Special Reference to Intense Intermittent Exercise." *Acta Physiol Scand Suppl*, *619*, 1–155.

Bangsbo, J., Marcello, Iaia. & Peter, Krustrup. (2008). "The Yo-Yo Intermittent Recovery Test : A Useful Tool for Evaluation of Physical Performance in Intermittent Sports." *Sports Medicine*, *38*, 37–51.

Bellenger, Clint R., Joel, T. Fuller., Rebecca, L. Thomson., Kade, Davison., Eileen, Y. Robertson. & Jonathan, D. Buckley. (2016). "Monitoring Athletic Training Status Through Autonomic Heart Rate Regulation: A Systematic Review and Meta-Analysis." *Sports Medicine*, *46*, 1461–86. doi: 10.1007/s40279-016-0484-2.

Bentley, David J., John, Newell. & David, Bishop. (2007). "Incremental Exercise Test Design and Analysis: Implications for Performance Diagnostics in Endurance Athletes." *Sports Medicine*, *37*, 575–86. doi: 10.2165/00007256-200737070-00002.

Borresen, Jill. & Mike, I. Lambert. (2007). "Changes in Heart Rate Recovery in Response to Acute Changes in Training Load." *European Journal of Applied Physiology*, *101*, 503–11. doi: 10.1007/s00421-007-0516-6.

Bosquet, Laurent., Francois, X. Gamelin. & Serge, Berthoin. (2008). "Reliability of Postexercise Heart Rate Recovery." *International Journal of Sports Medicine*, *29*, 238–43.

Bradley, Paul S., Christopher, Carling., Antonio, Gomez., Peter, Hood., Chris, Barnes., Jack, D. Ade., Mark, Boddy., Peter, Krustrup. & Magni, Mohr. (2013). "Match Performance and Physical Capacity of Players in the Top Three Competitive Standards of English Professional Soccer." *Human Movement Science*, *32*, 808–21. doi: 10.1016/j.humov.2013.06.002.

Bradley, Paul S., Michele, Di Mascio., Dan, Peart., Peter, Olsen. & Bill, Sheldon. (2010). "High-Intensity Activity Profiles of Elite Soccer

Players at Different Performance Levels." *Journal of Strength and Conditioning Research*, *24*, 2343–2351. doi: 10.1519/ JSC.0b013e 3181aeb1b3.

Buchheit, Martin., Arnaud, Chivot., Jonathan, Parouty., Dan, Mercier., Hani, Al Haddad., Paul, B. Laursen. & Said, Ahmaidi. (2010). "Monitoring Endurance Running Performance Using Cardiac Parasympathetic Function." *European Journal of Applied Physiology*, *108*, 1153–67. doi: 10.1007/s00421-009-1317-x.

Buchheit, Martin. & Cyrille, Gindre. (2006). "Cardiac Parasympathetic Regulation: Respective Associations with Cardiorespiratory Fitness and Training Load." *American Journal of Physiology-Heart and Circulatory Physiology*, *291*, H451-8. doi: 10.1152/ ajpheart. 00008.2006.

Buchheit, Martin., Ben, Simpson., Hani, Al Haddad., Pitre, C. Bourdon. & Alberto, Mendez-Villanueva. (2012). "Monitoring Changes in Physical Performance with Heart Rate Measures in Young Soccer Players." *European Journal of Applied Physiology*, *112*, 711–723. doi: 10.1007/ s00421-011-2014-0.

Buchheit, Martin., Roberto, Solano. & Gregory, Millet. (2007). "Heart-Rate Deflection Point and the Second Heart-Rate Variability Threshold during Running Exercise in Trained Boys." *Pediatric Exercise Science*, *19*, 192–204.

Carling, Christopher., Franck, Le Gall. & Gregory, Dupont. (2012). "Analysis of Repeated High-Intensity Running Performance in Professional Soccer." *Journal of Sports Sciences*, *30*, 325–36. doi: 10.1080/02640414.2011.652655.

Carnethon, Mercedes R., David, R. Jr Jacobs., Stephen, Sidney., Barbara, Sternfeld., Samuel, S. Gidding., Christiana, Shoushtari. & Kiang, Liu. (2005). "A Longitudinal Study of Physical Activity and Heart Rate Recovery: CARDIA, 1987-1993." *Medicine and Science in Sports and Exercise*, *37*, 606–12. doi: 10.1249/01.mss.0000158190.56061.32.

Carter, J. (1982). *Physical Structure of Olympic Athletes. Part I: The Montreal Olympic Games Anthropological Project*. Basel: Karger.

Casamichana, David. & Julen, Castellano. (2010). "Time-Motion, Heart Rate, Perceptual and Motor Behaviour Demands in Small-Sides Soccer Games: Effects of Pitch Size." *Journal of Sports Science*, *28*, 1615–23. doi: 10.1080/02640414.2010.521168.

Casamichana, David., Esther, Morencos., Blanca, Romero-Moraleda. & Tim, J. Gabbett. (2018). "The Use of Generic and Individual Speed Thresholds for Assessing the Competitive Demands of Field Hockey." *Journal of Sports Science and Medicine*, *17*, 366–71.

Chamari, Karim. & Johnny, Padulo. (2015). "'Aerobic' and 'Anaerobic' Terms Used in Exercise Physiology: A Critical Terminology Reflection." *Sports Medicine - Open*, *1*, 1–4. doi: 10.1186/s40798-015-0012-1.

Christou, Demetra D. & Douglas, R. Seals. (2008). "Decreased Maximal Heart Rate with Aging Is Related to Reduced Beta-Adrenergic Responsiveness but Is Largely Explained by a Reduction in Intrinsic Heart Rate." *Journal of Applied Physiology*, *105*, 24–29. doi: 10.1152/japplphysiol.90401.2008.

Darr, Kevin C., David, R. Bassett., Barbara, J. Morgan. & David, P. Thomas. (1988). "Effects of Age and Training Status on Heart Rate Recovery after Peak Exercise." *The American Journal of Physiology*, *254*, 340-3. doi: 10.1152/ajpheart.1988.254.2.H340.

Deprez, Dieter., Job, Fransen., Matthieu, Lenoir., Renaat, M. Philippaerts. & Roel, Vaeyens. (2015). "The Yo-Yo Intermittent Recovery Test Level 1 Is Reliable in Young High-Level Soccer Players." *Biology of Sport*, *32*, 65–70. doi: 10.5604/20831862.1127284.

Du, Na., Siqin, Bai., Kazuo, Oguri., Yoshihiro, Kato., Ichie, Matsumoto., Harumi, Kawase. & Toshio, Matsuoka. (2005). "Heart Rate Recovery after Exercise and Neural Regulation of Heart Rate Variability in 30-40 Year Old Female Marathon Runners." *Journal of Sports Science & Medicine*, *4*, 9–17.

Engström, Elise., Elin, Ottosson., Björn, Wohlfart., Nils, Grundström. & Anita, Wisén. (2012). "Comparison of Heart Rate Measured by Polar RS400 and ECG, Validity and Repeatability." *Advances in Physiotherapy*, *14*, 115–22. doi: 10.3109/14038196.2012.694118.

Esco, Michael R., Henry, N. Williford. & Michele, S. Olson. (2011). “Skinfold Thickness Is Related to Cardiovascular Autonomic Control as Assessed by Heart Rate Variability and Heart Rate Recovery.” *Journal of Strength and Conditioning Research*, *25*, 2304–10. doi: 10.1519/JSC.0b013e3181f90174.

Garcia-Lopez, Juan., Jose, A. Rodriguez-Marroyo., Juan, C. Morante., José, L. Gonzalez-Montesinos., Jesús, Mora. & José, G. Villa-Vicente. (2004). “Validación Lactica de un Test de Esfuerzo Interválico (Test de Probst) para Determinar el Umbral Anaeróbico del Futbolista.” [“Lactic Validation of an Interval Effort Test (Probst Test) to Determine the Anaerobic Threshold of the Soccer Player.”] *Revista Internacional de Fútbol y Ciencia*, *2*, 3–19.

Garcia-Lopez, Juan., Jose, G. Villa-Vicente., Jose, A. Rodriguez-Marroyo., Juan, C. Morante., Eduardo, Alvarez. & Ramiro, Jover. (2003). “Aplicación de Un Test de Esfuerzo Interválico (Test de Probst) Para Valorar La Cualidad Aeróbica En Futbolistas de La Liga Española.” [“"Application of an Interval Effort Test (Probst Test) to Assess Aerobic Quality in Soccer Players of the Spanish League.”] *Apunts: Educación Física y Deportes*, *71*, 80–81.

Glassbrook, Daniel J., Tim, L. A. Doyle., Jacqueline, A. Alderson. & Joel, T. Fuller. (2019). “The Demands of Professional Rugby League Match-Play: A Meta-Analysis.” *Sports Medicine - Open*, *5*, 24. doi: 10.1186/s40798-019-0197-9.

Haraldsdottir, Kristin., Stacey, Brickson., Jennifer, Sanfilippo., Warren, Dunn. & Andrew, Watson. (2018). “In-Season Changes in Heart Rate Recovery are Inversely Related to Time to Exhaustion but Not Aerobic Capacity in Rowers.” *Scandinavian Journal of Medicine & Science in Sports*, *28*, 418–24. doi: 10.1111/sms.12934.

Harry, Khavish. & Marc, J. Booysen. (2019). “Faster Heart Rate Recovery Correlates With High-Intensity Match Activity in Female Field Hockey Players-Training Implications.” *Journal of Strength and Conditioning Research*. https://doi.org/10.1519/ JSC.000000000000 3073.

Haydar, Bachar., Hani, al Haddad., Said, Ahmaidi. & Martin, Buchheit. (2011). "Assessing Inter-Effort Recovery and Change of Direction Ability with the 30-15 Intermittent Fitness Test." *Journal of Sports Science and Medicine*, *10*, 346–54.

Hopkins, Will G. (2000). "Measures of Reliability in Sports Medicine and Science." *Sports Medicine*, *30*, 375–81. doi: 10.2165/00007256-200030050-00006.

Javorka, Michal., Ivn, Zila., Tomás, Balharek. & Kamil, Javorka. (2002). "Heart Rate Recovery after Exercise: Relations to Heart Rate Variability and Complexity." *Brazilian Journal of Medical and Biological Research*, *35*, 991–1000.

Krustrup, Peter., Magni, Mohr., Tommas, Amstrup., Torben, Rysgaard., Johnny, Johansen., Aadam, Steensberg., Preben, K. Pedersen. & Jeans, Bangsbo. (2003). "The Yo-Yo Intermittent Recovery Test: Physiological Response, Reliability, and Validity." *Medicine & Science in Sports & Exercise*, *35*, 697–705. doi: 10.1249/01.MSS.0000058441.94520.32.

Kuipers, Henry., Frank, Verstappen., Harry, Keizer., Paul, Geurten. & Gregor, van Kranenburg. (1985). "Variability of Aerobic Performance in the Laboratory and Its Physiologic Correlates." *International Journal of Sports Medicine*, *6*, 197–201. doi:10.1055/s-2008-1025839.

Lamberts, Robert P., Jeroen, Swart., Benoit, Capostagno., Timothy, D. Noakes. & Mike, I. Lambert. (2010). "Heart Rate Recovery as a Guide to Monitor Fatigue and Predict Changes in Performance Parameters." *Scandinavian Journal of Medicine and Science in Sports*, *20*, 449–57. doi: 10.1111/j.1600-0838.2009.00977.x.

Lamberts, Robert P., Jeroen, Swart., Timothy, D. Noakes. & Michael, I. Lambert. (2009). "Changes in Heart Rate Recovery after High-Intensity Training in Well-Trained Cyclists." *European Journal of Applied Physiology*, *105*, 705–13. doi: 10.1007/s00421-008-0952-y.

Lucia, Alejandro., Oscar, Sanchez., Alfredo, Carvajal. & José, López-Chicharro. (1999). "Analysis of the Aerobic-Anaerobic Transition in Elite Cyclists during Incremental Exercise with the Use of

Electromyography." *British Journal of Sports Medicine*, *33*, 178–85. doi: 10.1136/bjsm.33.3.178.

Mahon, Anthony D., Cindy, S. Anderson., Molly, J. Hipp. & Kindal, A. Hunt. (2003). "Heart Rate Recovery from Submaximal Exercise in Boys and Girls." *Medicine and Science in Sports and Exercise*, *35*, 2093–97. doi: 10.1249/01.MSS.0000099180.80952.83.

Midgley, Adrian W., Sean, Carroll., David, Marchant., Lars, R. McNaughton. & Jason, Siegler. (2009). "Evaluation of True Maximal Oxygen Uptake Based on a Novel Set of Standardized Criteria." *Applied Physiology, Nutrition, and Metabolism*, *34*, 115–23. doi: 10.1139/H08-146.

Midgley, Adrian W., Lars, R. McNaughton. & Sean, Carroll. (2006). "Verification Phase as a Useful Tool in the Determination of the Maximal Oxygen Uptake of Distance Runners." *Applied Physiology, Nutrition, and Metabolism*, *31*, 541–48. doi: 10.1139/h06-023.

Midgley, Adrian W., Lars, R. McNaughton., Remco, Polman. & David, Marchant. (2007). "Criteria for Determination of Maximal Oxygen Uptake: A Brief Critique and Recommendations for Future Research." *Sports Medicine*, *37*, 1019–28.

Mikulic, Pavle., Vlatko, Vucetic. & Davor, Sentija. (2011). "Strong Relationship Between Heart Rate Deflection Point and Ventilatory Threshold in Trained Rowers." *Journal of Strength and Conditioning Research*, *25*, 360–66. doi: 10.1519/JSC.0b013e3181bf01f7.

Mourot, Laurent., Nicolas, Fabre., Erik, Andersson., Sarah, Willis., Martin, Buchheit. & Hans-Christer, Holmberg. (2015). "Cross-Country Skiing and Postexercise Heart-Rate Recovery." *International Journal of Sports Physiology and Performance*, *10*, 11–16. doi: 10.1123/ijspp.2013-0445.

Nagashima, Junzo., Haruki, Musha., Hideomi, Takada., Kumiko, Takagi., Toshiharu, Mita., Takashi, Mochida. & Takeshi, Yoshihisa. (2010). "Three-Month Exercise and Weight Loss Program Improves Heart Rate Recovery in Obese Persons along with Cardiopulmonary Function." *Journal of Cardiology*, *56*, 79–84. doi: 10.1016/ j.jjcc. 2010.03.001.

Narazaki, Kenji., Kris, Berg., Nicholas, Stergiou. & Boli, Chen. (2009). "Physiological Demands of Competitive Basketball." *Scandinavian Journal of Medicine & Science in Sports*, *19*, 425–32. doi: 10.1111/j.1600-0838.2008.00789.x.

Noakes, Timothy D. (2008). "Testing for Maximum Oxygen Consumption Has Produced a Brainless Model of Human Exercise Performance." *British Journal of Sports Medicine*, *42*, 551–55. doi: 10.1136/bjsm.2008.046821.

Ostojic, Sergej M., Julio, Calleja-Gonzalez., Djordje, G. Jakovljevic., Vlatko, Vucetic. & Facundo, Ahumada. (2010). "Ultra Short-Term Heart Rate Recovery in Athletes of Different Sports." *Medicina Dello Sport*, *63*, 145–52.

Ostojic, Sergej M., Marko, D. Stojanovic. & Julio, Calleja-Gonzalez. (2011). "Ultra Short-Term Heart Rate Recovery after Maximal Exercise: Relations to Aerobic Power in Sportsmen." *Chinese Journal of Physiology*, *54*, 105–10.

Otsuki, Takeshi., Seiji, Maeda., Motoyuki, Iemitsu., Yoko, Saito., Yuko, Tanimura., Jun, Sugawara., Ryuichi, Ajisaka. & Takashi, Miyauchi. (2007). "Postexercise Heart Rate Recovery Accelerates in Strength-Trained Athletes." *Medicine and Science in Sports and Exercise*, *39*, 365–70. doi: 10.1249/01.mss.0000241647.13220.4c.

Palucci, Vieira., Luiz, Henrique., Christopher, Carling., Fabio, A. Barbieri., Rodrigo, Aquino. & Paulo, R. Pereira. (2019). "Match Running Performance in Young Soccer Players: A Systematic Review." *Sports Medicine*, *49*, 289–318. doi: 10.1007/s40279-018-01048-8.

Pichot, Vincent., Frederic, Roche., Jean, M. Gaspoz., Franck, Enjolras., Anestesis, Antoniadis., Pascal, Minini., Frederic, Costes., Thierry, Busso., Jean, René Lacour. & Jean, C. Barthelemy. (2000). "Relation between Heart Rate Variability and Training Load in Middle-Distance Runners." *Medicine & Science in Sports & Exercise*, *32*, 1729–36.

Rabbani, Alireza. & Martin, Buchheit. (2015). "Heart Rate-Based versus Speed-Based High-Intensity Interval Training in Young Soccer Players." *International Research in Science and Soccer II*.

Robinson, Salomon., Mark, Pearcy., Frank, R. Brueckman., John, R. Nicholas. & David, I. Miller. (1953). "Effects of Atropine on Heart Rate and Oxygen Intake in Working Man." *Journal of Applied Physiology*, *5*, 508–12. doi: 10.1152/jappl.1953.5.9.508.

Rodríguez-Fernández, Alejandro., Javier, Sanchez-Sanchez., Rodrigo, Ramirez-Campillo., Jose, A. Rodríguez-Marroyo., Fabio, Y. Nakamura, & Jose, G. Villa-Vicente. (2019). "Relationship between Repeated Sprint Ability, Aerobic Capacity, Intermittent Endurance and Heart Rate Recovery in Youth Soccer Players." *Journal of Strength and Conditioning Research*, *33*, 3406-3413. doi: 10.1519/JSC.0000000000002193.

Saltin, Bruce. & Louis, B. Rowell. (1980). "Functional Adaptations to Physical Activity and Inactivity." *Federation Proceedings*, *39*, 1506–13.

Silva, Joao R., Michael, C. Rumpf., Maxime, Hertzog., Carlo, Castagna., Abdulaziz, Farooq., Olivier, Girard. & Karim, Hader. (2018). "Acute and Residual Soccer Match-Related Fatigue: A Systematic Review and Meta-Analysis." *Sports Medicine.*, *48*, 539-583. doi: 10.1007/s40279-017-0798-8.

Suarez-Arrones, Luis., Ignacio, Torreno., Bernardo, Requena., Eduardo, Saez de Villarreal., David, Casamichana., José, C. Barbero-Alvarez. & Diego, Munguia-Izquierdo. (2014). "Match-Play Activity Profile in Professional Soccer Players during Official Games and the Relationship between External and Internal Load." *Journal of Sports Medicine and Physical Fitness*, *55*, 1417-1422

Suzic, Lazic., Jelena, Milica, Dekleva., Ivan, Soldatovic., Roman, Leischik., Slavica, Suzic., Dragan, Radovanovic., Biljana, Djuric., Dejan, Nesic., Milivoje, Lazic. & Sanja, Mazic. (2017). "Heart Rate Recovery in Elite Athletes: The Impact of Age and Exercise Capacity." *Clinical Physiology and Functional Imaging*, *37*, 117–23. doi: 10.1111/cpf.12271.

Thomson, Rebecca L., Clint, R. Bellenger., Peter, R. C. Howe., Laura, Karavirta. & Jonathan, D. Buckley. (2016). "Improved Heart Rate Recovery despite Reduced Exercise Performance Following Heavy

Training: A within-Subject Analysis." *Journal of Science and Medicine in Sport*, *19*, 255–59. doi: 10.1016/j.jsams.2015.02.010.

Tomlin, Dona L. & Howard, A. Wenger. (2001). "The Relationship between Aerobic Fitness and Recovery from High Intensity Intermittent Exercise." *Sports Medicine*, *31*, 1–11.

Trevizani, Gabriela A., Paulo, R. Benchimol-Barbosa. & Jurandir, Nadal. (2012). "Effects of Age and Aerobic Fitness on Heart Rate Recovery in Adult Men." *Arquivos Brasileiros de Cardiologia*, *99*, 802–10. doi: 10.1590/s0066-782x2012005000069.

Turner, Antony N. & Perry, F. Stewart. (2014). "Strength and Conditioning for Soccer Players." *Strength & Conditioning Journal*, *36*, 1–13. doi: 10.1519/SSC.0000000000000054.

Vaquera Jiménez, Alejandro., Juan, C. Morante., Juan, García-López., Jose, A. Rodríguez-Marroyo., Maria, C. Ávila., Paulo, R. Mendonca. & José, G. VillaVicente. (2007). "Design and Application of the Field Test TIVRE-Basket for the Evaluation of the Aerobic Resistance in Basketball Players." *European Journal of Human Movement*, *18*, 19-40.

Villa-Vicente, Jose G., Juan, García-López., Juan, C. Morante. & Zósimo, San Román. (2000). "Validation of the Probst Specific Resistance Test in Professional Soccer Players." *Sports Medicine Archives*, *17*, 185–86.

Vucetic, Vlatko., Davor, Sentija., Goran, Sporis., Nebojsa, Trajkovic. & Zoran, Milanovic. (2014). "Comparison of Ventilation Threshold and Heart Rate Deflection Point in Fast and Standard Treadmill Test Protocols." *Acta Clinica Croatica*, *53*, 190–203.

Whitehead, Sarah., Kevin, Till., Dan, Weaving. & Ben, Jones. (2018). "The Use of Microtechnology to Quantify the Peak Match Demands of the Football Codes: A Systematic Review." *Sports Medicine*, *48*, 2549–75. doi: 10.1007/s40279-018-0965-6.

In: An Essential Guide to Sports Performance ISBN: 978-1-53617-608-7
Editors: Daniel Castillo Alvira et al.

Chapter 6

TRAINING LOAD PERIODIZATION IN SOCCER WITH ONE OFFICIAL MATCH A WEEK: A SYSTEMATIC REVIEW

Markel Rico-González[1], Alberto Mendez-Villanueva[2] and Asier Los Arcos[1,*]

[1]Department of Physical Education and Sport,
University of Basque Country, Vitoria-Gasteiz, Spain
[2]ASPIRE, Academy for Sports Excellence, Doha, Qatar

ABSTRACT

In competitive soccer, the organization of the weekly training load (TL) should warrant peak performance in the official match The aim of the study was to review the weekly training load (TL) that players are exposed to during in the competitive period while playing one-match a week. Three electronic databases (Pubmed, SPORTdiscus and ProQuest Central) were searched for research articles published up to February

[*] Corresponding Author's Email: asierlosarcos@gmail.com.

2018. Articles were considered when one-match weekly TL quantification included training and match loads and players´participation level on both sessions were specified during the regular competitive period in male soccer players. TL arising from the match represented 38% of the weekly differenciated sRPE-TL, being almost the exclusive source of weekly high-speed and sprinting (90-97%) in professional soccer players. The number of weekly training sessions carried out by the team does not seem to influence weekly TL in both professional and young soccer players. TL progressively increased up 4 days after the previous match (i.e., 3 days before the next match) to get reduced up to the day before the competition in professional soccer players, but a clear trend for weekly TL distribution was not apparent for young soccer players. Finally, inter-players training, match and weekly TL variability was lower for young soccer players in comparison to professional soccer players.

Keywords: team sport, football, periodization, training, competition

INTRODUCTION

Depending on the level of the competition and team, soccer players should be prepared to carry out 3-7 training sessions and compete 1-2 times per week during the 9-10 months of the competition period (i.e., domestic league). Despite that some high-level soccer teams often compete twice a week, most young, amateur and the vast majority of professional soccer teams have to play one match a week. Regardless of the competition level and match fixtures, the organization of the weekly training load should warrant peak performance in the most important session of the week: the official match. Since accumulated external and/or internal training load (TL) has been shown to be related, at least partially, to changes in players' physical fitness performance (Jaspers et al. 2017) and injury occurrence (Bowen et al. 2017; Owen et al. 2015), its quantification is of interest for soccer teams. Moreover, optimal weekly TL distribution is pivotal to ensure the sufficient after-game recovery and prevent pre-match fatigue (Malone et al. 2015; Coutinho et al. 2015; Jeong et al. 2011; Akenhead, Harley, and Tweddle 2016; Fessi et al. 2016). However, the complex nature of soccer competition and training complicates the individual prescription of the weekly TL, which results in considerably TL differences between soccer players of the same team (Akubat et al. 2012; Gil-Rey, Lezaun, and Los Arcos 2015).

A training week is typically designed to ensure readiness to play in the next official match, but regulations only allow the participation of, at most, 14 players. The remaining players of the squad cannot participate in the most physical/physiological demanding session of the week (Anderson et al., 2016; Arcos et al. 2014; Los Arcos, Mendez-Villanueva, and Martínez-Santos, 2017). Even though compensatory training strategies are implemented to compensate for the missing match, weekly TL for the starters players is largely greater than for the non-starters (Azcárate, Yanci, and Los Arcos, 2018; Los Arcos, Mendez-Villanueva, and Martínez-Santos, 2017). Moreover, *strategical* (e.g., playing system and positions), *competition* (e.g., opponent team level, playing at home/away, period of the season) and *game internal* (e.g., temporary score) *factors* (Sarmento et al. 2014; Castellano, Alvarez-Pastor, and Bradley 2014) can substantially influence match loads and produce a high match-to-match load variability and considerably differences among participating players (Bush et al. 2015; Carling et al. 2016; Gregson et al. 2010; Los Arcos et al. 2016).

In addition to match, weekly training strategies can also produce substantial differences on TL accumulation between players of the same team (Malone et al. 2015; Akenhead, Harley, and Tweddle 2016; Fessi et al. 2016). Soccer coaches typically use group exercises in order to improve players' technical and tactical dimensions in relation to the forthcoming fixtures (O'Connor, Larkin, and Williams 2018; Ford, Yates, and Williams 2010). This reduces considerably the capacity to prescribe individual TL and can produce high inter-players variability depending on the structural traits (Parlebas 2002) of the tasks (Halouani et al. 2014; Hill-Haas et al. 2011; Lacome et al. 2018; Los Arcos et al. 2014), strategical instructions applied (e. g. playing positions and systems, with or without man-marking) (Ngo et al. 2012), teaching organization used (Cushion, Ford, and Williams 2012; Partington and Cushion 2013) and the training style of the coach (Rampinini et al. 2007).

Therefore, the aim of the study was to assess the TL that players are exposed to during the whole week in the competitive period while playing one-match a week, including both the training sessions and the match.

METHODS

Search Strategy

The systematic review was reported in accordance with the Preferred Reporting Items for Systematic Reviews and Meta Analyses (PRISMA) guidelines (Moher et al. 2009). The protocol was not registered prior to initiation of the project and did not require Institutional Review Board approval. A systematic search of three electronic databases (Pubmed, SPORTdiscus and ProQuest Central) was performed until 22 February 2018 by the two authors (MR, ALA). The search was limited to full texts and the English language. The authors were not blinded to journal names or manuscript authors. We created a Boolean phrase to include European football players (*population*), and search terms relevant to team-sport periodization (*temporal units*) and physical or psycho-physiological response of the players (*training load*). Groups of keywords (*population, temporal unit* and *training load*) were connected with OR within each group and using AND to combine the three groups (Table 1).

Table 1. Database search strategy

Search Term	Keywords
European football	"*soccer*" OR "*football*"
Temporal unit	"*season**" OR "*week**" OR "*training**" OR "*session**" OR "*match**" OR "*game**"
Training load	"l*oad**" OR "*workload**" OR *intensity* OR *intensities* OR "*effort**" OR "*exertion**" OR *velocity* OR *velocities*

Screening Strategy and Study Selection

After confirming that the two authors found the same number of articles in each electronic databases, one of the authors (MR) exported the electronic search results to an Excel spreadsheet (Microsoft Excel, Microsoft, Redmond, USA) and removed the duplicate records. Then, the same authors screened remaining records against the inclusion-exclusion criteria using a hierarchical approach (Table 2) in two phases: Phase 1, titles and abstracts were screened and excluded by the two authors (MR, ALA) against criteria 1–4 where applicable; Phase 2, full texts of the remaining papers were then accessed and screened against inclusion criteria 1–9 also by the two authors (MR, ALA). Any disagreements on the final inclusion-exclusion status were resolved through discussion in both screening and excluding phases (Phase 1, n = 120; Phase 2, n = 35). Moreover, not identified relevant articles were also screened in an identical manner and the studies that complied with inclusion-exclusion criteria were included and labelled as 'not identified from search strategy'. If we have any question about the application of the inclusion-exclusion criteria, we requested further information from the authors. The additional information provided by the authors was considered during the screening process. Lack of additional forthcoming information led to the article being excluded.

Since the aim of this systematic review was to assess weekly TL in all male soccer competition level teams, we considered the most frequent type week, that is, one-match weeks. Pre-competitive and off-season period, tournaments and international cups were excluded because they are special periods. We omitted any intervention studies that compared the effects of different training programs on the same team or on different teams because this could affect on the accumulated total TL by the players. Therefore, we considered the studies that assessed weekly TL during the habitual training regimen of the soccer team (i.e., competitive period). We did not considered studies dealing with injured or returning from injury players. Only studies providing mean weekly TL from at least two players were considered.

Table 2. Study inclusion-exclusion criteria

Criteria	Inclusion	Exclusion	Phases
1	Male soccer players	Females No athletes: referees, coaches, spectators, emergency department or police officer.	Title/ Abstract
		Physical education students Other sports players: For example: rugby, futsal, hockey, fencing, contact sport Other football codes players: American football, Canadian football Australian football, Gaelic football, Tag football, soccer-7, beach soccer…	Full-text
2	Federated footballers which are healthy, not injured and are not returning from injury	Non-athletic players, and recreational or former soccer players. Athletes considered to be injured or returning from injury. Special populations: clinical patients, athletes with a physical or mental disability.	Full-text
3	Weekly TL is quantified during the regular season	Independent training sessions, several training drills (e.g., small-sided games), physical fitness tests, official, friendly and simulated matches, or during match warm-up.	Full-text
		Pre-competitive and off-season period, tournaments or international Cups.	
		Intervention studies: comparing the effects of several additional training programs	
4	Team analysis	One case study	Full-text
5	Weekly TL includes training sessions and match loads	Match load is not included	Full-text
6	One-match week	Two- and three-match a week	Full-text
7	The week type and organization were detailed in the study	The week type and organization were *not* detailed in the study	Full-text
8	Players' participation level on training sessions and matches were specified in the study	Players' participation level on training sessions and matches were *not* specified in the study	Full-text
9	At least two players were considered to calculate weekly TL	TL data of only one players was provided	Full-text

TL: training load

Inter-player variation in one-match weekly and session (trainings and official matches) TLs were quantified by means of the coefficient of variation (CV) (Atkinson and Nevill 1998). In order to compare the results between studies, practical significance was assessed by calculating Cohen's *d* effect size (Cohen 1988). Effect sizes (d) of above 0.8, between 0.8 and 0.5, between 0.5 and 0.2 and lower than 0.2 were considered as large, moderate, small and trivial, respectively.

RESULTS

A total of 2901 studies were initially retrieved from the three databases, of which 916 were duplicates. Thus, a total of 1985 articles were screened. Despite that the search was limited to full texts and the English language, 30 and 6 reports were abstracts and conferences or congress reports, respectively, and one article was not written in English. Moreover, a study was a letter and 3 were not found. After screening the titles and abstracts against criteria 1–4 where applicable, and full texts of the remaining papers against inclusion criteria 1–9, 5 studies met the inclusion criteria. Moreover, one additional article was identified through additional sources (Figure 1). Four articles assessed Spanish or English professional players (Anderson et al., 2016; Azcárate et al., 2018; Los Arcos, Mendez-Villanueva, and Martínez-Santos, 2017; Thorpe et al., 2016) and 2 English or Portuguese young teams (Rebelo et al., 2012; Wrigley et al. 2012). Analysed weeks ranged from 1 to 10 according to the training week type (Saturday-Saturday, Saturday-Sunday, Sunday-Saturday and Sunday-Sunday). In order to quantify weekly TL, session rating of perceived exertion TL (sRPE-TL) was used 5 times (Azcárate et al., 2018; Los Arcos, Mendez-Villanueva, and Martínez-Santos, 2017; Rebelo et al., 2012; Thorpe et al., 2016; Wrigley et al., 2012). One study used portable global positioning system (GPS) units (Viper pod 2, STATSports, Belfast, UK) for quantifying training sessions TL and computerised semi-automatic video match-analysis image recognition system (Prozone Sports Ltd®, Leeds, UK) for match load (Anderson et al. 2016). Moreover, only one study (Rebelo et al., 2012) used heart rate based methods (i.e., Edwards' TL method (Edwards 1993), and the TRIMP method (Banister 1991)) to quantify TL.

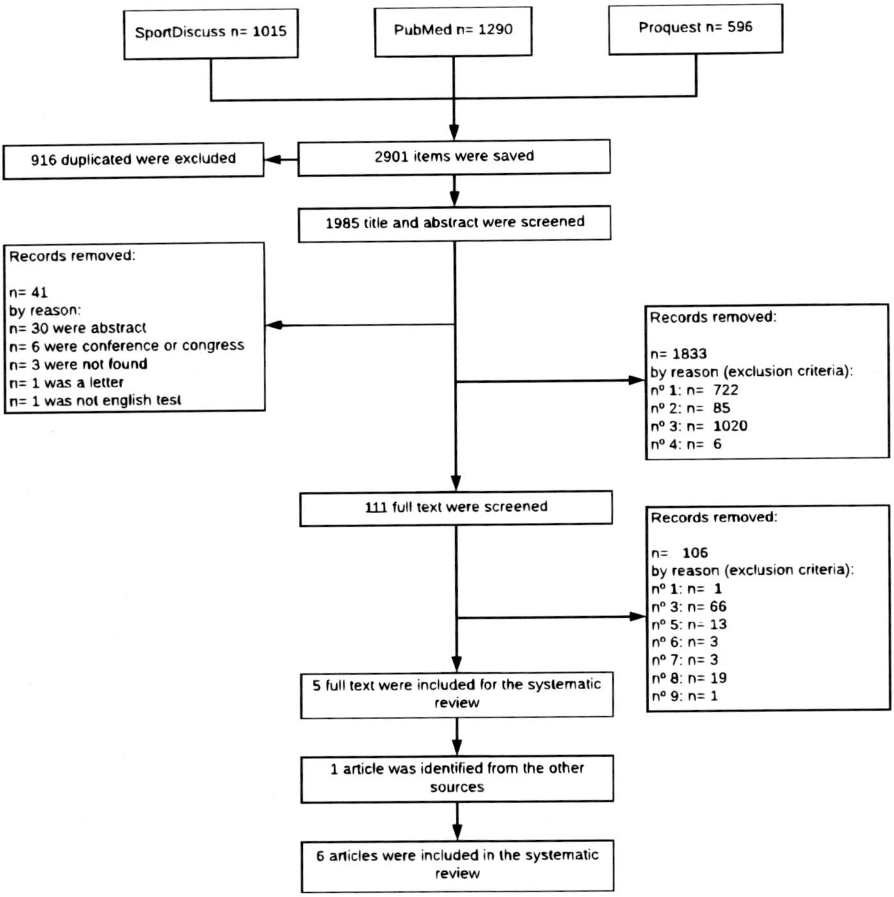

Figure 1. Flow diagram.

Overall TL

After 6 training sessions plus a match and 5 training sessions plus a match, weekly differentiated sRPE-TL was of ~1200 and ~1600 AUs for Spanish 2nd division players (Azcárate et al., 2018) and elite reserve team players (Los Arcos, Mendez-Villanueva, and Martínez-Santos 2017), respectively, and after 5 training sessions plus a match, weekly overall sRPE-TL (sRPEo-TL) of ~1580 AUs for Premier League players (Thorpe et al. 2016) (Table 3a). One match weekly differentiated sRPE-TL ranged from 965 ± 138 to 1117 ± 227 AUs for professional non-*starters* players and from 800 ± 174 to 856 ± 181 AUs for professional soccer players that did not participate at all in the match (Azcárate et al., 2018) (Table 3b). After 3 training sessions plus a match, 7 training sessions plus a match, 5 training sessions plus a match and 5 training sessions plus a match, one-match VAS-TL was of 2661-3103 AUs, and sRPEo-TL of 3984 ± 222, 2919 ± 136 and 2524 ± 128 AUs for regional level Portuguese youth soccer players (Rebelo et al. 2012) and U18, U16 and U14 elite English players (Wrigley et al. 2012) (Table 4). Only one study quantified one-match weekly external load in professional soccer players (Anderson et al. 2016) (Table 5).

Match vs Training Sessions TL

Official match represented the greatest session TL of the week for the professional *starters* soccer players, accounting for one third of the weekly TL (Tables 6a and 6b). Top level English soccer players accumulated significantly greater sRPEo-TL (Thorpe et al. 2016) (Table 6a) and covered significantly greater distances at different speed thresholds (Anderson et al. 2016) (Table 6b) during the match than during the any of the training sessions. Moreover, match differentiated sRPE-TL (i.e., sRPEres- and sRPEmus-TL) was substantially greater than the most demanding training session of the week for Spanish elite reserve team players (Los Arcos, Mendez-Villanueva, and Martínez-Santos 2017) (Table 6a). TL arising from the match represented 38% of the total weekly overall (Thorpe et al. 2016) and 32-36% of the total weekly differentiated sRPE-TL (Los Arcos, Mendez-Villanueva, and Martínez-Santos 2017) (Table 6a). Moreover, match-derived TL equated to 40% of the total distance covered during all the training sessions (excluding the match) and was almost the exclusive source of weekly high-speed (90%) and sprinting (97%) (Anderson et al. 2016) (Table 6b) in Premier League players.

Table 3a. One-match weekly training load (TL) for professional soccer players that completed all training sessions of the week and participated in at least 45 min of the official (starters) during competitive weeks

Study	Number (n), competition level and age (mean ± SD) of the players	Season period	Wks analysed	Wk type	Number of training sessions per wk and its organization	Method to quantify TL	Mean (±SD) TL (AUs) and its variability (CV [%])
Azcárate, Yanci, and Los Arcos (2018)	21 Spanish professional soccer players, 27 (3) years	1st competitive period	3 (33 occurrences)	Sa- Su (8 days)	Training sessions: 6 Mo/We (2ss) /Th/Fr/Sa	sRPE-TL Foster's 0-10 scale (Foster et al. 2001)	*sRPEres-TL* 1157 ± 185 (CV = 16%) *sRPEmus-TL* 1271 ± 222 (CV = 17%)
			4 (46 occurrences)	Sa-Sa (7 days)	Training sessions: 6 Mo/Tu (2ss)/We/Th/ Fr		*sRPEres-TL* 1151 ± 223 (CV = 19%) *sRPEmus-TL* 1240 ± 254 (CV = 20%)
			3 (34 occurrences)	Su-Su (7 days)	Training sessions: 6 Mo/We (2ss)/Th/Fr/ Sa		*sRPEres-TL* 1201 ± 237 (CV = 20%) *sRPEmus-TL* 1314 ± 242 (CV = 18%)
			3 (35 occurrences)	Su-Sa (6 days)	Training sessions: 6 Mo/Tu (2ss)/We/Th /Fr		*sRPEres-TL* 1102 ± 217 (CV = 20%) *sRPEmus-TL* 1203 ± 249 (CV = 21%)
Los Arcos, Mendez-Villanueva, and Martínez-Santos. (2017)	24 reserve team professional soccer players, 20.3 (2.0) years	All competitive period	10 (3-9 weeks per player)	Sa- Su (8 days)	Training sessions: 5 Mo/We/Th/Fr/Sa	sRPE-TL Foster's 0-10 scale (Foster et al. 2001)	*sRPEres-TL* 1600 ± 293 (CV = 18%) *sRPEmus-TL* 1639 ± 320 (CV = 20%)
Thorpe et al. (2016)	29 English Premier League soccer players, 21 (5.1) years	All competitive period	Median duration of 3 weeks per player (range: 1-13)	Su-Su (7 days)	Training sessions: 5 Mo/Tu/Th/Fr/Sa	sRPE-TL Foster's 0-10 scale (Foster et al. 2001)	*sRPEo-TL* ≈1580

Mo: Monday; Tu: Tuesday; We: Wednesday; Th: Thursday; Fr: Friday; Sa: Saturday; Su: Sunday; Wk(s): week(s); 1° competitive period: from September to December;; 2nd competitive period: from January to May; All competitive period: from September to May; sRPE-TL: perceived TL; sRPEres-TL: respiratory sRPE-TL; sRPEmus-TL: muscular sRPE-TL; sRPEo-TL: overall sRPE-TL; CV: Coefficient of variation.

Table 3b. One-match weekly differentiated perceived training load (TL) for professional soccer players that completed all training sessions of the week and participated for less than 45 min (Non-Starters) or did not participate (Non participants) in the official match during competitive weeks

Study	Number (n), competition level and age (mean ± SD) of the players	Season period	Wks analysed	Wk type	Number of training sessions per wk and its organization	Method to quantify TL	Mean (±SD) TL (AUs) and its variability (CV [%])
Non-Starters							
Azcárate, Yanci, and Los Arcos (2018)	21 Spanish professional soccer players, 27 (3) years	1st competitive period	3 (8 occurrences)	Sa-Su (8 days)	Training sessions: 6 Mo/We (2ss)/Th/Fr/Sa	Differentiated sRPE-TL. Foster's 0-10 scale (Foster et al. 2001)	*sRPEres-TL* 965 ± 138 (CV = 14%) *sRPEmus-TL* 971 ± 202 (CV = 21%)
			4 (11 occurrences)	Sa-Sa (7 days)	Training sessions: 6 Mo/Tu (2ss)/We/Th/Fr		*sRPEres-TL* 984 ± 141 (CV = 14%) *sRPEmus-TL* 1054 ± 197 (CV = 19%)
			3 (8 occurrences)	Su-Su (7 days)	Training sessions: 6 Mo/We (2ss)/Th/Fr/Sa		*sRPEres-TL* 993 ± 235 (CV = 24%) *sRPEmus-TL* 1065 ± 258 (CV = 24%)
			3 (7 occurrences)	Su-Sa (6 days)	Training sessions: 6 Mo/Tu (2ss)/We/Th/Fr		*sRPEres-TL* 966 ± 117 (CV = 12%) *sRPEmus-TL* 1053 ± 171 (CV = 16%)
Los Arcos, Mendez-Villanueva, and Martínez-Santos (2017)	24 reserve team professional soccer players, 20.3 (2.0) years	All competitive period	10 (3-9 weeks per player)	Sa-Su (8 days)	Training sessions: 5 Mo/We/Th/Fr/Sa	Differentiated sRPE-TL. Foster's 0-10 scale (Foster et al. 2001)	*sRPEres-TL* 1117 ± 227 (CV = 20%) *sRPEmus-TL* 1089 ± 259 (CV = 24%)
Non-participants							
Azcárate, Yanci, and Los Arcos (2018)	21 Spanish professional soccer players, 27 (3) years	1st competitive period	3 (20 occurrences)	Sa-Su (8 days)	Training sessions: 6 Mo/We (2ss)/Th/Fr/Sa	Differentiated sRPE-TL. Foster's 0-10 scale (Foster et al. 2001)	*sRPEres-TL* 829 ± 175 (CV = 21%) *sRPEmus-TL* 800 ± 174 (CV = 22%)
			4 (24 occurrences)	Sa-Sa (7 days)	Training sessions: 6 Mo/Tu (2ss)/We/Th/Fr		*sRPEres-TL* 852 ± 159 (CV = 19%) *sRPEmus-TL* 845 ± 169 (CV = 20%)
			3 (20 occurrences)	Su-Su (7 days)	Training sessions: 6 Mo/We (2ss)/Th/Fr/Sa		*sRPEres-TL* 808 ± 213 (CV = 26%) *sRPEmus-TL* 864 ± 238 (CV = 28%)
			3 (18 occurrences)	Su-Sa (6 days)	Training sessions: 6 Mo/Tu (2ss)/We/Th/Fr		*sRPEres-TL* 856 ± 181 (CV = 21%) *sRPEmus-TL* 826 ± 202 (CV = 24%)

Mo: Monday; Tu: Tuesday; We: Wednesday; Th: Thuesday; Fr: Friday; Sa: Saturday; Su: Sunday; Wk(s): week(s); 1° competitive period: from September to December; All competitive period: from September to May; sRPE-TL: perceived TL; sRPEres-TL: respiratory sRPE-TL; sRPEmus-TL: muscular sRPE-TL; sRPEo-TL: overall sRPE-TL; 2ss: two sessions that day: CV: Coefficient of variation.

Table 4. One-match weekly training load (TL) for young soccer players that completed all training sessions and the official match (Starters) during competitive weeks

Study	Number (n), competition level and age (mean ± SD) of the players	Season period	Wks analysed	Wk type	Number of training sessions per wk and its organization	Method to quantify TL	Mean (±SD) TL (AUs) and its variability (CV [%])
Rebelo et al. (2012)	51 Portuguese youth soccer players, 16 (0) years	2nd competitive period	2 (occurrences not defined)	- Su	Training sessions: 3 Tu/Th/Fr/Su (Ma 80 min)	VAS questionnaire for rating perceived exertion, TRIMP (Banister 1991) and Edward´s (Edwards 1993)	*VAS1-TL* 3103 ± 172 (CV = 6%) *VAS2-TL* 2661 ± 151 (CV = 6%) *TRIMP* 80 ± 1 (CV = 1%) *Edward's* 627 ± 19 (CV = 5%)
Wrigley et al. (2012)	8 U18 English elite players, 17(1)	1st competitive period	2 (16 occurrences)	- Sa	Training sessions: 7 Mo (2ss)/Tu (2 ss)/Th (2s)/Fr/Sa (Ma, 90 min)	sRPEo-TL Modified 10-point Borg scale (Borg 1998)	*sRPEo-TL* 3984 ± 222 (CV = 6%)
	8 U16 English elite players, 15 (1)	1st competitive period	2 (16 occurrences)	- Sa	Training sessions: 5 Mo/Tu (2ss)/Th (2ss)/Sa (Ma, 80 min)		*sRPEo-TL* 2919 ± 136 (CV = 5%)
	8 U14 English elite players, 13 (1)	1st competitive period	2 (16 occurrences)	- Su	Training sessions: 5 Mo (2ss)/We (2ss)/Th/Su (Ma, 80 min) Starters: 80 min		*sRPEo-TL* 2524 ± 128 (CV = 5%)

Mo: Monday; Tu: Tuesday; We: Wednesday; Th: Thursday; Fr: Friday; Sa: Saturday; Su: Sunday; Ma: Match; wk(s): week(s); 1° competitive period: from September to December;; 2nd Competitive period: from January to May; sRPE-TL: perceived TL; sRPEres-TL: respiratory sRPE-TL; sRPEmus-TL: muscular sRPE-TL; sRPEo-TL: overall sRPE-TL; VAS-TL: Visual analogue scale (VAS1, "How do you classify the effort made during the training session (or match) today?" and VAS2-TL: How physically demanding did you perceive the training session (or match) today?''); TRIMP: Training impulse; CV: Coefficient of variation; 2ss: two sessions that day.

Table 5. One-match weekly external training load (TL) (distance covered [m]) for professional soccer players that completed all weekly training sessions and participated at least 75 min in the official match

Study	Number (n), competition level and age (mean ± SD) of the players	Season period	Wk(s) analysed	Wk type	Number of training sessions per wk and its organization	Method to quantify TL	Mean (±SD) distance covered (m) and its variability (CV [%])
Anderson et al. (2016)[1]	10 English Premier League players, 25 (5)	2nd competitive period	1	Su-Su	Training sessions: 4 We/Th/Fr/Sa	GPS and computerised tracking system.	*Standing* 26 ± 6 (CV = 23%) *Walking* 12635 ± 195 (CV = 2%) *Jogging* 9647 ± 303 (CV = 3%) *Running* 2439 ± 125 (CV = 5%) *HSR* 784 ± 62 (CV = 8%) *Sprinting* 298 ± 26 (CV = 9%)

We: Wednesday; Th: Thursday; Fr: Friday; Sa: Saturday; Su: Sunday; wk(s): week(s); 2nd competitive period: from January to May; GPS: Global Positioning System; Standing: 0–0.6 $km \cdot h^{-1}$; Walking: 0.7–7.1 $km \cdot h^{-1}$; Jogging: 7.2–14.4 $km \cdot h^{-1}$; Running: 4.4–19.7 $km \cdot h^{-1}$; High Speed Running (HSR): 19.8–25.2 $km \cdot h^{-1}$; Sprinting: >25.2 $km \cdot h^{-1}$;CV: Coefficient of variation. [1]Training load was quantified by: portable global positioning system (GPS) units (Viper pod 2, STATS ports, Belfast, UK) and match load by computerised semi-automatic video match-analysis image recognition system (Prozone Sports Ltd®, Leeds, UK)

Table 6a. One-match weekly training load (TL) distribution along the competitive weeks for the players that completed all weekly training sessions

Study	Number (n), competition level and age (mean ± SD) of the players. Season period. Wks analysed	Sa	Su	Mo	Tu	We	Th	Fr	Sa	Su	
Starters: participated for at least 45 min in the official match											
Los Arcos, Mendez-Villanueva, and Martínez-Santos (2017)	24 reserve team professional soccer players, 20.3 (2.0) years. All competitive period. 10 Wks.	Ma	-	*sRPEres-TL* 255 ± 82 (CV = 32%) *15% of the Wk* *46% of the Ma*	-	*sRPEres-TL* 291 ± 92 (CV = 32%) *17% of the Wk* *53% of the Ma*	*sRPEres-TL* 316 ± 96 (CV = 30%) *18% of the Wk* *57% of the Ma*	*sRPEres-TL* 182 ± 103 (CV= 57%) *11% of the Wk* *33% of the Ma*	*sRPEres-TL* 119 ± 73 (CV = 61%) *7% of the Wk* *21% of the Ma*	*sRPEres-TL* 554 ± 170 (CV=31%) *32% of the Wk*	Mo<[a]Tu<[a] We>[c]Th>[b] Fr<[d]Ma
		Ma		*sRPEmus-TL* 246 ± 73 (CV = 30%) *15% of the Wk* *42% of the Ma*	-	*sRPEmus-TL* 242 ± 72 (CV = 30%) *15% of the Wk* *41% of the Ma*	*sRPEmus-TL* 326 ± 109 (CV = 33%) *20% of the Wk* *55% of the Ma*	*sRPEmus-TL* 186 ± 106 (CV = 57%) *11% of the Wk* *32% of the Ma*	*sRPEmus-TL* 126 ± 76 (CV=60%) *8% of the Wk* *21% of the Ma*	*sRPEmus-TL* 590 ± 189 (CV=32%) *36% of the Wk*	Mo<[a]Tu<[a] We>[c]Th>[a]Fr<[d]Ma
Rebelo et al. (2012)	51 regional level youth soccer players from 3 teams competing in the 1° division of the Portuguese soccer league. In the middle of the season. 4 Wks	Nd	Nd	-	*VAS1-TL* 955 ± 83 (CV = 9%) *19% of the Wk 45% of the Ma*	-	*VAS1-TL* 1299 ± 106 (CV = 8%) *26% of the Wk* *61% of the Ma*	*VAS1-TL* 656 ± 70 (CV = 11%) *13% of the Wk* *31% of the Ma*	-	*VAS1-TL* 2127 ± 143 (CV = 7%) *42% of the Wk*	Tu<Th>Fr <Ma
		Nd	Nd	-	*VAS2-TL* 764 ± 73 (CV = 10%) *15% of the Wk 35% of the Ma*	-	*VAS2-TL* 1315 ± 101 (CV = 8%) *26% of the Wk* *60% of the Ma*	*VAS2-TL* 582 ± 55 (CV = 9%) *12% of the Wk* *27% of the Ma*	-	*VAS2-TL* 2177 ± 115 (CV = 5%) *43% of the Wk*	Tu<Th>Fr <Ma

Study	Number (n), competition level and age (mean ± SD) of the players. Season period. Wks analysed	Sa	Su	Mo	Tu	We	Th	Fr	Sa	Su	
		Nd	Nd	-	*TRIMP* 23.6 ± 0.4 (CV = 2%) *21% of the Wk 75% of the Ma*	-	*TRIMP* 30.8 ± 0.6 (CV = 2%) *28% of the Wk 98% of the Ma*	*TRIMP* 25.5 ± 0.9 (CV = 3%) *23% of the Wk 81% of the Ma*	-	*TRIMP* 31.5 ± 0.1 (CV = 0%) *28% of the Wk*	Tu<Th>Fr <Ma
		Nd	Nd	-	*Edward´s TL* 189.2 ± 6.3 (CV = 3%) *20% of the Wk 56% of the Ma*	-	*Edward´s* TL 241.2 ± 8.0 (CV = 3%) *25% of the Wk 71% of the Ma*	*Edward´s TL* 196.6 ± 9.6 (CV = 5%) *20% of the Wk 58% of the Ma*	-	*Edward´s TL* 339.9 ± 9.0 (CV = 3%) *35% of the Wk*	Tu<Th>Fr <Ma
Thorpe et al. (2016)	29 English Premier league soccer players, 27 (5.1) years. All competitive period.	Nd	*sRPEo-TL* ~ 600 *38% of the Wk*	*sRPEo-TL* ~ 40 *3% of the Wk 7% of the Ma*	*sRPEo-TL* ~ 220 *14% of the Wk 37% of the Ma*	-	*sRPEo-TL* ~ 300 *19% of the Wk 50% of the Ma*	*sRPEo-TL*~ 240 *15% of the Wk 40% of the Ma*	*sRPEo-TL* ~ 180 *11% of the Wk 14% of the Ma*	Nd	Mo-Tu<Th>Fr >Sa<Ma
Wrigley et al. [2012]	8 U18 elite soccer players, 17 (1.0) years. 1° competitive period. 2 Wks. 8 U16 elite soccer players, 15 (1.0) years.1° competitive period. 2 Wks. 8 U14 elite soccer players 13 (1.0) years. 1° competitive period. 2 Wks.	Nd	Nd	*sRPEo-TL* (2ss) 650 ± 125 (CV = 19%) *19% of the Wk96% of the Ma*	*sRPEo-TL* (2ss) 1000 ± 100 (CV = 10%) *30% of the Wk148% of the Ma*	-	*sRPEo-TL* (2ss) 1025 ± 100 (CV = 10%) *31% of the Wk152% of the Ma*	-	*sRPEo-TL* 675 ± 125 (CV=18%) *20% of the Wk*	-	Mo<Tu<Th >Ma
		Nd	Nd	*sRPEo-TL* 1175 ± 50	*sRPEo-TL* (2ss)	-	*sRPEo-TL* (2ss) 800 ±	*sRPEo-TL* 650 ± 175	*sRPEo-TL* 775 ± 50 (CV	-	Mo>Tu<Th >Fr<Ma

Table 6a. (Continued)

Study	Number (n), competition level and age (mean ± SD) of the players. Season period. Wks analysed	Sa	Su	Mo	Tu	We	Th	Fr	Sa	Su	
				(CV = 4%) *28% of the Wk* *152% of the Ma*	775 ± 75 (CV = 10%) *19% of the Wk* *100% of the Ma*		100 (CV = 12%) *19% of the Wk* *103% of the Ma*	(CV=27%) *16% of the Wk* *84% of the Ma*	= 6%) *19% of the Wk*		
		Nd	Nd	*sRPEo-TL* (2ss) 1050 ± 100 (CV = 10%) *37% of the Wk* *150% of the Ma*	-	*sRPEo-TL* (2ss) 300 ± 100 (CV = 33%) *11% of the Wk* *43% of the Ma*	*sRPEo-TL* 800 ± 100 (CV = 12%) *28% of the Wk* *114% of the Ma*	-	-	*sRPEo-TL* 700 ± 100 (CV = 14%) *25% of the Wk*	Mo>We<Th>Ma
Non-Starters: did not participate, or played for less than 45 minutes in the official match											
Los Arcos, Mendez-Villanueva, and Martínez-Santos (2017)	24 reserve team professional soccer players, 20.3 (2.0) years. All competitive period. 10 Wks.	Ma	-	*sRPEres-TL* 255 ± 80 (CV = 32%) *19% of the Wk* *234% of the Ma*	-	*sRPEres-TL* 301 ± 85 (CV = 28%) *23% of the Wk* *376% of the Ma*	*sRPEres-TL* 341 ± 100 (CV = 29%) *41% of the Wk* *313% of the Ma*	*sRPEres-TL* 181 ± 134 (CV=74%) *14% of the Wk* *166% of the Ma*	*sRPEres-TL* 121 ± 68 (CV=56%) *9% of the Wk* *111% of the Ma*	*sRPEres-TL* 109 ± 72 (CV = 66%) *8% of the Wk*	Mo<[a]Tu<[a]We>[c]Th>[a]Fr-[c]Ma

Mo: Monday; Tu: Tuesday; We: Wednesday; Th: Thursday; Fr: Friday; Sa: Saturday; Su: Sunday; Ma: Match; Wk(s): week(s); 1° competitive period: from September to December; 2nd Competitive period: from January to May; All competitive period: from September to May; sRPE-TL: perceived TL; sRPEres-TL: respiratory sRPE-TL; sRPEmus-TL: muscular sRPE-TL; sRPEo-TL: overall sRPE-TL; VAS-TL: Visual analogue scale (VAS1, "How do you classify the effort made during the training session (or match) today?" and VAS2-TL: How physically demanding did you perceive the training session (or match) today?''); TRIMP: Training impulse; CV: Coefficient of variation; 2ss: two sessions that day; ES: Effect size a: ES small; b: ES moderate; c: ES large; d: ES very large; e: ES unclear; Nd: non-defined; >: significantly ($p < 0.05$) lower; -: no significant differences ($p > 0.05$).

Table 6b. One-match weekly external training load (TL) (distance covered [m]) distribution along the competitive weeks for the players that completed all weekly training sessions and participated for at least 75 min in the official match

Study	Number (n), competition level and age (mean ± SD) of the players. Season period. Wk(s) analysed	Sa	Su	Mo	Tu	We	Th	Fr	Sa	Su Official Match	Comparison between days
Anderson et al. (2016)[1]	10 English Premier League players, 25 (5). 2nd Competitive period. One wk.					*Standing* 0 (CV = %) *0% of the Wk* *0% of the Ma*	*Standing* 0 (CV = %) *0% of the Wk* *0% of the Ma*	*Standing* 0 (CV = %) *0% of the Wk* *0% of the Ma*	*Standing* 0 (CV = %) *0% of the Wk* *0% of the Ma*	*Standing* 26 ± 6 (CV = 23%) *100% of the Wk*	We-Th-Fr-Sa<Ma
						Walking 2422 ± 106 (CV = 4%) *19% of the Wk* *64% of the Ma*	*Walking* 2520 ± 171 (CV = 7%) *20% of the Wk* *67% of the Ma*	*Walking* 2043 ± 143 (CV = 7%) *16% of the Wk* *54% of the Ma*	*Walking* 1894 ± 117 (CV=6%) *15% of the Wk* *50% of the Ma*	*Walking* 3756 ± 438 (CV = 12%) *30% of the Accumulate W TL*	We-Th>Fr-Sa<Ma
						Jogging 1733 ± 171 (CV = 10%) *18% of the Wk* *43% of the Ma*	*Jogging* 2117 ± 388 (CV = 18%) *22% of the Wk* *53% of the Ma*	*Jogging* 918 ± 102 (CV = 11%) *9% of the Wk* *23% of the Ma*	*Jogging* 899 ± 131 (CV = 15%) *9% of the Wk* *23% of the Ma*	*Jogging* 3980 ± 726 (CV = 18%) *41% of the Accumulate W TL*	We-Th>Fr-Sa<Ma
						Running 176 ± 37 (CV = 21%) *7% of the Wk* *11% of the Ma*	*Running* 473 ± 129 (CV = 27%) *19% of the Wk* *30% of the Ma*	*Running* 130 ± 58 (CV = 45%) *5% of the Wk* *8% of the Ma*	*Running* 101 ± 46 (CV = 46%) *4% of the Wk* *6% of the Ma*	*Running* 1559 ± 357 (CV = 23%) *64% of the Accumulate W TL*	We<Th>Fr-Sa<Ma
						HSR 18 ± 13 (CV = 72%) *2% of the Wk* *3% of the Ma*	*HSR* 18 ± 13 (CV = 72%) *2% of the Wk* *3% of the Ma*	*HSR* 26 ± 28 (CV = 108%) *3% of the Wk* *4% of the Ma*	*HSR* 16 ± 11 (CV = 69%) *2% of the Wk* *2% of the Ma*	*HSR* 706 ± 246 (CV = 35%) *90% of the Accumulate W TL*	We-Th-Fr-Sa<Ma
						Sprinting 0 (CV = -) *0% of the Wk* *0% of the Ma*	*Sprinting* 6 ± 8 (CV = 133%) *2% of the Wk* *3% of the Ma*	*Sprinting* 0 ± 1 (CV = -) *0% of the Wk* *0% of the Ma*	*Sprinting* 2 ± 3 (CV = 150%) *1% of the Wk* *1% of the Ma*	*Sprinting* 290 ± 118 (CV = 41%) *97% of the Accumulate W TL*	We-Th-Fr-Sa<Ma

Mo: Monday; Tu: Tuesday; We: Wednesday; Th: Thursday; Fr: Friday; Sa: Saturday; Su: Sunday; Ma: Match; wk(s): week(s); 1° competitive period: from September to December;; 2nd Competitive period: from January to May; Standing: 0–0.6 km·h-[1]; Walking: 0.7–7.1 km·h-[1]; Jogging: 7.2–14.4 km·h-[1]; Running: 4.4–19.7 km·h-[1]; High Speed Running (HSR): 9.8–25.2 km·h-[1]; Sprinting: 25.2 km·h-[1]; CV: Coefficient of variation.[1]Training load was quantified by: portable global positioning system (GPS) units (Viper pod 2, STATS ports, Belfast, UK) and match load by computerised semi-automatic video match-analysis image recognition system (Prozone Sports Ltd®, Leeds, UK); <: significantly ($p < 0.05$) higher; >: significantly ($p < 0.05$) lower; -: no significant differences ($p > 0.05$).

The match was also the more demanding session of the week for Portuguese regional level youth soccer players (Rebelo et al. 2012). However, U18, U16 and U14 English elite player had a lower match sRPEo-TL compared to training sessions (Wrigley et al. 2012) (Table 6a). The match accounted for 20-23% of the total sRPEo-TL of the week (Wrigley et al. 2012).

Weekly TL Distribution

Substantial/significant TL differences were found between consecutive training sessions and match in elite reserve players (sRPEres-TL, Mo < Tu < We > Th > Fr < Match; sRPEmus-TL, Mo < Tu < We > Th > Fr < Match) (Los Arcos, Mendez-Villanueva, and Martínez-Santos 2017), and English Premier League players (sRPEo-TL; Mo-Tu < Th > Fr > Sa < Match) (Thorpe et al. 2016) (Tables 6a).

TL Variability

Match, training session and one-match weekly TL variability (CV) was of the 31-41%, 30-100% and 2-28%, respectively, for professional soccer players, and of the 0-18%, 2-27% and 6%, respectively, for young soccer players (Los Arcos, Mendez-Villanueva, and Martínez-Santos 2017; Thorpe et al. 2016; Rebelo et al. 2012; Wrigley et al. 2012; Anderson et al. 2016; Azcárate et al., 2018) (Tables 3a, 3b, 4, 5, 6a and 6b).

Discussion

Weekly TL quantification and its management along the training sessions and official matches are important to prepare soccer players to 40-45 weeks of competition. Despite that several studies have assessed TL to monitor changes in players' physical fitness performance (Jaspers et al.

2017; Arcos et al. 2014; Gil-Rey, Lezaun, and Los Arcos 2015; Akubat et al. 2012; Los Arcos et al. 2017), to investigate potential links with injury incidence (Bowen et al. 2017; Owen et al. 2015; Brink et al. 2010; Ehrmann et al. 2015) and to ensure the sufficient after-game recovery and prevent pre-match fatigue (Malone et al. 2015; Coutinho et al. 2015; Jeong et al. 2011; Akenhead, Harley, and Tweddle 2016; Fessi et al. 2016), few studies have analysed one-match weekly TL dynamics during the competitive period considering both training sessions and matches and providing detailed information about the practice time of the players.

Impact of Number of Training Sessions between Consecutive Games

Five of the six studies that quantified one-match weekly TL providing detailed information about the training and match practice time of the players (Los Arcos, Mendez-Villanueva, and Martínez-Santos 2017; Azcárate et al., 2018; Wrigley et al. 2012; Thorpe et al. 2016; Rebelo et al. 2012) used sRPE-TL (Foster et al. 1996). Only high-level soccer teams can access and use heart-rate and/or GPS devices during training sessions and until several years ago the use of these devices was prohibited during official games. Thus, overall (Foster et al. 2001) and differentiated (Ekblom and Goldbarg 1971; Pandolf, Burse, and Goldman 1975) perceived exertion (PE) has become an interesting alternative to quantify TL in young, amateur and professional soccer teams due to its simplicity, low cost (Borg 1973; Borg 1998), validity (Arcos et al. 2014; Impellizzeri et al. 2004; Scott et al. 2013; Casamichana et al. 2013) and versatility.

Professional Football

Two of the four studies that assessed TL in professional soccer players quantified weekly differentiated sRPE-TL (respiratory sRPE-TL [sRPEres-TL] and muscular sRPE-TL [sRPEmus-TL] (Los Arcos, Mendez-Villanueva, and Martínez-Santos 2017; Azcárate et al., 2018) and used the same scale (Foster's 0-10 scale (Foster et al. 2001)) and protocol (Table

3a). In order to calculate respiratory and muscular sRPE-TLs (Arcos et al. 2014; Los Arcos et al. 2015) (sRPE * volume (Foster et al. 2001)), training session volume included warm-up and recovery periods but excluded cool-down and stretching exercises and match duration was recorded excluding the warm-up and the half-time rest period (Azcárate, Yanci, and Los Arcos 2018; Los Arcos, Mendez-Villanueva, and Martínez-Santos 2017). Both studies quantified weekly training and match load during competitive period in Spanish soccer. While.Los Arcos, Mendez-Villanueva, and Martínez-Santos (2017) considered the week from the first training session of the week until the official match on weekend, Azcárate et al. (2018) from the official match until the last training session of the next week. Ten, Saturday-Sunday weeks were analysed in a reserve team (Los Arcos, Mendez-Villanueva, and Martínez-Santos 2017) and several Saturday-Sunday, Saturday-Saturday, Sunday-Sunday, and Sunday-Saturday weeks ($\geq$3 weeks of each type) in a Spanish 2nd division team (Azcárate et al., 2018). Interestingly, Azcárate et al. (2018) did not find significant differences ($p>0.05$) between Saturday-Sunday (i.e., 8 days), Saturday-Saturday (i.e., 7 days), Sunday-Sunday (i.e., 7 days), and Sunday-Saturday (i.e., 6 days) weeks on one-match weekly TL. This suggests that the length of the between-match microcycle have no effect on players' accumulated weekly TL (Azcárate, Yanci, and Los Arcos 2018). That is, a similar weekly TL is apparently distributed on the available training sessions. The lack of differences between the week types allows the comparison between Spanish 2nd division and elite reserve teams.

Despite that Spanish 2nd division players completed one session more than reserve team players (6 vs 5 training sessions), one-match weekly differentiated sRPE-TL was considerably lower for Spanish 2nd division *starters* soccer players in comparison to reserve team players (sRPEres-TL, ~ 1155 vs 1600 ± 293 AUs, Cohen's $d = 1.50 - 1.93$; sRPEmus-TL, ~ 1260 vs 1639 ± 320 AUs, Cohen's $d = 1.34 - 1.52$) (Table 3a). Similarly, high-level *non-starters* players accumulated considerably lower sRPEres-TL (~ 980 vs ± 1127 ± 227 AUs, Cohen's $d = 0.58 - 0.90$) than elite reserve team players, although the magnitude of the difference was lower for sRPEmus-TL (~1040 vs 1089 ± 259 AUs, Cohen's $d = 0.09 - 0.51$) (Table 3b). In comparison to English Premier league *starters* players (Thorpe et al. 2016) (5 training sessions, one-match weekly overall sRPE-TL [sRPEo-TL], ~ 1580 AUs), elite reserve team players accumulated a similar differentiated sRPE-TL (~ 1620 AUs) (Los Arcos, Mendez-Villanueva, and Martínez-Santos 2017) but substantially less (~ 25%) than Spanish 2nd division players (~ 1200 AUs) (Azcárate et al., 2018) (Table 3a). Even though more studies are required, the observed differences between teams suggest that one-match weekly sRPE-TL does not depend on the competition level of the players and number of training sessions carried out by their team during the week. The structural traits (Parlebas 2002) and strategical instructions (Ngo et al. 2012) of the applied tasks and their organization during the week, and the teaching organization (Cushion, Ford, and Williams 2012; Partington and Cushion 2013) and style (Rampinini et al. 2007) could explain these differences. Thus, in addition to the number of weekly training sessions and applied training strategies, intervention studies should provide players' accumulated TL because this can affect, at least partially, on the physical fitness performance of professional soccer players (Arcos et al., 2014; Fitzpatrick, Hicks, and Hayes, 2018; Jaspers et al., 2017; Los Arcos, Mendez-Villanueva, and Martínez-Santos, 2017). Since only one study quantified one-match weekly external load in professional soccer players (Anderson et al., 2016) (Table 5), the impact of number of training sessions on the weekly running demand cannot be assessed.

Youth Football

Similar to professional soccer players, the two studies that assessed weekly TL in young *starters* soccer players used perceived TL (sRPE-TL or Visual Analogue Scale [VAS-TL]). Although they used different scales, all of them considered overall exertion (Foster et al. 2001; 1996), ranging from 0 to 10 points (or it was a 100-mm horizontal line (Rebelo et al., 2012)) and TL was calculated multiplying PE by training or match volume (min) (Foster et al. 2001) (Table 4). Only Rebelo et al. (2012) used heart rate based methods to determine TL (HR-based TL) in Portuguese youth soccer players. Specifically, they used Edwards' training load method

(Edwards 1993), and the TRIMP method (Banister 1991). Wrigley et al. (2012) considered warm-up and cool down to define training volume in English teams and Rebelo et al. (2012) considered warm-up to define training and match training volume in Portuguese teams. TL was quantified only in *starters* players from a English elite soccer academy (U14, U16 and U18 teams (Wrigley et al. 2012)) and in 3 youth teams (16 ± 0 years) competing in the first division of the Portuguese soccer league (Rebelo et al. 2012). All studies considered the week from the first training session of the week until the official match on weekend (Wrigley et al. 2012; Rebelo et al. 2012).

One-match weekly perceived TL varied considerably (until ~ 35%) between young soccer teams (Table 4), ranging from 2524 ± 128 to 3984 ± 222 AUs (Wrigley et al. 2012; Rebelo et al. 2012) (Table 4). It seems that oldest players accumulated greater perceived TL than youngest players (U18 vs U17, Cohen d = 4.4 - 7.0; U17 vs U16, Cohen d = 1.8/- 1.2; U16 vs U14, Cohen d = 3.0). Those differences were not due to the number of training sessions carried out during the week. While U17 Portuguese youth soccer players trained three times a week, U16 and U14 English elite soccer players trained 5 times per week, being TL assesses with VAS1-TL considerably greater for Portuguese soccer players (Table 4). Moreover, the number of weekly training sessions was equal for U16 and U14 players but substantial differences were found between both groups (Cohen d = 3.0). Since the three teams were from different European countries, cultural factors could affect the training strategies and in consequence total weekly TL. For example, young English U18, U16 and U14 soccer players carried out two extra gym sessions targeting strength factors. Unfortunately, we cannot compare the HR-based one-match weekly TL to other studies, but, at least we might have a benchmark for young soccer players: TRIMP TL, 80 AUs and Edward's TL, 627 ± 19 AUs (Rebelo et al. 2012).

Impact of Official Match-Play on Weekly TL

Even though several studies have assessed match internal and external TLs in professional (Bradley et al. 2016; Bush et al. 2015; Bush et al. 2015; Carling et al. 2016; Di Salvo et al. 2013; Fessi and Moalla 2018; Los Arcos et al. 2016) and young (Mendez-Villanueva et al. 2013; Buchheit, Simpson, and Mendez-Villanueva 2013; Buchheit et al. 2010; Harley et al. 2010; Goto, Morris, and Nevill 2015; Rebelo et al. 2014; Saward et al. 2016; Vigh-Larsen, Dalgas, and Andersen 2018) soccer players, the lack of information about the accumulated TL during the training sessions prevents assessing the impact of the official match-play on weekly TL. Moreover, some studies quantified both training and match TLs, but detailed information about the practice time of the players was not provided.

Professional Football

Match participation is likely to be the main factor in determining players' weekly TL (Azcárate et al., 2018; Los Arcos, Mendez-Villanueva, and Martínez-Santos 2017). After analysing 10 Saturday-Sunday (i.e., 8 days) weeks and using the typical differentiation between players (i.e., *starters* vs *non-starters* (Anderson et al. 2016; Morgans, Di Michele, and Drust 2018; Los Arcos et al. 2016; Kraemer et al. 2004)),Los Arcos, Mendez-Villanueva, and Martínez-Santos 2017) reported that reserve team *starters* accumulated a substantial greater one-match weekly TL than *non-starters* (sRPEres-TL, 1600 ± 293 vs 1117 ± 227 AUs, Cohen's $d = 1.84$; sRPEmus-TL, 1639 ± 320 vs 1089 ± 259 AUs, Cohen's $d = 1.89$) (Table 3a). Similarly, during the same type of week (i.e., Saturday-Sunday) and Saturday-Saturday, Sunday-Sunday, and Sunday-Saturday weeks, Spanish 2nd division *starters* players accumulated significant higher weekly differentiated sRPE-TL in comparison to *non-starters* players (sRPEres-TL, ~1150 vs ~980 AUs, Cohen's $d = 0.78\text{-}1.18$); sRPEmus-TL, ~1260 vs ~1040 AUs, Cohen's $d = 0.70\text{-}1.41$) (Azcárate et al., 2018). In addition, Azcárate et al. (2018) accounted for a third group: the players that not participated on the match at all. They found that those players accumulated substantial lower weekly TL (sRPEres-TL, ~836; sRPEmus-TL, ~ 834) than *starters* (vs sRPEres-TL, ~ 1155 AUs, Cohen's *d = 1.23 -1.82; vs sRPEms-TL, ~ 1260* AUs, Cohen's *d = 1.66 - 2.36)* and *non-starters* (vs sRPEres-TL, ~ 980 AUs, Cohen's *d = 0.72 - 0.83; vs sRPEms-TL, ≈ 1040* AUs, Cohen's *d = 0.81 - 1.21)* (Table 3b). That is, players who did not participated in the match at all accumulated around 30% and 17% lower weekly TL than *starters* and *non-starters*, respectively. Thus, it is suggested that professional soccer coaches should design weekly training strategies contemplating, at least, three groups of players (i.e., *starters*, *non-starters* and *non-participants*). In this regard, since weekly TL variation magnitude (e.g., acute: chronic load ratio (Hulin et al. 2014)) might have an impact on injury incidence in professional soccer players (Jaspers et al. 2018) and weekly TL varies considerably between *starters*, *non-starters* and *non-participants*, soccer coaches should give special attention to these last two groups of players.

Even though training week organization was very different between the four professional soccer teams (Tables 6a and 6b), all studies show that official match impose the greatest session TL of the week for the *starters* (Thorpe et al. 2016; Anderson et al. 2016; Los Arcos, Mendez-Villanueva, and Martínez-Santos 2017). The distances covered at different speed thresholds (0–0.6 $km \cdot h^{-1}$, 0.7–7.1 $km \cdot h^{-1}$, 7.2–14.4 $km \cdot h^{-1}$, 14.5–19.7 $km \cdot h^{-1}$, 19.8–25.2 $km \cdot h^{-1}$, and > 25.2 $km \cdot h^{-1}$) were significantly ($p < 0.05$) greater during the match in comparison to any of the 4 training sessions for English Premier players (Anderson et al. 2016). Also in top level English soccer players, sRPEo-TL was significantly higher ($p < 0.05$) during the match than during any of the 5 training sessions of the week (Thorpe et al. 2016). In addition, match differentiated sRPE-TL (i.e., sRPEres- and sRPEmus-TL) was substantially greater than the most demanding training session of the week (i.e., Wednesday, three days before match) for Spanish elite reserve team players (Los Arcos, Mendez-Villanueva, and Martínez-Santos 2017). TL arising from the match equated to 40% of the total distance covered during all the training sessions (excluding the match) of the week and 100%, 30%, 41%, 64%, 90% and the 97% of the distance covered at 0–0.6 $km \cdot h^{-1}$, 0.7–7.1 $km \cdot h^{-1}$, 7.2–14.4 $km \cdot h^{-1}$, 14.5–19.7 $km \cdot h^{-}$

^{1}, 19.8–25.2 km·h^{-1}, and > 25.2 km·h-^{1}, respectively, during the one-match week (Anderson et al. 2016). Of special interest is the fact that the official match was almost the exclusive source of weekly high-speed (90%) and sprinting (97%) TL. Considering the impact that high-speed running distances can have on the risk of hamstring injury (Malone et al. 2018), which is the most common injury subtype in soccer, carefully monitoring of high-speed running session during official matches is warranted. Moreover, the match represented 38% of the total weekly overall (Thorpe et al. 2016) and 32-36% of the total weekly differentiated sRPE-TL (Los Arcos, Mendez-Villanueva, and Martínez-Santos 2017). Thus, the official match is the most demanding session of the week representing, at least, one third of the weekly TL for *starters* professional soccer. However, this was not the case for *non-starters* players. The only study that assessed one-match weekly TL for *non-starters* found that the match was not, unsurprisingly, the highest session TL of the week (Los Arcos, Mendez-Villanueva, and Martínez-Santos 2017). Match differentiated sRPE-TL was substantially lower (Cohen's $d > -2.2$) in comparison to the most demanding training session of the week (i.e., Wednesday, three days before match) for *non-starters*. The match only represented 7-8% of the total weekly differentiated sRPE-TL (Los Arcos, Mendez-Villanueva, and Martínez-Santos 2017).

Youth Football

Similar to professional soccer players (Los Arcos, Mendez-Villanueva, and Martínez-Santos 2017; Thorpe et al. 2016; Anderson et al. 2016), the game was the more demanding session of the week for Portuguese regional level youth soccer players (Rebelo et al. 2012). With exception of the 2nd training session *vs* match for TRIMP TL, match perceived (i.e., VAS-TL) and HR-based (i.e., Edwards' TL and TRIMP methods) TLs were significantly ($p < 0.05$) greater than the training sessions (Rebelo et al. 2012). Specifically, the match represented 42% and 28-35% of the total weekly perceived and HR-based TL of the *starters* players, respectively. However, U18, U16 and U14 English elite player had a lower match sRPEo-TL compared to training (combined field and gym) and field-based training ($p < 0.05$) with the U18 group having the largest difference in both cases (Wrigley et al. 2012). The match accounted for 20-23% of the total sRPEo-TL of the week. Thus, the impact of match-play on weekly TL varied considerably between young soccer teams.

Training Load Distribution along the Week

Several studies have assessed weekly TL distribution along the competitive week in soccer teams (Coutinho et al. 2015; Fessi et al. 2016; Brito, Hertzog, and Nassis 2016; Akenhead, Harley, and Tweddle 2016; Jeong et al. 2011; Malone et al. 2015; Impellizzeri et al. 2004; Arcos et al. 2014; Scott et al. 2014; Owen et al. 2017). However, few assessed TL of all training sessions and official match and, in addition, provided detailed information about the practice time of the players during each week (Los Arcos, Mendez-Villanueva, and Martínez-Santos 2017; Anderson et al. 2016; Rebelo et al. 2012; Wrigley et al. 2012; Thorpe et al. 2016). Four of these were carried out in professional soccer players and other two in young soccer teams. Only a study assessed weekly TL distribution for *non-starters* soccer players (Los Arcos, Mendez-Villanueva, and Martínez-Santos 2017) (Table 6a). The most used TL quantification method was perceived TL. Only Anderson et al. (2016) quantified external TL to assess training and match load (Table 6b).

Professional Football

Anderson et al. (2016), Los Arcos, Mendez-Villanueva, and Martínez-Santos (2017) and Thorpe et al. (2016) found that coaches periodized training contents to attain the highest weekly TL in the middle of the week. TL increased until 4 days following the previous match (i.e., 3 days before the next match) and later decreases up to the day before the competition ((Los Arcos, Mendez-Villanueva, and Martínez-Santos 2017 2017; Thorpe et al., 2016). In addition, Los Arcos, Mendez-Villanueva, and Martínez-Santos (2017) described substantial TL differences (effect sizes ranging from small to very large) between consecutive training sessions and matches (sRPEres-TL, Mo < Tu < We > Th > Fr < Match; sRPEmus-TL, Mo < Tu < We > Th > Fr < Match) in elite reserve team players. Similarly, except between Monday and Tuesday training days, Thorpe et al. (2016) also found significant TL differences between consecutive training sessions and match (Mo-Tu < Th > Fr > Sa < Match) (Tables 6a). Despite that no TL differences were described between consecutive training sessions in the majority of the speed bands in Premier League players (Anderson et al., 2016), maybe due to the week type was somewhat special (four consecutive training sessions before official match) (Tables 6b), it is suggested an *increasing-decreasing* TL trend during the training week until the most demanding session of the week, the official match, in professional soccer players. In this way, a sufficient after-game recovery is expected (Ascensão et al. 2008; Ispirlidis et al. 2008; Rampinini et al. 2011; Doeven et al. 2018; Silva et al. 2013) and pre-match fatigue can be managed.

However, TL accumulation until the most demanding training session of the week, typically occurring in the middle of the week, varied between teams. While elite reserve team players (Los Arcos, Mendez-Villanueva, and Martínez-Santos., 2017) accumulated 30-32% and the 18-19% of the total weekly differentiated sRPE-TL before and after the most demanding training session of the week, respectively, Premier League players (Thorpe et al. 2016) accumulated 26% and 17% before and after the central session of the week, respectively (Tables 6a). In addition, Anderson et al. (2016) found that the external TL accumulated after the most demanding training session of the week was similar or higher than the accumulated TL before (standing, 0–0.6 $km \cdot h^{-1}$: 0% vs 0%; walking, 0.7–7.1 $km \cdot h^{-1}$: 19% vs 31%; jogging, 7.2–14.4 $km \cdot h^{-1}$: 18% vs 18%; running, 14.4–19.7 $km \cdot h^{-1}$:7% vs 9%; high speed running (HSR), 19.8–25.2 $km \cdot h^{-1}$: 2% vs 5%; sprinting, 25.2 $km \cdot h^{-1}$: 0% vs 1%) (Table 6b). The substantial weekly TL distribution differences between studies can be due to the training week organization, with special relevance to the location of the first training day of the week following the match. Elite reserve team players had an off day straight after the match day and, in addition, they had another day off straight after the first training session of the week two days after the match (Los Arcos,

Mendez-Villanueva, and Martínez-Santos, 2017). Premier League players had either two consecutives training sessions (Thorpe et al. 2016) or two rest days (Anderson et al., 2016) immediately after the match.

Each training session represented a relative load ranging from 3 to 20% of the total weekly sRPE-TL (Los Arcos, Mendez-Villanueva, and Martínez-Santos, 2017; Thorpe et al., 2016) and 0% to 22% of the total weekly external load depending of the speed band evaluated (Thorpe et al. 2016) (Tables 6a and 6b). Thus, the most demanding training session represented, at most, two-thirds of the match load, suggesting that professional soccer coaches prevent a similar effort to the match during one-match weeks. While the reduction of the sRPE-TL during the day before the competition was usual, the accumulated TL of the first session of the week represented a greater TL in elite reserve players (15-16% of the total weekly TL) (Los Arcos, Mendez-Villanueva, and Martínez-Santos, 2017) in comparison to English Premier League players (3% of the total weekly TL) (Thorpe et al. 2016) (Tables 6a and 6b). This was likely due to the fact that elite reserve players had a rest day after match while English Premier League players trained on the next day following the match. Thus, studies should provide previous and next match days in order to assess weekly TL in soccer.

Youth Football

TL distribution during the week did not show a clear trend in young soccer players. Similar to professional soccer teams, Rebelo et al. (2012) found that perceived TL increased until 3 days before the next match and decreased the day before the competition. In addition, they also found significant TL differences between consecutive training sessions (VAS1-TL, Tu < Th > Fr < Ma; VAS2, Tu < Th > Fr < Ma; TRIMP, Tu < Th > Fr < Ma; Edward's TL, Tu < Th > Fr < Ma) (Table 6a). However, maybe due to the organization of double training sessions (i.e., implementation of gym sessions), the previously identified in adult players TL increasing-decreasing trend was not found in U18, U16 and U14 English elite players and training days represented between 16 to 37% of the weekly TL (Wrigley et al. 2012) (Table 6a). Sometimes training day's TL (i.e., two training sessions a day) was greater than the official match TL. In addition, the reduction of the perceived TL during the day before the competition was not clear and the accumulated TL of the first session of the week was considerably greater than the reported in other young (Rebelo et al., 2012) and professional (Anderson et al., 2016; Los Arcos, Mendez-Villanueva, and Martínez-Santos, 2017; Thorpe et al., 2016) soccer players.

Each training session typically represented a higher percentage of the weekly TL in young soccer players than in professional soccer teams (12-28% *vs* 3-20%), suggesting that the preparation of the next game was less important than the training sessions for young soccer coaches. In addition, with the exception of TRIMP (session TL represented 78-98% of the match TL), each training session represented from 27% to 71% of the match TL for regional level Portuguese youth soccer players. However, due to the double training sessions schedule, these values ranged from 96 to 152%, 84 to 152% and 43 to 150% in U18, U16 and U14 English elite soccer players, respectively. In comparison to professional soccer players (Los Arcos, Mendez-Villanueva, & Martínez-Santos 2017; Thorpe et al. 2016; Anderson et al. 2016) (training session represented, at most, two-thirds of the match load), young soccer players are exposed to a higher TL during the training sessions, sometimes exceeding match TL. Due to the different training week organization, more studies are required in order to assess one-match weekly TL distribution in young soccer teams.

Weekly Training Load Variability

Interestingly, young soccer players (Rebelo et al., 2012; Wrigley et al., 2012) accumulated greater weekly TL than professional soccer players (Azcárate et al., 2018; Los Arcos, Mendez-Villanueva, and Martínez-Santos, 2017; Thorpe et al., 2016). This might be, at least partially, related to the fact that the importance of the official match is less for the development, under-age teams and soccer coaches prioritize the optimization of training contents even though this could potentially compromise readiness to play. In addition to compare accumulated weekly

TL, the analysis of inter-players TL variability seems interesting in order to assess the ability to accurately prescribe TL prescription in professional and young soccer players.

Professional Soccer

Previous studies found relatively large match-to-match perceived TL (Fessi and Moalla, 2018; Los Arcos et al., 2016) and external load (i.e., high-intensity running demand) (Bush et al. 2015; Carling et al. 2016; Gregson et al. 2010) inter-players variability (coefficient of variation [CV] = 10.2% - 32.3%) in professional *starters* soccer players. After considering only the players that participated in full in the entire week (training plus match), an elevated match inter-players sRPEres-TL, sRPEmus-TL and high intensity running demand variability, ranging from the 31% to the 41% (Anderson et al., 2016; Los Arcos, Mendez-Villanueva, and Martínez-Santos, 2017) (Tables 6a and 6b). In addition, the differentiated training sessions sRPE-TL (CV = 30-61%) and external TL (CV = 30%-100%, depending of the speed band considered) variability was considerably greater than the match TL variability (Tables 6a and 6b). That is, training sessions demand less than matches but produce more differences between players, which complicates the prescription of the TL. Regarding the *non*-starters, this review and a previous study (Los Arcos et al., 2016) found that differentiated sRPE-TL match variability ranged from the 23% to the 71% depending on the playing time, being lower the longer the players participated in the match (Los Arcos et al., 2016). These match perceived TL CV values were considerably greater than the reports for *starters* players, although TL variability was similar for both groups of players (CV = 28%-74% vs 30-61%). Since match load can only be managed by player substitutions, soccer coaches should adjust TL of the players with insufficient or excessive match time during the training. Among other strategies, soccer coaches could implement extra individual training contents for the players with insufficient TL and reduce training volume or use different roles (p.e., floaters (Lacome et al. 2017)) during the soccer tasks for the players with excessive TL.

Even though only players that completed all weekly training sessions were considered and players were classified according to the match playing time, one-match weekly differentiated sRPE-TL TL variability was relatively high (CV > 10% (Atkinson and Nevill 1998)) in all groups. This ranged from the 16% to the 21% for *starters*, from the 12% to the 24% for *non-starters* and from the 19% to the 28% for the players that did not participate in the match (Tables 3a). Regarding external TL, the variability ranged from 2% to 23% depending on the speed band examined. Since this classification did not consider the players that could not participate or completed some training session due to mild illnesses and injuries, the actual between-players weekly TL variability during competitive period in professional soccer players is expected to be higher than what is reported in this systematic review. This reinforces the importance of the quantification of the individual's TL (Alexiou and Coutts 2008) in soccer. Practically, from the individual TL values, a team weekly TL benchmark (and its variability) can be obtained, which would allow the identification of players with insufficient or excessive TL allowing potential adjustments of training strategies at individual level.

Youth Soccer

In comparison to professional soccer players (CV = 2-28%), weekly TL variability was considerably lower in young *starters* soccer players (CV < 6%) (Table 4). This was was due to both match (CV = 0-18%) and training sessions (CV = 2-27%) TL variability was substantially lower for young soccer players than for professional soccer players (match, CV = 31-41%, training sessions, CV = 30-100%). Thus, young soccer players accumulated a greater weekly TL than professional soccer players, but their response during the matches and training sessions was more homogenous and in consequence between-players accumulated one-match weekly TL was more similar.

Conclusion

Professional soccer players accumulate lower (around 1200-1600 AUs) one-match perceived weekly TL than young soccer players (around 2500-4000 AUs) during in-season period. Moreover, inter-players training, match and weekly TL variability are greater for professional soccer players in comparison to young soccer players.

Match participation is the main contributor of the one-match weekly TL (> 32-36% of the total internal and external weekly TL) and almost the exclusive source of weekly high-speed and sprinting running in professional soccer players. However, the impact of the match on the one-match weekly TL is less clear in young soccer teams.

It seems that number of training sessions carried out by the teams during the week do not influence the global weekly TL in both professional and young soccer players. TL progressively increase up to 4 days after the previous match (i.e., 3 days before the next match) to get reduced up to the day before the competition in professional soccer players, but a clear trend for weekly TL distribution along the week in young soccer players is not apparent.

References

Akenhead, Richard, Jamie A. Harley & Simon P. Tweddle. (2016). "Examining the External Training Load of an English Premier League Football Team With Special Reference to Acceleration." *Journal of Strength and Conditioning Research*, *30*, 2424-32. https://doi.org/10.1519/JSC.0000000000001343.

Akubat, Ibrahim, Ebrahim Patel, Steve Barrett & Grant Abt. (2012). "Methods of Monitoring the Training and Match Load and Their Relationship to Changes in Fitness in Professional Youth Soccer Players". *Journal of Sports Sciences*, *30*, 1473-80. https://doi.org/10.1080/02640414.2012.712711.

Alexiou, Helen & Aaron J. Coutts. (2008). "A Comparison of Methods Used for Quantifying Internal Training Load in Women Soccer Players". *International Journal of Sports Physiology and Performance*, *3*, 320-30.

Anderson, Liam, Patrick Orme, Rocco Di Michele, Graeme L. Close, Ryland Morgans, Barry Drust & James P. Morton. (2016). "Quantification of seasonal long physical load in soccer players with different starting status from the English Premier League: Implications for maintaining squad physical fitness". *International Journal of Sports Physiology and Performance*, *11*, 1038-46. https://doi.org/10.1123/ijspp.2015-0012.

Anderson, Liam, Patrick Orme, Rocco Di Michele, Graeme L. Close, Ryland Morgans, Barry Drust & James P. Morton. (2016). "Quantification of Training Load during One-, Two- and Three-Game Week Schedules in Professional Soccer Players from the English Premier League: Implications for Carbohydrate Periodisation". *Journal of Sports Sciences*, *34*, 1250-59. https://doi.org/10.1080/ 02640414.2015.1106574.

Arcos Asier, Javier Yanci, Jurdan Mendiguchia & Esteban M. Gorostiaga. (2014). "Rating of Muscular and Respiratory Perceived Exertion in Professional Soccer Players". *Journal of Strength and Conditioning Research*, *28*, 3280-88. https://doi.org/10.1519/ JSC.0000000000000540.

Ascensão, António, António Rebelo, Eduardo Oliveira, Franklim Marques, Laura Pereira & José Magalhães. (2008). "Biochemical Impact of a Soccer Match - Analysis of Oxidative Stress and Muscle Damage Markers throughout Recovery". *Clinical Biochemistry*, *41*, 841-51. https://doi.org/10.1016/j.clinbiochem.2008.04.008.

Atkinson, Greg & Alan Michael Nevill. (1998). "Statistical Methods for Assessing Measurement Error (Reliability) in Variables Relevant to Sports Medicine". *Sports Medicine*, *26*, 217-38.

Azcárate, Unai, Javier Yanci & Asier Los Arcos. (2018). "Influence of match playing time and the length of the between-match microcycle in

Spanish professional soccer players' perceived training load". *Science and Medicine in Football*, *2*, 23-28.

Banister, Erik. (1991). "Modeling elite athletic performance". In *Physiological testing of the high-performance athlete*, 403-24. Illinois: Human Kinetics Books.

Borg, Gunnar. (1973). "Perceived Exertion: A Note on "History" and Methods". *Medicine and Science in Sports*, *5*, 90-93.

Borg Gunnar. (1998). *Borg's perceived exertion and pain scales*. USA: Human Kinetics.

Bowen, Laura, Aleksander Stefan Gross, Mo Gimpel & François-Xavier Li. (2017). "Accumulated Workloads and the Acute:Chronic Workload Ratio Relate to Injury Risk in Elite Youth Football Players". *British Journal of Sports Medicine*, *51*, 452-59. https://doi.org/10.1136/bjsports-2015-095820.

Bradley, Paul S., David T. Archer, Bob Hogg, Gabor Schuth, Michael Bush, Chris Carling & Chris Barnes. (2016). "Tier-Specific Evolution of Match Performance Characteristics in the English Premier League: It's Getting Tougher at the Top". *Journal of Sports Sciences*, *34*, 980-87. https://doi.org/10.1080/02640414.2015.1082614.

Brink, Michel S., Chris Visscher, Suzanne Arends, Johannes Zwerver, Wendy J. Post & Koen Apm Lemmink. (2010). "Monitoring Stress and Recovery: New Insights for the Prevention of Injuries and Illnesses in Elite Youth Soccer Players". *British Journal of Sports Medicine*, *44*, 809-15. https://doi.org/10.1136/bjsm.2009.069476.

Brito, Joao, Maxime Hertzog & George P. Nassis. (2016). "Do Match-Related Contextual Variables Influence Training Load in Highly Trained Soccer Players?" *Journal of Strength and Conditioning Research*, *30*, 393-99. https://doi.org/10.1519/ JSC.0000000000001113.

Buchheit, Martin., Alberto Mendez-Villanueva, Ben M. Simpson & Pitre C. Bourdon. (2010). "Match Running Performance and Fitness in Youth Soccer". *International Journal of Sports Medicine*, *31*, 818-25. https://doi.org/10.1055/s-0030-1262838.

Buchheit, Martin., Ben M. Simpson & Alberto Mendez-Villanueva. (2013). "Repeated High-Speed Activities during Youth Soccer Games in Relation to Changes in Maximal Sprinting and Aerobic Speeds". *International Journal of Sports Medicine*, *34* (1), 40-48. https://doi.org/10.1055/s-0032-1316363.

Bush, Michael, Chris Barnes, David T. Archer, Bob Hogg & Paul S. Bradley. (2015). "Evolution of Match Performance Parameters for Various Playing Positions in the English Premier League". *Human Movement Science*, *39*, 1-11. https://doi.org/10.1016/ j.humov. 2014.10.003.

Bush, Michael D., David T. Archer, Robert Hogg & Paul S. Bradley. (2015). "Factors influencing physical and technical variability in the english premier league". *International Journal of Sports Physiology and Performance*, *10*, 865-72. https://doi.org/10.1123/ijspp.2014-0484.

Carling, Christopher, Paul Bradley, Alan McCall & Gregory Dupont. (2016). "Match-to-Match Variability in High-Speed Running Activity in a Professional Soccer Team". *Journal of Sports Sciences*, *34*, 2215-23. https://doi.org/10.1080/02640414.2016.1176228.

Casamichana, David, Julen Castellano, Julio Calleja-Gonzalez, Jaime San Román & Carlo Castagna. (2013). "Relationship between Indicators of Training Load in Soccer Players". *Journal of Strength and Conditioning Research*, *27*, 369-74. https://doi.org/10.1519/ JSC. 0b013e3182548af1.

Castellano, Julen, David Alvarez-Pastor & Paul S. Bradley. (2014). "Evaluation of Research Using Computerised Tracking Systems (Amisco and Prozone) to Analyse Physical Performance in Elite Soccer: A Systematic Review". *Sports Medicine*, *44*, 701-12. https://doi.org/10.1007/s40279-014-0144-3.

Cohen, Jacob. (1988). *Statistical power analysis for the behavioral sciences*. Second Edition. L. Erlbaum Associates.

Coutinho, Diogo, Bruno Gonçalves, Bruno Figueira, Eduardo Abade, Rui Marcelino & Jaime Sampaio. (2015). "Typical Weekly Workload of under 15, under 17, and under 19 Elite Portuguese Football Players".

Journal of Sports Sciences, *33*, 1229-37. https://doi.org/10.1080/02640414.2015.1022575.

Cushion, Chris, Paul R. Ford. & Andrew Mark Williams. (2012). "Coach Behaviours and Practice Structures in Youth Soccer: Implications for Talent Development". *Journal of Sports Sciences*, *30*, 1631-41. https://doi.org/10.1080/02640414.2012.721930.

Di Salvo, Valter, Pigozzi, Carlos González-Haro, Moore Stephens Laughlin & John K. De Witt. (2013). "Match Performance Comparison in Top English Soccer Leagues". *International Journal of Sports Medicine*, *34*, 526-32. https://doi.org/10.1055/s-0032-1327660.

Doeven, Steven H., Michel S. Brink, Silke J. Kosse & Koen A. P. M. Lemmink. (2018). "Postmatch Recovery of Physical Performance and Biochemical Markers in Team Ball Sports: A Systematic Review". *BMJ Open Sport & Exercise Medicine*, *4*, e000264. https://doi.org/10.1136/bmjsem-2017-000264.

Edwards, Sebastian. (1993). "High performance training and racing". En *The Heart Rate Monitor Book*, 113 – 123. Sacramento: Feet Fleet Press.

Ehrmann, Fabian E., Craig S. Duncan, Doungkamol Sindhusake, William N. Franzsen & David A. Greene. (2016). "GPS and Injury Prevention in Professional Soccer". *Journal of Strength and Conditioning Research*, *30*, 360-7. https://doi.org/10.1519/JSC.0000000000001093.

Ekblom, Björn & Alberto N Goldbarg. (1971). "The Influence of Physical Training and Other Factors on the Subjective Rating of Perceived Exertion". *Acta Physiologica Scandinavica*, *83*, 399-406. https://doi.org/10.1111/j.1748-1716.1971.tb05093.x.

Fessi, Mohamed Saifeddin. & Wassim Moalla. (2018). "Postmatch Perceived Exertion, Feeling, and Wellness in Professional Soccer Players". *International Journal of Sports Physiology and Performance*, mayo, 1-7. https://doi.org/10.1123/ijspp.2017-0725.

Fessi, Mohamed Saifeddin, Sabeur Nouira, Alexandre Dellal, Adam Owen, Mohamed Elloumi & Wassim Moalla. (2016). "Changes of the Psychophysical State and Feeling of Wellness of Professional Soccer Players during Pre-Season and in-Season Periods". *Research in Sports*

Medicine, *24*, 375-86. https://doi.org/10.1080/ 15438627.2016. 1222278.

Fessi, Mohamed Saifeddin, Nidhal Zarrouk, Valter Di Salvo, Cristoforo Filetti, Alan R. Barker & Wassim Moalla. (2016). "Effects of Tapering on Physical Match Activities in Professional Soccer Players". *Journal of Sports Sciences*, *34*, 2189-94. https://doi.org/10.1080/ 02640414. 2016.1171891.

Fitzpatrick, John F., Kirsty M. Hicks & Philip R. Hayes. (2018). "Dose-Response Relationship between Training Load and Changes in Aerobic Fitness in Professional Youth Soccer Players". *International Journal of Sports Physiology and Performance*, mayo, 1-22. https://doi.org/10.1123/ijspp.2017-0843.

Ford, Paul R., Ian Yates & Andrew Mark Williams. (2010). "An Analysis of Practice Activities and Instructional Behaviours Used by Youth Soccer Coaches during Practice: Exploring the Link between Science and Application". *Journal of Sports Sciences*, *28*, 483-95. https://doi.org/10.1080/02640410903582750.

Foster, Carl, Erin Daines, Lisa Hector, Ann C. Snyder & Ralph S. Welsh. (1996). "Athletic Performance in Relation to Training Load". *Wisconsin Medical Journal*, *95*, 370-74.

Foster, Carl, Jessica A. Florhaug, Jodi Franklin, Lori Gottschall, Lauri A. Hrovatin, Suzanne Parker, Pamela Doleshal & Christopher Dodge. (2001). "A New Approach to Monitoring Exercise Training". *Journal of Strength and Conditioning Research*, *15*, 109-15.

Gil-Rey, Erreka, Alejandro Lezaun & Asier Los Arcos. (2015). "Quantification of the Perceived Training Load and Its Relationship with Changes in Physical Fitness Performance in Junior Soccer Players". *Journal of Sports Sciences*, *33*, 2125-32. https://doi.org/ 10.1080/02640414.2015.1069385.

Goto, Heita, John G. Morris & Mary E. Nevill. (2015). "Motion Analysis of U11 to U16 Elite English Premier League Academy Players". *Journal of Sports Sciences*, *33*, 1248-58. https://doi.org/10.1080/ 02640414.2014.999700.

Gregson, Warren, Barry Drust, Greg Atkinson & Valter Di Salvo. (2010). "Match-to-match variability of high-speed activities in premier league soccer". *International Journal of Sports Medicine*, *31*, 237-42. https://doi.org/10.1055/s-0030-1247546.

Halouani, Jamel, Hamdi Chtourou, Tim Gabbett, Anis Chaouachi & Karim Chamari. (2014). "Small-Sided Games in Team Sports Training: A Brief Review". *Journal of Strength and Conditioning Research*, *28*, 3594-3618. https://doi.org/10.1519/JSC.0000000000000564.

Harley, Jamie A., Christopher A. Barnes, Matthew Portas, Ric Lovell, Stephen Barrett, Darren Paul & Matthew Weston. (2010). "Motion Analysis of Match-Play in Elite U12 to U16 Age-Group Soccer Players". *Journal of Sports Sciences*, *28*, 1391-97. https://doi.org/10.1080/02640414.2010.510142.

Hill-Haas, Stephen V., Brian Dawson, Franco M. Impellizzeri & Aaron J. Coutts. (2011). "Physiology of Small-Sided Games Training in Football: A Systematic Review". *Sports Medicine*, *41*, 199-220. https://doi.org/10.2165/11539740-000000000-00000.

Hulin, Billy T., Tim J. Gabbett, Peter Blanch, Paul Chapman, David Bailey & John W. Orchard. (2014). "Spikes in Acute Workload Are Associated with Increased Injury Risk in Elite Cricket Fast Bowlers". *British Journal of Sports Medicine*, *48*, 708-12. https://doi.org/10.1136/bjsports-2013-092524.

Impellizzeri, Franco M., Ermanno Rampinini, Aaron J. Coutts, Aldo Sassi & Samuele M. Marcora. (2004). "Use of RPE-Based Training Load in Soccer". *Medicine and Science in Sports and Exercise*, *36*, 1042-47.

Ispirlidis, Ioannis, Ioannis G Fatouros, Athanasios Z Jamurtas, Michalis G Nikolaidis, Ioannis Michailidis, Ioannis Douroudos, Konstantinos Margonis., et al. (2008). "Time-Course of Changes in Inflammatory and Performance Responses Following a Soccer Game". *Clinical Journal of Sport Medicine: Official Journal of the Canadian Academy of Sport Medicine*, *18*, 423-31. https://doi.org/10.1097/ JSM.0b013e3181818e0b.

Jaspers, Arne, Michel S. Brink, Steven G. M. Probst, Wouter G. P. Frencken & Werner F. Helsen. (2017). "Relationships Between

Training Load Indicators and Training Outcomes in Professional Soccer". *Sports Medicine*, *47*, 533-44. https://doi.org/10.1007/s40279-016-0591-0.

Jaspers, Arne, Jurian P. Kuyvenhoven, Filip Staes, Wouter G. P. Frencken, Werner F. Helsen & Michel S. Brink. (2018). "Examination of the External and Internal Load Indicators' Association with Overuse Injuries in Professional Soccer Players". *Journal of Science and Medicine in Sport*, *21*, 579-85. https://doi.org/10.1016/ j.jsams.2017. 10.005.

Jeong, Tae-Seok, Tom Reilly, James Morton, Sang-Won Bae & Barry Drust. (2011). "Quantification of the Physiological Loading of One Week of "Pre-Season" and One Week of "in-Season" Training in Professional Soccer Players". *Journal of Sports Sciences*, *29*, 1161-66. https://doi.org/10.1080/02640414.2011.583671.

Kraemer, William J., Duncan N. French, Nigel J. Paxton, Keijo Häkkinen, Jeff S. Volek, Wayne J. Sebastianelli, Margot Putukian., et al. (2004). "Changes in Exercise Performance and Hormonal Concentrations over a Big Ten Soccer Season in Starters and Nonstarters". *Journal of Strength and Conditioning Research*, *18*, 121-28.

Lacome, Mathieu, Ben M. Simpson, Yannick Cholley & Martin Buchheit. (2017). "Locomotor and Heart Rate Responses of Floaters During Small-Sided Games in Elite Soccer Players: Effect of Pitch Size and Inclusion of Goal Keepers". *International Journal of Sports Physiology and Performance*, septiembre, 1-13. https://doi.org/ 10.1123/ijspp.2017-0340.

Los Arcos, Asier, Alberto Mendez-Villanueva & Raúl Martínez-Santos. (2017). "In-season training periodization of professional soccer players". *Biology of Sport*, *34*, 149-55. https://doi.org/10.5114/ biolsport.2017.64588.

Los Arcos, Asier, Alberto Mendez-Villanueva, Javier Yanci & Raúl Martinez-Santos. (2016). "Respiratory and muscular perceived exertion during official games in professional soccer players". *International Journal of Sports Physiology and Performance*, *11*, 301-4.

Los Arcos, Asier, Raúl Martínez-Santos, Javier Yanci, Juan Martín & Carlo Castagna. (2014). "Variability of Objective and Subjective Intensities during Ball Drills in Youth Soccer Players". *Journal of Strength and Conditioning Research*, *28*, 752-57. https://doi.org/10.1519/JSC.0b013e3182a47f0b.

Los Arcos, Asier, Raúl Martínez-Santos, Javier Yanci & Alberto Mendez-Villanueva. (2017). "Monitoring perceived respiratory and muscular exertions and physical fitness in young professional soccer players during a 32-weeks period". *Kinesiology*, *49*, 153-60.

Los Arcos, Asier, Raul Martínez-Santos, Javier Yanci, Jurdan Mendiguchia & Alberto Méndez-Villanueva. (2015). "Negative Associations between Perceived Training Load, Volume and Changes in Physical Fitness in Professional Soccer Players". *Journal of Sports Science & Medicine*, *14*, 394-401.

Malone, James J., Rocco Di Michele, Ryland Morgans, Darren Burgess, James P. Morton & Barry Drust. (2015). "Seasonal Training-Load Quantification in Elite English Premier League Soccer Players". *International Journal of Sports Physiology and Performance*, *10*, 489-97. https://doi.org/10.1123/ijspp.2014-0352.

Malone, Shane, Adam Owen, Bruno Mendes, Brian Hughes, Kieran Collins & Tim J. Gabbett. (2018). "High-Speed Running and Sprinting as an Injury Risk Factor in Soccer: Can Well-Developed Physical Qualities Reduce the Risk?" *Journal of Science and Medicine in Sport*, *21*, 257-62. https://doi.org/10.1016/j.jsams.2017.05.016.

Mendez-Villanueva, Alberto, Martin Buchheit, Ben M. Simpson & Pitre C. Bourdon. (2013). "Match Play Intensity Distribution in Youth Soccer". *International Journal of Sports Medicine*, *34*, 101-10. https://doi.org/10.1055/s-0032-1306323.

Moher, David, Alessandro Liberati, Jennifer Tetzlaff, Douglas G. Altman & PRISMA Group. (2009). "Preferred Reporting Items for Systematic Reviews and Meta-Analyses: The PRISMA Statement". *PLoS Medicine*, *6*, e1000097. https://doi.org/10.1371/journal.pmed.1000097.

Morgans, Ryland, Rocco Di Michele & Barry Drust. (2018). "Soccer Match Play as an Important Component of the Power-Training

Stimulus in Premier League Players". *International Journal of Sports Physiology and Performance*, *1*, 1-3. https://doi.org/10.1123/ ijspp. 2016-0412.

Ngo, Jake K., Man-Chung Tsui, Andrew W. Smith, Christopher Carling, Gar-Sun Chan & Del P. Wong. (2012). "The Effects of Man-Marking on Work Intensity in Small-Sided Soccer Games". *Journal of Sports Science & Medicine*, *11*, 109-14.

O'Connor, Donna, Paul Larkin & Andrew Mark Williams. (2018). "Observations of Youth Football Training: How Do Coaches Structure Training Sessions for Player Development?" *Journal of Sports Sciences*, *36*, 39-47. https://doi.org/10.1080/02640414.2016.1277034.

Owen, Adam L., Jacky J. Forsyth, Del P. Wong, Alexandre Dellal, Sean P. Connelly & Karim Chamari. (2015). "Heart Rate-Based Training Intensity and Its Impact on Injury Incidence among Elite-Level Professional Soccer Players". *Journal of Strength and Conditioning Research*, *29*, 1705-12. https://doi.org/10.1519/ JSC.0000000000000 810.

Owen, Adam L., Carlos Lago-Peñas, Miguel-Ángel Gómez, Bruno Mendes & Alexandre Dellal. (2017). "Analysis of a training mesocycle and positional quantification in elite European soccer players". *International Journal of Sports Science & Coaching*, *12*, 665-76. https://doi.org/10.1177/1747954117727851.

Pandolf, Kent B., Richard L. Burse & Ralph F. Goldman. (1975). "Differentiated Ratings of Perceived Exertion during Physical Conditioning of Older Individuals Using Leg-Weight Loading". *Perceptual and Motor Skills*, *40*, 563-74.

Parlebas, Pierre. (2002). "Elementary mathematic modelization of games and sports." En *The Explanatory Power of Models. Bridging the gap between empirical sciences and theoretical research in the social sciences*, 197-228. Boston, London, Dordrecht: Kluwer Academic Publishers.

Partington, Mark & Christopher Cushion. (2013). "An Investigation of the Practice Activities and Coaching Behaviors of Professional Top-Level Youth Soccer Coaches". *Scandinavian Journal of Medicine & Science in Sports*, *23*, 374-82. https://doi.org/10.1111/j.1600-0838.2011.01383.x.

Rampinini, Ermanno, Andrea Bosio, Ivan Ferraresi, Andrea Petruolo, Andrea Morelli & Aldo Sassi. (2011). "Match-Related Fatigue in Soccer Players". *Medicine and Science in Sports and Exercise*, *43*, 2161-70. https://doi.org/10.1249/MSS.0b013e31821e9c5c.

Rampinini, Ermanno, Franco M. Impellizzeri, Carlo Castagna, Grant Abt, Karim Chamari, Aldo Sassi & Samuele M. Marcora. (2007). "Factors Influencing Physiological Responses to Small-Sided Soccer Games". *Journal of Sports Sciences*, *25*, 659-66. https://doi.org/10.1080/02640410600811858.

Rebelo, Antonio, João Brito, André Seabra, José Oliveira, Drust & Peter Krustrup. (2012). "A New Tool to Measure Training Load in Soccer Training and Match Play". *International Journal of Sports Medicine*, *33*, 297-304. https://doi.org/10.1055/s-0031-1297952.

Rebelo, António, João Brito, André Seabra, José Oliveira & Peter Krustrup. (2014). "Physical Match Performance of Youth Football Players in Relation to Physical Capacity". *European Journal of Sport Science*, *14*, S148-56. https://doi.org/10.1080/17461391.2012.664171.

Sarmento, Hugo, Rui Marcelino, M. Teresa Anguera, Jorge Campaniço, Nuno Matos & José Carlos Leitao. (2014). "Match Analysis in Football: A Systematic Review". *Journal of Sports Sciences*, *32*, 1831-43. https://doi.org/10.1080/02640414.2014.898852.

Saward, Chris, John Morris, Mary E. Nevill, Alan Michael Nevill & Caroline Sunderland. (2016). "Longitudinal Development of Match-Running Performance in Elite Male Youth Soccer Players". *Scandinavian Journal of Medicine & Science in Sports*, *26*, 933-42. https://doi.org/10.1111/sms.12534.

Scott, Brendan R., Robert G. Lockie, Samantha J. G. Davies, Andrew C. Clark, David M. Lynch & Xanne A. K. Janse de Jonge. (2014). "The physical demands of professional soccer players during in-season field-based training and match-play". *The Journal of Australian Strength and Conditioning*, *22* (4), 7-15.

Scott, Brendan R., Robert G. Lockie, Timothy J. Knight, Andrew C. Clark & Xanne A. K. Janse de Jonge. (2013). "A Comparison of Methods to Quantify the In-Season Training Load of Professional Soccer Players". *International Journal of Sports Physiology and Performance*, *8*, 195-202.

Silva, João R., António Ascensão, Franklim Marques, André Seabra, António Rebelo & José Magalhães. (2013). "Neuromuscular Function, Hormonal and Redox Status and Muscle Damage of Professional Soccer Players after a High-Level Competitive Match". *European Journal of Applied Physiology*, *113*, 2193-201. https://doi.org/10.1007/s00421-013-2633-8.

Thorpe, Robin T., Anthony J. Strudwick, Martin Buchheit, Greg Atkinson, Barry Drust & Warren Gregson. (2016). "Tracking Morning Fatigue Status Across In-Season Training Weeks in Elite Soccer Players". *International Journal of Sports Physiology and Performance*, *11*, 947-52. https://doi.org/10.1123/ijspp.2015-0490.

Vigh-Larsen, Jeppe F., Ulrik Dalgas & Thomas B. Andersen. (2018). "Position-Specific Acceleration and Deceleration Profiles in Elite Youth and Senior Soccer Players". *Journal of Strength and Conditioning Research*, *32*, 1114-22. https://doi.org/10.1519/JSC.0000000000001918.

Wrigley, Russell, Barry Drust, Gareth Stratton, Mark Scott & Warren Gregson. (2012). "Quantification of the Typical Weekly In-Season Training Load in Elite Junior Soccer Players". *Journal of Sports Sciences*, *30*, 1573-80. https://doi.org/10.1080/02640414.2012.709265.

In: An Essential Guide to Sports Performance ISBN: 978-1-53617-608-7
Editors: Daniel Castillo Alvira et al. © 2020 Nova Science Publishers, Inc.

Chapter 7

METHODOLOGY OF MUSCLE FORCE DEVELOPMENT IN SPIKE IN ELITE VOLLEYBALL PLAYERS

Milos Milosevic[1], *Morteza Jourkesh*[2] *and Milenko Milosevic*[3,*]
[1]Faculty of Physical Education and Sports Management, Singidunum University, Belgrade, Serbia
[2]Department of Physical Education and Sports Science, Islamic Azad University, Shabestar Branch, Iran
[3]Center for diagnostics and training design CEDIP, Belgrade, Serbia

ABSTRACT

The aim of this study is to discover the mechanisms of muscle force generation in spike and to determine the methodology of its development in the training course of the elite volleyball players. To this purpose, the

* Corresponding Author's Email: mlsvc2010@gmail.com.

biomechanical and functional analyses of muscle force generation in isometric and dynamic muscle working mode were performed. The methodology of its development was proposed based on the analysis results. The study was conducted on a sample of 21 top volleyball players. To generate muscle force in spike in landing, eccentric contraction is used, however, in all other cases one uses a reversible contraction. To achieve good results in spike, one must have developed all dimensions from which the force depends, that is, muscle force generation of all muscle groups involved in the realization of spike, motor units recruitment velocity and a synchronization of their work, the maximum force of certain groups of motor units, muscle force generation change velocity, inter and intramuscular coordination. The maximum values of the specified parameters in the elite volleyball players are achieved in the time interval ranging from 0.005 s to 0.082 s. The maximum muscle force production velocities in the elite volleyball players are ranging from 3440.00 daN.s-1 do 14988.69daN.s-1 at the motor units recruitment velocity ranging from 22.00 IU to 95.0 IU. The force of certain groups of motor units of the knee extensors in elite volleyball players ranges from 1.09 daN to 105.14 daN. During the vertical-landing jumps the elite volleyball players synchronize up to 94.7% of the leg extensors motor units. The greatest impact on the enormous increase in muscle force along with the shortening time of its generation in reversible contractions in service is attributed to the disinhibition process at all levels. In accordance with the results of the analysis a muscle force development methodology is suggested in which, in addition to mastering the disinhibition process, the whole set of required parameters is devised, on which the level and muscle force generation velocity depend, on a daily, weekly, monthly and annual basis, applying the appropriate resources and methods for each particular parameter. Within the proposed methodology, a mathematical model of managing training changes in the domain of force is defined.

Keywords: volleyball, muscle force generation velocity, motor units recruitment and synchronization velocity, intra and intermuscular coordination, disinhibition

INTRODUCTION

Successful performance in volleyball often depends on the ability of the individuals to perform high enough high jumps, a good spike and a good landing. High jump precedes service, block and spike. These spike features require adequate preparedness and high sports performance. Each jump ends up in a good landing. Good landing eliminates the risk of injury [1] and provides a good preparation for the generation of muscle force for the next vertical jump [2-12]. At the elite volleyball players' matches 71% of high jumps is realized during spike, 20% in service and 9% in the block [13]. Since a spike is the most frequently used technique during the game it is quite natural that the spike is analyzed for the production of muscle force and its development by training, which is the focus of this paper. The main problem to be solved in this paper, in relation to the training of muscle force is to discover the adaptation mechanisms which cause changes in neuromuscular apparatus and to determine its technology of development. Therefore, the aim of this study is to discover the mechanisms of force generation in spike and to determine the methodology for its development by training. In addition, the goal is to define a mathematical model for managing training changes in the domain of force.

Biomechanical Analysis of Spike

Spike realization can be divided into 4 stages: initial, preparatory, primary and final stage in which following elements are alternating: initial diagonal position, run-up, takeoff, flight and landing [14-16]. In the initial phase a volleyball player can be in the front or back zone in a high diagonal position [14, 16]. Position height is slightly higher when a player is in the back zone [13-16]. In the initial phase, immediately before the onset of the preparation phase, volleyball players shift the center of mass onto the front part of their feet by moving the shoulder forward [14, 16]. From this position on starts the preparation phase, the spike run-up. Right-handed persons use the usual 4 steps volleyball approach pattern R-L-(RL) or R-L- R-L [13-16]. The main task of the run-up is for the volleyball player to achieve the highest possible horizontal velocity and blend the approach with the takeoff [13-18]. Explanation for the set task can be found in that the level of the horizontal velocity is conditioned by the fact that muscles protagonists of amortization and takeoff do not generate immediately the maximum level of muscle force, but by the exponential function in a time whose form it is:

$$F_m(t) = F_{\max} \times \left(1 - e^{-k \times \Delta t}\right) \tag{1}$$

where: Fm - is a level of 1%, 2%,....,99% of the maximum muscle force expressed in daN; Fmax - maximum force generated by leg extensors expressed in dekanewtons (daN); k - is a constant that characterizes the speed of the motor units recruitment expressed in index units (IU); t - is the time in which the appropriate level is achieved from the maximum muscle force expressed in seconds (s) [8-10,14]. This function shows that the run-up horizontal velocity is conditioned by the maximum velocity of the muscle force generation (in elite volleyball players 7666.42 ± 1105.42 $daN.s^{-1}$ - 14988.69 ± 1795.46 $daN.s^{-1}$ for a period ranging from 0.063 ± 0.007 s up to 0.082 ± 0.020 s) and the motor units recruitment velocity (in elite volleyball players 64.9 ± 7.14 IU - 79.6 ± 6.85 IU) of the leg extensors muscles to absorb (an eccentric phase of the reversible contraction) the run-up horizontal velocity and immediately perform the adequate high jump (concentric phase of the reversible contraction) [4-10, 18-21]. Maximum velocity of the muscle force generation that leg extensors achieve up to 0.100 s directly depends both on the motor units recruitment velocity and on the level of the motor units synchronization (Figure 3), as well as on the level of muscle force produced by certain groups of motor units (Figure 1) and the intramuscle coordination [4-10, 18-21].

That is to say that the bigger the muscle force generation velocity of the leg extensors in elite volleyball players, the quicker they will perform amortization with higher run-up velocity in a shorter time and will attain faster transition into the concentric phase of the muscle force generation, which will in turn increase the height of the vertical spike jump and vice versa. The run-up protagonists are the plantar flexors in the upper ankle joint, then the muscle group of the knee extensors, extensors and flexors of the hip joint (m. triceps surae, m. quadriceps, m. iliopsoas and m. gluteus maximus) functioning in the reverse regime [4, 6, 10, 12, 17]. Run-up velocity is increased in the first three steps and is the largest in the third step [13-15]. In the elite volleyball players horizontal velocity of the take-off in the third step ranges from 3.8 to 4.2 m.s^{-1} [13-15]. Preparation for the blending of the approach phase and take-off begins in step 4, whereupon the extension of the last step and planting on both feet occur, reducing the horizontal velocity from 1.8 up to 2.4 m.s^{-1} and lowering the center of mass at the expense of reducing the angle in the knee joint, which at the moment before the vertical jump varies, depending on the volleyball players constitution from 118° up to 143° [13-16].

The protagonists of reducing the horizontal velocity are the knee and hip extensors (m. quadriceps, m. gluteus maximus) that function in an eccentric mode regime - the first phase of the reversible contraction [4, 6, 10, 17, 21]. At the moment of amortization (first phase of the reversible contraction), knee and hip extensors accompanied by the plantar flexors in the upper ankle joint, move into the second concentric phase of the reversible contraction, generate the force by the maximum velocity that amounts up to 14988.69 ± 1795.46 daN.s^{-1} [4, 7, 10, 19, 21]. Its vertical component conditions volleyball players' body movement into the vertical jump with a starting velocity of 2.5 up to 2.9 m.s^{-1} [4, 10, 1-15]. During the vertical jump spinal column extensors maintain their stability working in the isometric regime whereby achieving a maximum velocity of the motor units recruitment of 27.0 IU at a time of 0.005 s with a force of 23.60 daN and the muscle force generation velocity of 4720.4 daN/s. Extensors of the knee joint as protagonists of the vertical jump are trying to shorten the time of transition from the eccentric into the concentric phase of the reversible contraction [4, 6, 7, 10, 12, 19, 20, 22].

The volleyball player would swing both arms back to the waist and then swing the arms forward and upward and with each run up step will use retroflexors in the shoulder joint in an effort to generate power for the spike [13-15]. In a moment of take-off volleyball player's body pulls up and inclines slightly forward with both hands forward. While the volleyball player's body lifts up vertically after the take off he raises his right hand in a distinctive attacking spike position (elbow angle ranging from 44^0 to 47^0) thus activating first m. deltoideus, then m. supraspinatus and finally m. biceps brachii [13-15, 17]. At the same time shoulders are rotated to the right. This movement includes first m. biceps brachii and then m. wrist extensor. In addition, at the same time trunk rotates to the right (m. obliquus internus abdominus and m. psoas major et minor). Thus, the first (eccentric) phase of the reversible contraction in spike is being implemented simultaneously in torso, shoulder, elbow and finally, ankle joints.

Implementation of the second (concentric) phase of the reversible contractions in spike is carried out successively. It is first realized in the trunk joint angle (trunk rotators to the left) whereby the motor units recruitment velocity is 22.00 IU in the interval of 0.005 s, at the force of 17.20 daN, and the maximum Muscle force generation velocity change of 3440.00 daN.s^{-1} of shoulders (anteflexsors in the shoulder joint - m. deltoideus and m. pectoralis major), then the elbow (elbow extensors - m. triceps brachii) whereby the maximum motor units recruitment velocity is 34.00 IU, in the interval of 0.005 s, at the force of 43.55 daN, and the motor units recruitment velocity of 8710.0 daN.s^{-1}, and finally in the hand wrist (right fist flexors) whereby the motor units recruitment velocity is 95.0 IU, in the interval of 0.003 s, at the force of 14.40 daN, and the maximum muscle force generation velocity of 4800.1 daN.s^{-1} [4, 8, 9, 12-20]. In each joint it is strong, lightning rapid, timely (perfect intra and intermuscular coordination) [4, 6, 8-10, 12]. Successive series of muscle contractions produce a force that allows the ball flight velocity of 21.5 m.s^{-1} and even higher [13-15]. The elbow angle at the moment of spiking the ball from the back zone is 146° and in spiking the ball from the front zone it is 159° [14].

After a realized spike there follows a final phase, landing on the toes of both feet at the same time, in which plantar flexors in the upper ankle joint, knee and hip joint extensors work in the eccentric regime performing the amortization, whereas the spinal column extensor, by isometric contraction, maintain a stability of the trunk. The elite volleyball players achieve the maximum muscle force generation velocity of the leg extensors

7666.42 ± 1105.42 daN.s^{-1} in the interval of amortization of 0.082 ± 0.020 s, at the knee joint angle of 132.20 ± 10.850, level of muscle force of 628.65 ± 91.68 daN, and the motor units recruitment velocity of 64.9 ± 7.14 IU [4, 6, 8, 10]. If, after landing immediately follows take-off the leg extensors of the elite volleyball players again work in the reverse regime (the eccentric and concentric phase are connected with the aim to shorten as much as possible the interval between the phases) whereby they achieve the maximum motor units recruitment velocity of 14988.69 ± 1795.46 daN.s^{-1} in a time interval of transition from the eccentric to concentric contraction of 0.063 ± 0.007 s, muscle force level of 944.26 ± 113.11 daN, and the motor units recruitment velocity of 79.6 ± 6.85 IU, in order to achieve the necessary vertical jump height from which to successfully perform a spike or block [4-10, 12, 19, 20].

Physiological Analysis of Muscle Force Production in Spike

In all movements in the realization of spike, except in landing, muscle force production is enabled by the reversible muscle contractions. Reversible contractions consist of the eccentric and concentric phases in which the shortening of muscles is preceded by their sudden elongation [4-6, 9-12, 22]. A combination of the eccentric concentric contraction (a cycle) in the described spike movements is called a reversible contraction [4-6, 9, 10, 22]. In the eccentric concentric cycle, during shortening phase (concentric contraction) a greater force is produced than individually in the eccentric or concentric muscle contraction for several reasons. First, at the highest point of the cycle, at the moment when the elongation stops and shortening of a muscle begins, force is developed in isometric conditions [4-6, 9, 10, 22]. Second, considering the fact that the force begins to increase in the eccentric phase, the time at which it is possible to generate a force in a reversible contraction is extended [4-6, 8-12, 22]. Third, the level of muscle force is affected by the muscle tendon elasticity (accumulation of elastic energy in the phase of muscles and tendons elongation), and fourth, reflex muscle contraction [4, 8-10, 22]. It has already been said that the length of all the muscles involved in spike changes causing the same abrupt changes of their level of muscle force. This is particularly pronounced in the knee extensors after contact with the ground in landings or jump landings.

Thus, the muscles are forcingly elongated and at the same time their tension is greatly increased [4-6, 8-12, 22]. Those changes are simultaneously controlled and partly held in balance by the common function of the two motor reflexes: elongation reflex, maintaining optimal muscle length, and Golgi tendon organ reflex, preventing the extreme and damaging muscle strain. Eccentric discharge to the muscle in the elongation phase is modified by the joint action of the two reflexes, elongation reflex and Golgi tendon organ reflex. Stretch reflex has a positive effect (increasing discharge) while Golgi reflex has a negative (inhibitory) efferent effect, and their effect is manifested by the muscle force measure. What is important to learn about reversible contractions during the large muscle strains in volleyball is that the activation of the Golgi tendon organ inhibits further muscle activity, i.e., concentric contraction because it prevents efferent inflow into the muscle. However, in landing with amortization or block, jump landing with rapid elongation due to the possibility of the body integrity violation CNS reacts by the amplification and disinhibition effects at different levels. In this case, the reticular system begins to operate by amplification increasing the efferent inflow. Then, there occurs central inhibition of the Renshaw's inhibitory interneurons resulting in the free passage of the increased efferent consecutive inflow of impulses.

Also, Golgi tendon organ is inhibited peripherally thus removing the last obstacle to an increased influx of the efferent impulses to the muscle. The neural disinhibition, from the above mentioned conditions, causes the increase in stretch reflex (shortens the reflex latency time and increases the velocity and level of muscle force produced in a reflex). Furthermore, neural disinhibition causes an increase in the motor units recruitment velocity by controlling the release and diffuse rate of Ca++ ions and inhibition of the troponin - tropomyosin complex in muscle fibers, which essentially represents a muscle fiber disinhibition; then, there is increase in the level of the synchronization of the muscle motor units functioning, change in the motor units recruitment pattern, whereby the first involved are the highest firing rate motor units and muscle force, (intramuscular coordination). Also, increased is the intramuscular coordination and reprogramming (by increasing) the limits of muscle force of all motor units above the maximum measured on standard tests. By increasing the motor units recruitment velocity, their synchronization, intra and intermuscular coordination and muscle force level of the individual groups of motor units, muscle force generation velocity and level are increased, as well as the velocity of its generation changes. Thus, the greatest impact on the enormous increase in muscle force along with the shortening time of its generation in a reversible contraction in all phases of service and spike, is attributed to the neural component of muscle contraction, primarily to the disinhibition process at all levels [4-6, 8-12, 22]. The biggest challenge to the mind of the elite volleyball players in learning and mastering a reversible contraction is learning how to master disinhibition. Those volleyball players who are bad at mastering disinhibition process in a reversible contraction, in spite of achieving much higher levels of maximal muscle force in tests, as compared to those who have mastered reversible contraction, as a rule, have a weaker serve, spike, jumps and landings, due to the lack of training and mastering the knowledge of the effects of the Golgi tendon reflex in the concentric contraction phase.

METHODS

Participants

The force generated by all muscle groups participating in the realization of spike, or the realization of exercises designed for its development, is measured in isometric and dynamic mode of muscle functioning on a sample of 21 top volleyball players whose average weight was 85.5 ± 5.21 kg and height 198.5 ± 5.86 cm.

Testing Procedure

The force in isometric mode (Table 3) is measured by specially designed and certified hardware and software system (Programme Engineering, Belgrade). Peripheral equipment for isometric muscle force measuring are tensiometric probes with measurement range from 0 to 15000 daN and measurement accuracy of 0.0002 daN. For muscle force measuring, for all muscle groups Belt method is used [5, 8, 10, 18-20]. The force Fm(t) to a level of 1%, 2%...., 99% of maximum muscle force expressed in daN and the time intervals of their generation (s) are measured. Then the maximum muscle force Fmax also expressed in daN and the time intervals of their generation are measured [5, 8, 18-20]. Thus, designed system allows during isometric measurement the control and varying of the muscle length (the angle at which the muscle works), time and manner of its work (smooth and twitch) and the number of muscles and joints involved in measurement (one joint, two or more joints). Each test is repeated three times and the best result is selected.

Muscle force measurement in dynamic mode is performed by the optoelectronic system (Figure 2), force plate and a certified hardware and software (Bioengineering VAC) system, which consists of free weights with equipment allowing time measurement (s), vertical and horizontal weights bar change positions every 1 mm in the whole lifting range [4, 9-12, 18-20, 23, 24]. Force plate and optoelectronic systems measure muscle force production during different types of jump landing, landings, vertical jumps and run-up vertical jumps. Piezoelectric sensors built into the platform register at high speed (1000 Hz) compression muscle forces during the execution of jump landing, landings, individual or serial jumps and provide for a detailed dynamic analysis of all the phases of the jump and the high validity of every single performed movement. In addition to standard parameters, force plate allows for the monitoring of dynamics and transitivity development of muscle force, the jump execution velocity, the degree of the take-off and landing depth, the stretching effects, the abilities of rapid alternation of the eccentric and concentric contraction and elastic energy transfer [23] and numerous other parameters.

Hardware Software (Bioengineering VAC) system is used to measure muscle force in weightlifting (Table 1, 2 and 3). It allows for measurements to be controlled and varied: muscle length (angle), the time, the weight of the length and speed of work, shortening velocity (concentric contraction) and elongation of muscles (eccentric contraction), the time of transition from eccentric to concentric contraction (reversible contraction). When lifting all weights vertical and horizontal bar position changes time is measured, vertical on each 5.8 mm and horizontal on each 1 mm, spanning the whole range of muscle work. Each test was repeated three times and the best result was selected. The attempts whose horizontal barbell displacement is not permitted in the allowed zone (4-5 cm) were disregarded. On average, 100 points are observed per measurement. Based on the data length vs time one calculates vertical velocity and acceleration for each monitored sample as the first and the second performance per time. Results of velocity and acceleration to are fitted before the muscle force is calculated. Then, based on the fitted results, one calculates force in each measurement in the entire range of lifting according to the following formula [9-12, 18, 19]:

$$F = m\,(a + 9.81)/10 \tag{2}$$

where F - is the force expressed in daN, m - is the mass of the barbell expressed in kg, and a is the acceleration ($m.s^{-2}$) observed in a certain measurement. In both working regimes, there were measured ratio of force time on each 1% of the maximum muscle force, and maximum force and the time during which it is generated. From the obtained data for muscle force and time, one calculates the muscle force production velocity as their sums per time for all the muscle groups involved in the testing. From the data obtained for muscle force and time one calculates muscle force production velocity as their performance per time for all the muscle groups involved in the testing.

Force in vertical jumps in spike, which are performed during the match can be calculated through the vertical jump height, body height and body weight of each volleyball player. Once the results are known for the vertical jump in spike, body weight and body height of the volleyball player the force is calculated using this function [18-20]:

$$F = [(G \, . \, VJh) \, . \, BH^{-1}] \, . \, 10^{-1} \tag{3}$$

where F - is the level of muscle force expressed in decanewtons (daN) G - is the body weight expressed in newtons (N), VJh – is a vertical jump height expressed in centimeters (cm), BH - is the body height in meters (m).

The force of torso, shoulder girdle and hand rotators in spike is calculated using partialization method [18-20].

In isometric and dynamic measurement regime, in the entire range of muscle force generation, for every 1%, one calculates muscle force generation velocity according to the formula:

$$RFD = F/t \tag{4}$$

where RFD - is muscle force development rate expressed in decanewtons in seconds ($daN.s^{-1}$), F - is an adequate level of muscle force expressed in decanewtons (daN) and t - is the time of muscle force observation expressed in seconds (s).

From the data force time for both measurement regimes changes of muscle force generation velocity are calculated according to the formula:

$$CRFD = (F_2\text{-}F_1)/(t_2\text{-}t_1) \tag{5}$$

where CRFD - is change in muscle force generation velocity expressed in decanewtons in second ($daN.s^{-1}$), for each % of the measured muscle force, force (F) from 1% to 100% and time (t) expressed in seconds (s) when it happens, F_1 and F_2 - are adequate levels of k force expressed in decanewtons (daN), and t_1 and t_2 -are the time of muscle force observation expressed in seconds (s).

From the data force time, obtained by means of the Belt method and weight lifting (Table 1, 2 and 3) motor units recruitment velocity was calculated for each Ft according to the formula [3, 5, 8, 10, 18-20]:

$$k = - (1/t) * \ln ((1 - F_t/Fmax)) \quad (6)$$

where: F_t - is a level of 1%, 2% .... 99% of the maximum muscle force expressed in decanewtons (daN); Fmax - is a maximum force generated by the actual muscles expressed in decanewtons (daN); k - is a constant which characterizes the motor units recruitment velocity expressed in index units (IU); t - is the time in which to achieve the appropriate level of the maximum muscle force expressed in seconds (s).

When using force plate for measuring muscle force in landings, landing blocks, landing jumps, run-up take-off, motor units recruitment velocity is calculated by the following formula (Figure 2, 4) [5, 10, 18-20, 24]:

$$k = Ln\ (1 - F_{exp}/A/e^{B\ X\ \beta\ exp})\ \Delta\ t_{exp} \quad (7)$$

where k - is a constant which characterizes the motor units recruitment velocity expressed in index units (IU); F_{exp} – is the level of muscle force registered in the dynamic conditions of muscle functioning during the period when a muscle strains under isometric conditions expressed in decanewtons (daN), β_{exp} - is the angle of the knee joint in which the angular velocity is zero, expressed in degrees (^{0}); Δt_{exp} – is the time interval elapsed since contact with force plate until the moment in which the angular velocity of the knee joint is equal to zero, expressed in seconds (s).

Data Analysis

The RFD depends directly on the certain groups of motor units force and the rate of their involvement (k) [5, 7-9, 18-21]. From this relationship, it follows that the value of the certain groups of motor units force, for each of the 100 surveyed points, for each participant, represents quotient of the rate of force development and the speeds of recruitment for motor units

$$F_{MU} = (F/t)/[- (1/t) * \ln ((1 - F_t/Fmax))] \quad (8)$$

expressed in daN [5, 7-9, 18-21]. On these data the descriptive and cluster statistics analysis were performed [21] (Figure 1).

Based on the relationships between the force time, recruitment velocity and the level of muscle force of the individual motor units in the whole range of muscle force generation, it is possible to calculate the level of motor units work synchronization using cluster analysis [5, 7, 8, 18-21] (Figure 3).

Fitting the data on the level of muscle force of the individual motor units and the time of its achievement in the entire range of muscle force generation for one or more muscles, the optimization of their work is calculated on the intra or intermuscular level [5, 7, 8, 18-21] (Figure 4).

All statistical analysis was done by the application of software package SPSS for Windows, Release 22.0.

METHODOLOGY OF MUSCLE FORCE DEVELOPMENT IN SPIKE IN ELITE VOLLEYBALL PLAYERS

The main problem in relation to the muscle force training is still nowadays present [4-12, 18-22] as it was many years ago [25-27] and it is a discovery of the mechanism of adaptation that causes changes in neuromuscular apparatus in accordance with the expressed needs of sports, and consequently, determining technology for its development. Friedebolit et al. [25-27] locates adaptation mechanism at the level and method of motor units activation. Friedebolit et al., 1957 [25], assumes that the increased level of the motor units work synchronization explains the muscle force generation velocity, while Duntsh and Stoboy [27] explain this phenomenon by the increased number of active motor units and (or) increased frequency of the impulses reaching the muscle. Neural disinhibition causes an increase in the motor units recruitment velocity by controlling the release and diffuse rate of the Ca^{++} ions and controlling inhibition of the troponin - tropomyosin complex in muscle fibers, which essentially represents a muscle fiber disinhibition; then, there is an increase in the level of synchronization of the muscle motor units functioning, change in the motor units recruitment pattern, whereby the first involved are the highest firing rate motor units, and muscle force, (intramuscular coordination). Also, increased is the intramuscular coordination and reprogramming (by increasing) the limits of muscle force of all the motor units above the maximum measured on standard tests. [4-12, 18-22, 28, 29]. By increasing the motor units recruitment velocity, their synchronization, intra and disinhibition and muscle force level of the individual groups of motor units, muscle force generation velocity and level are increased, as well as the velocity of its generation changes. The above mentioned increases cause an increase in the maximum muscle force production velocity and its production change velocity. In addition to initiating disinhibition mechanism in the course of training, listed parameters on which the force depends can be developed by initiating the specific mechanisms of their adaptation thus achieving their high intensity and arrangement in a time interval ranging from 0.005 s to 0.082 s, which is determined by the spike characteristics [4-12, 18-22, 25-28]. The best results in the development of muscle force generation velocity, the maximum muscle force of certain groups of motor units, motor units recruitment velocity, muscle force generation velocity change, motor units work synchronization are achieved through training using maximum work speed, lifting free weights (load), through jumps, leaps, landings, landing jumps, and sprints with direction changes [4-12, 18-20], in the reversible contraction in landing jumps from 60 cm, then in landing block (brutal plyometrics) from the height of 120 to 200 cm, and weight training 80% and 100% of 1RM most intensively develops maximum muscle force generation velocity (Table 1 and Figure 2).

Development of the maximum muscle force (Figure 1) of the muscle groups as well as the maximum muscle force of the certain groups of motor units is achieved in a reversible contraction using weights and applying different training methods [4-12, 18-20]. The most commonly used weights are those of 30%, 40%, 50%, 70%, 75%, 80%, 85%, 90%, 95%, 97%, 100%, 130% and 150% of the 1RM which are lifted at the maximum velocity in different combinations [8-12, 18-20]. To develop the maximum muscle force of all groups of motor units following weights are used of 90%, 95%, 97% to 100%, 130% and 150% [8-12, 18-20]. To develop the maximum muscle force of a group of motor units of the high and the highest level of muscle force generation weights of 80%, 85%, 90 and 95% or 100%, 95% and 85% are used [8-12, 18.20]. To develop the maximum muscle force of the motor units of the medium, large and maximum levels of muscle force generation weights of 75%, 80%, 85%, 95% are used [8-12, 18-20]. Only for the motor units of the maximum level of muscle force generation the weights of 80%, 85%, 90%, 95% are used, and for the lowest level of motor unit muscle force generation the weights of 30% to 50% of 1RM are used [8-12, 18-20].

Table 1. The analysis of parameter changes in leg extensor velocity, force and its dimensions were measured by lifting different weights (50%, 70%, 80%, 90% and 100% of maximal weight) at medium (V3), high (V2) and maximal (V1) velocity from deep squat in the entire leg extension range

	50%			70%			80%			90%		100%
	V3	V2	V1	V3	V2	V1	V3	V2	V1	V2	V1	V1
Fmax	151	176	163	165	191	217	271	298	305	186	181	239
tmax	0.19	0.14	0.12	0.24	0.2	0.23	1.36	1.41	145	0.8	1.16	0.81
CRFD	1133	1863	1136	699	1328	2178	5682	7579	18372	497	607	897
RFD	424	583	635	471	652	939	355	816	1266	518	765	961
FRFD	93.1	105	89.4	132	163	216	135	204	228	166	153	202
tRFD	0.21	0.18	0.14	0.28	0.25	0.23	0.38	0.25	0.18	0.32	0.2	0.21

Note: F - is an adequate level of muscle force expressed in decanewtons (daN), RFD - is muscle force development rate expressed in decanewtons in seconds (daN.s-1), CRFD- is change in muscle force generation velocity expressed in decanewtons in second (daN.s-1), t- is the time of muscle force observation expressed in seconds (s). All variables are at the level of average values.

In the reversible contraction landing jump from the height of 76 cm and weight lifting 70% of 1RM most intensively develop the motor units recruitment velocity (Figure 2 and Table 2) [6, 10, 18-20].

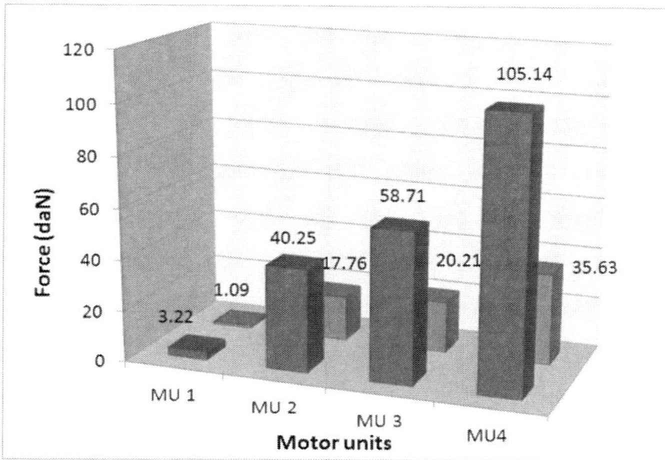

Figure 1. Muscle force of some motor unit groups of the knee extensors in two elite volleyball players during vertical jump expressed in decanewtons daN.

Table 2. Rate of change of leg extensors motor units recruitment during various load in weight lifting with maximal speed

Weight load	50%	70%	80%	90%	100%
Maximal units recruitment speed MU (k)	9.89	16.61	3.09	8.45	12.27
Time from k(s)	0.159	0.218	1.436	0.195	0.16
Force Fk (daN)	162	211	300	149	219

Note: All variables are at the level of average values.

With 85% of the maximum weight lifted in one elevation (1RM), at a maximum speed of lifting and in landing jumps from the height of 80 cm (Table 1, 3 and Figure 2) most intensive changes in the muscle force generation occur, together with the most intense process of creating proteins actin and myosin, but there is also an increases in both inter and intramuscular muscle coordination and the level of changes in the muscle force generation [6, 10, 18-20, 30].

The highest level of motor units work synchronization is achieved in landing drop jump-block (brutal plyometrics) from the heights of 120 to 200 cm, lifting the maximum weights (100% 1RM), at the maximum speed, and movement direction changes from sprints (Figure 3 and Table 1) [6, 10, 18-20].

Training optimization (Figure 4) of motor units functioning in intermuscular and intramuscular level is achieved using weights and varying the speed of lifting and weight of barbells in a series [8-2, 18-20]. The most commonly used weights are those of 30%, 40%, 50%, 70%, 75%, 80%, 85%, 90%, 95% and 100%. The excellent results of the optimization of motor units work in the intermuscular and intramuscular level and development of the maximum muscle force for certain groups of motor units are achieved by various combinations of the leaps, jumps, landings, landing drop jumps [10, 18-20]. The most common combinations in jumps or leaps are the heights of 60% to 100% and lengths from 40% to 100% of the maximum. In landing release heights of 30 to 80 cm are combined, in landing spring upward height of 100 to 170 cm are combined. In optimization conditions, with the aim of achieving disinhibition effect landings from the height of 100 to 200 cm and landing jumps -block from a height of 120-200 cm are used (Figure 2) [10, 18-20].

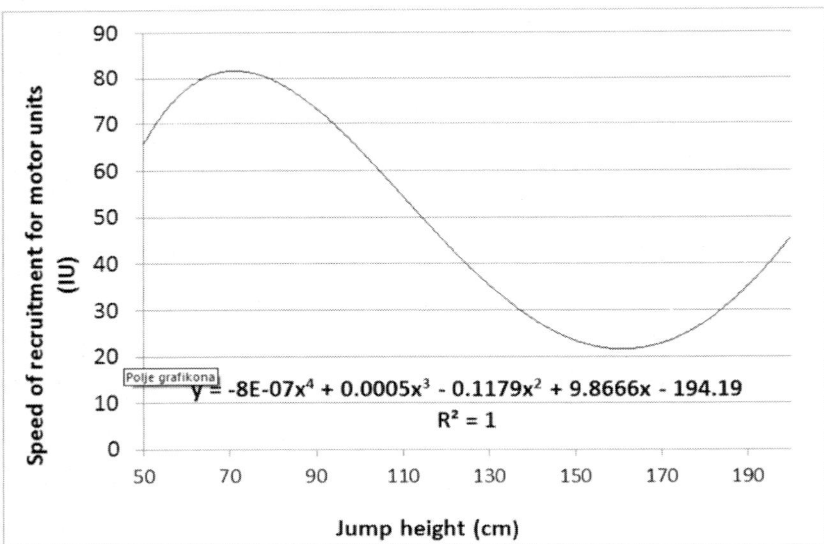

Figure 2. Rate of change of moment units recruitment with height change in depth jump/hop off (Reversible contraction).

Table 3. The comparative analysis of force generation velocity and its dimensions at maximal voluntary contractions in isometric and dynamic muscle work regime

	Fmax	tmax	kmax	tkmax	Fkmax	RFD	CRFD	FCRFD	tCRFD
I	545	1.36	3.99	0.089	164.2	1743	6303.8	93.3	0.061
D	239.1	0.81	11.5	0.22	219.8	898	1095.8	215.2	0.196

Note: I - Isometric mode, D - Dynamic mode (Half-Squat), F - adequate level of muscle force (daN), RFD - muscle force development rate (daN.s-1), CRFD - change in muscle force generation velocity (daN.s-1), t - the time of muscle force observation (s). All variables are at the level of average values.

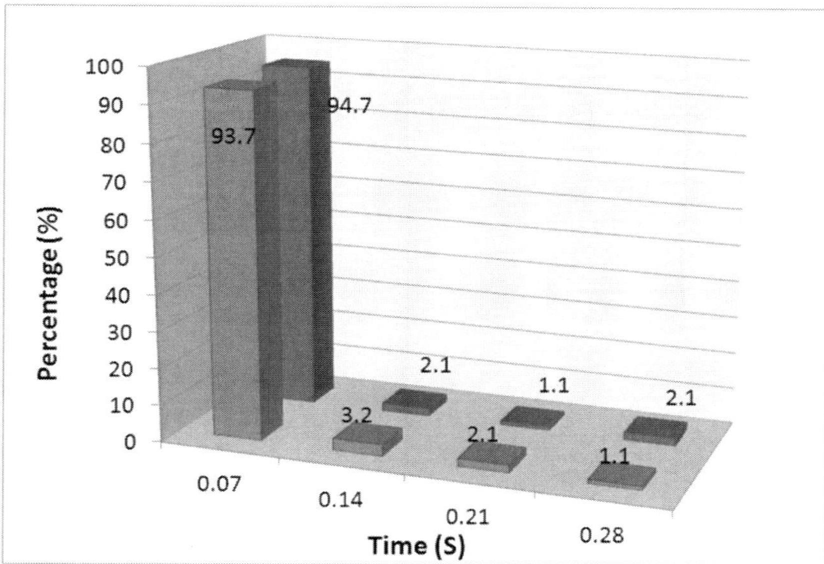

Figure 3. Leg extensors motor units work synchronization in two elite volleyball players during vertical jump expressed in percentages (%).

The best training results are achieved if presented laws are used and if the training is programmed specifically for each individual athlete [4-12, 18-20]. Training sessions are programmed to last for four weeks on the basis of the current state of each volleyball player [4-12, 18-20]. After each month of the training application regardless of how it is directed, diagnostics should be repeated and the existing training reprogrammed, that is the new one should be designed, suitable to the current status with the potential to result in the planned changes. During each training session all the relevant muscle groups are treated. Monthly training sessions are designed in such a way to develop motor units recruitment velocity in the first week, the muscle force generation velocity and optimization of motor units at the intramuscular level and increase in the level of diffusion speed of Ca ++ ions and their removal [9-12, 18-20]. In the second week the maximum force of certain groups of motor units, that is muscle groups, is developed, as well as the muscle force generation velocity and optimization of the motor units at the intramuscular level [9-12, 18-20]. In the third week disinhibition mechanisms are developed, then the optimization of motor units in the intramuscular level, muscle density and the speed of Ca ++ ions diffusion are also increased [9-12, 18-20]. In the fourth week the work on the development of motor units synchronization is emphasized, also the optimization of the motor units at the inter and intramuscular level as well as the disinhibition mechanisms are focused on [9-12, 18-20]. The amount of work for any athlete per training session is designed in relation to his or her current status [7, 18-20], capacity [11, 12], functions by which to develop or maintain force [7-10, 18-20] the effects and the changes that are meant to occur, that is, the definition of the objectives of training one wants to achieve [7, 18-20].

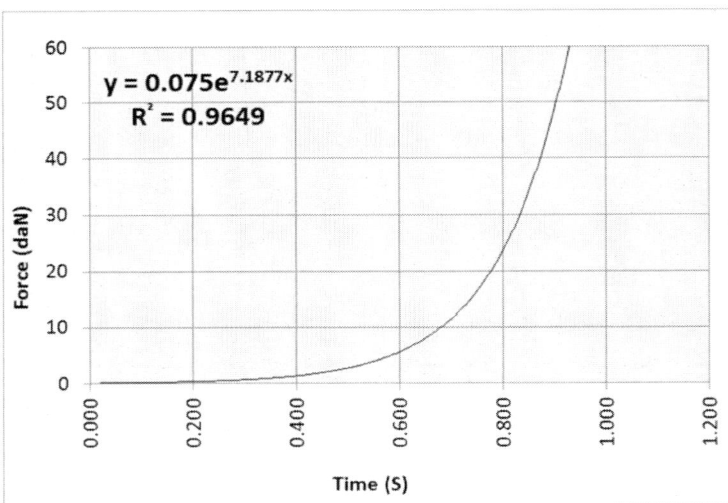

Figure 4. Model of force distribution of motor units of leg extensor muscles.

To have the force training designed in most successful way, it is necessary to know which categories are describing muscle straining (intensity of muscle straining, duration of muscle contraction, rest intervals between series) and what type of training effects and changes they cause.

Intensity of muscle straining is defined through maximum result in a single exercise-means with percentage. In weight lifting, that is % of maximum weight lifted in 1 attempt, in jumping it is % of maximum height or length of jump, in drop depth jumps it is a height from which a jump is made, in running it is % of maximum running speed (high, sub-maximum, maximum), etc. [7, 18-20].

Duration of contraction is implicitly defined with the speed of realization of exercise, except in cases of isometric contractions where duration of contraction is explicitly defined. The research [7, 18-20] have shown that the best results in development of maximum force of muscles or individual group of motor units, speed of activation of motor units, density of muscles, speed of change of force creation and synchronization of motor units is achieved with maximum work speed in the exercise. Synchronizing and optimizing work of motor units except with use of weights is done by varying speed, distance and direction of movement, using running as training means. By varying speed at the same distance, following effects are being accomplished. Running in high speed activates not only motor units of the lowest threshold of initiation and the lowest force level (group I). Running in sub-maximum speed activates motor units of higher threshold of initiation with higher force level (group II). Running in maximum speed activates not only the motor units of even higher threshold of initiation and higher force level (group III). Running in maximum speed with change of running direction synchronizes work of all motor units with activation of motor units with the highest threshold of initiation too, and with highest quantity of force (group IV) in a direction change phase. Increasing the distance in running the same speed activates more and more motor units of the same group. Speed as vary from high to sub-maximum to maximum so that all types of distances motor units are activated to have activated all motor units from the same group. Using accelerations at the same distance a continuous change of activation of groups of motor units occurs from those with the lowest force to those with highest force. The same effect is accomplished when the weight plate weight and the speed of its lifting varies.

A character of contraction is determined by change of length of muscle in contraction. Contraction may last without changing length of a muscle. That type of contraction is called isometric and the work regime is called static. The contraction may be realized during shortening of a muscle and it is called concentric and the work regime is called overcoming or myometric. and finally, a contraction may manifest during extension of a muscle and it is called eccentric and the work regime amortizing or plyometric. Large number of exercises is done in a combined work regime as well as large number of sports activities. Work in eccentric conditions is used as particularly good way for development of speed of force creation and the speed of activation of motor units, for optimizing their work at into-muscular and inter-muscular level, as well as disinhibitory mean with purpose of breaking barriers in creating force. Working in concentric and mixed conditions gives good results at creation of suitable configuration of force dimensions. Isometric work regime gives the weakest results in force development and is used only in conditions of extreme demands of a sport.

Total number of contractions of one muscle group at one training is determined by number of series, by number of repetitions in a series, influence of certain force dimension to development (training goal) and all that conditional to individual characteristics and capabilities of an athlete, by intensity of work and rest intervals between series [7, 18-20]. Each of these elements is individually determined for each athlete for each muscle group, at each training, through intensity control (quantity of load, height of drop jump, etc.), work speed and length of rest intervals between series. On a well-designed training, that number varies between 90 and 150 muscle contractions for all muscle groups treated at one training with weights and from 10 to 180 muscle contractions if various types of jumps and drop jumps are used.

Number of series depends on features developed, work intensity and individual characteristics of an athlete. It was shown that in controlled conditions it is not possible nor necessary to do more than 5 series for one muscle group (one exercise) and no need to do more than 6 exercises (six muscle groups) per training, applying parallel work [7, 18-20].

The best results in developing force and its dimensions are accomplished during 3-minute rest intervals between series [7, 18-20]. So defined rest interval with clearly defined speed and order of realization of exercise (muscle group), rationalizes training, and brings it to duration of 1 hour including warming up and loosening up. With this way of work, we avoid unnecessary and contra-productive large number of repetitions, that most often develop the muscle tissue that does not contribute to better results in a sport but slows down athlete and if he invested enormous amount of time for training.

Muscle force development lasts each year for eleven months of the annual cycle [7, 18-20]. In principle, the development of muscle force takes years and years of work [7, 18-20], that is until the achievement and realization of the volleyball players genetic capacity is accomplished [11, 12] according to the dynamics specific to each individual. Once this capacity is reached one starts programming of the training with the aim to maintain the achieved level of muscle force.

In elite volleyball players, along with other training sessions, to develop muscle force two sessions a week are needed, between which there is a break of 72 hours [7-12, 18-20]. Each training last up to one hour with lots of work (an average weight lifted is 11609 kg, 491 kcal and 104.9 liters of oxygen spent, and 44.24 kw of strength created) [7-12, 18-20]. This approach is used when athletes have no competitions or have one competition (match) a week. When they have to or three competitions (matches) a week, one training for force development a week, one hour in total, in enough. These types of training are either developing or maintaining. After the rest period of one month, a training directed at re-establishing previous status in force is used if necessary, and if not, we continue with force maintenance, when necessary.

MANAGING EDUCATIONAL AND TRAINING CHANGES

From the moment we define tools and methods, and when we finished determining transitive and final states, we have to determine rules according to which the dimensions of an individual's state will change under the influence of the implemented activities, because individuals may have similar adaptations and transformations when exposed to different training operators Educational and training tools for achieving previously determined goals are viewed primarily through two components: energy and information. The energy component is presented with a vector whose components are force that needs to be developed into activities, speed of performance for the mentioned activities and the duration of activities [18-20]:

$$E = a_{11}\, S + a_{12}\, B + a_{13}\, T \tag{9}$$

Information component is represented with the vector whose dimensions are the quantity of information brought by applied tools and methods, entropy of decoded information and information emission duration [18-20]:

$$Ij = a_{21}\, H(E) + a_{22}\, H(D) + a_{23}\, H(T) \tag{10}$$

We also have to ask ourselves what is the ratio of applying energy and information component and when this ratio changes the state of system, i.e., when are we supposed to change that ratio in order to get to the projected transitive or final state of the system.

Earlier, the general status of an individual was described with an equation of the state of system, i.e., an equation representing the dynamics of the system [18-20]:

$$\dot{X} = Ax + Bu \tag{11}$$

and an equation describing the output

$$y + Cx + Du \tag{12}$$

for

$$x(t_0) = x_0 \tag{13}$$

where $x \in X$ (space of state of the system), $y \in Y$ (space of output reactions) i $u \in U$ (space of input stimuli) having in mind that

$A{:}x \rightarrow X$ (training operator),
$B{:}u \rightarrow U$ (management operator),
$C{:}x \rightarrow Y$ (observation operator),
$D{:}u \rightarrow Y$ (operator of input output reaction),
$X_0 \rightarrow$ initial state.

Changes in the state of the system X can be described with a gradient form of the equation of state [18-20]:

$$\dot{X} = - \Delta X\ V, \tag{14}$$

where V represents a potential function of training operator A, with:

$$V{:}\ R^2 * R^1 \rightarrow R^1, \tag{15}$$

for

$$V/x,i,c/ = x^4/4 - ix^2 - cx,\ i \in I,\ c \in E \tag{16}$$

where I represent information and E represents energy component of the training operator, while Rn represents an n-dimensional Euclidean space.

The gradient of training operator's potential function is defined with the following relation:

$$\Delta\, x\ V = x^3 - ix - e, \tag{17}$$

and represents two-dimensional smooth manifolds $M \subset R3$.

The geometry of training process is represented in the following graphic:

The balance of training process is determined by the following relation [19, 20]:

$$\Delta \, x \, V = 0, \quad (18)$$

while local stable state can be achieved if [18-20]:

$$\Delta^2 \, x \, V = 0. \quad (19)$$

As we can see on the drawing, educational and training process is presented with the trajectory of the coordinates of an individual on a two-dimensional manifold (surface) M. In that context, in order to optimize training and educational process, we have to find two-dimensional training operators with a maximal difference in the state presented in the graphic with xi and x_0 (corresponding to final and initial state, respectively). The final position represents the "desired" training or educational state the final position represents the "desired" training or educational state.

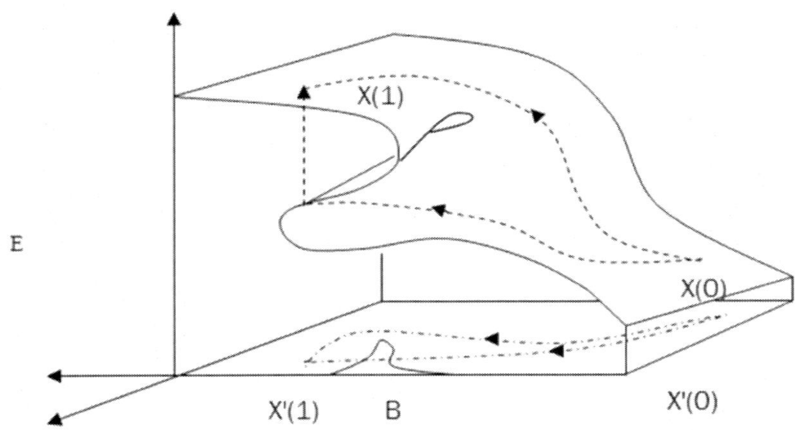

Figure 5. Model of state of training changes.

Besides this, the trajectory from x_0 to x_i has to be the shortest possible or we have to minimize the transfer from one state to the other [18-20]. The space-time geodesic equation will show an increase on the transition to the bifurcation space or on the exit from the bifurcation space (B), which depends on the system's history. In the case we decided to discuss here, optimization would be possible if the training procedure would include an increase in information demand with constant energy requirements in the beginner phase of the exercise, in order to jump to the desired, final state with an increase in energy requirements later on [18-20].

CONCLUSION

Based on the biomechanical and functional analyses performed on a sample of 21 top volleyball players, it can be concluded that for the muscle force production in spike and landing one uses eccentric contraction but in all other cases a reversible contraction is used. Also, it was found that in order to achieve good results in spike elite volleyball, players need to have a developed muscle force production of all muscle groups involved in the realization of spike, furthermore, they have to develop the recruitment velocity and synchronization of the motor units work, the maximum force of certain groups of motor units, the muscle force production velocity change, inter and intramuscular coordination. The maximum values of the cited values in spike in elite volleyball players are achieved in a time interval of 0.005 s to 0.082 s. The maximal muscle force production velocities in spike in elite volleyball players range from 3440.00 daN.s^{-1} to 14988.69 daN.s^{-1} at motor units recruitment velocities from 22.00 IU to 95.0 IU. The force of certain groups of the knee extensors motor units in elite volleyball players ranges from 1.09 daN to 105.14 daN. In landing vertical jumps elite volleyball players synchronize up to 94.7% of the leg extensors motor units. The greatest impact on the enormously large muscle force production along with the shortening of the time of its generation in a reversible contraction, in all stages of the service and the spike, is attributed to a neural component of the muscle contraction, primarily to the disinhibition process at all levels. Finally, in accordance with the results of the analyses, a methodology of the muscle force development is suggested whereby besides learning how to master disinhibition process one composes a set of all required parameters on which the level and velocity of muscle force generation depends, concerning a daily, weekly, monthly and annual basis, by utilising special means and methods. The mathematical model of managing change in the force domain is also defined as part of the given methodology.

REFERENCES

[1] Milosevic, Milenko., Miroljub, Blagojevic., Bratislav, Tosic. & Stevan, Pilipovic. (2000). "The Behavior of Muscles in External Instantaneous Force Fields." Paper presented at *the XVIII Iinternacional symposium of biomechanics in sport, Hong Kong*, June 25-30.

[2] Amasay, Tal. (2008). "Static Block Jump Techniques in Volleyball: Upright Versus Squat Starting Positions." *Journal of Strength and Conditioning Research*, *22*, 1242-1248. doi: 10.1519/ JSC.0b013e31816d5a7f.

[3] Amanovic, Djurica., Milenko, Milosevic., Radomir, Mudric., Milivoj, Dopsaj. & Dusan, Peric. (2006). "Modeling Variability of the Assigned Level of Force During Isometric Contractions of the Arms Extensor Muscles in Untrained Males." *Facta universitatis – Series: Physical Education and Sport*, *4*, 35-48.

[4] Milosevic, Milenko., Miroljub, Blagojevic., Stevan, Pilipovic. & Bratislav, Tosic. (2000). The muscle contraction and the force production. Paper presented at *the XVIII Iinternacional symposium of biomechanics in sport*, Hong Kong, June 25-30

[5] Milošević, Milenko., Radomir, Mudrić., Milivoj, Dopsaj., Miroljub, Blagojević. & Elleni, Papadimitriou. (2004). "The control of force creating in function of the muscle contraction intensity." *Paper*

presented at 4th International Conference on Strength Training., Thessaloniki, May 14-16.

[6] Milosevic, Milos., Milos, Mudrić., Radomir, Mudrić. & Milenko, Milošević. (2012). "Using the Mind in Reprogramming the Limits of Muscle Force in the Process of Creating Champions." *Sport Science & Practice*, *2*, 39-58.

[7] Milosevic, Milenko. & Milos, Milosevic. (2013). "Model for Assessing the Physical Status, as Well as Prediction and Programming of Training and Sports Performance of a Soccer Player." *Journal of Physical Education and Sport*, *13*, 479 – 488. doi:10.7752/jpes.2013.04076.

[8] Milosevic, Milenko., Predrag, Nemec., Dragan, Zivotic., Milos, Milosevic. & Rajko, Rajovic. (2014). "Force Distribution Model of Motor Units of Leg Extensor Muscles." *Journal of Sports Sciences*, *2*, 195-199. doi:10.17265/2332-7839/2014.04.004.

[9] Milosevic, Milenko., Milos, Milosevic., Predrag, Nemec., Dragan, Zivotic. & Ismet, Radjo. (2014). "A New Approach to Development of Human Maximal Muscle Force." *Journal of Exercise Physiologyonline*, *17*, 70-80.

[10] Milosevic, Milenko., Eleonora, Džoljić., Milos, Milošević., Morteza, Yourkesh. & David, Behm. (2014). "The Analysis of Muscle Force Development with Trained and Elite Athletes." *Physiology*, *24*, 5-12.

[11] Milosevic, Milenko., Vesna, Nemec., Morteza, Yourkesh., Predrag, Nemec., Milos, Milosevic. & David, Behm. (2016). "Determination of Capacity and Rules of the Variability of Maximum Force Using Nonlinear Mathematical Models: A Case Study." *Central European Journal of Sport Sciences and Medicine*, *16*, 91-101. doi: 10.18276/cej.2016.4-10.

[12] Nemec, Predrag., Milos, Milosevic., Vesna, Nemec. & Milenko, Milosevic. (2016). "Production and Development of Muscle Force in Elite Male Volleyball Players' Spike." *Sport Science*, *9*, 32-40.

[13] Wagner, Herbert., Markus, Tilp., Serge, Von Duvillard. & Erich, Muller. (2009). "Kinematic Analysis of Volleyball Spike Jump."

International Journal of Sports Medicine, *30*, 760-5. doi: 10.1055/s-0029-1224177.

[14] Djurovic, Tomislav., Nenad, Marelic., Zeljko, Hraski. & Ljiljana, Sikanja. (2005). "Kinematic Analisysis of the Front and Back Zone Spike in Volleyball." *Športskomed Vjesn*, *20*, 20-25.

[15] Tillman, Mark., Chris, Hass., Denis, Brunt. & Gregg, Bennett. (2004). "Jumping and Landing Techniques in Elite Women's Volleyball." *Journal of Sports Science and Medicine*, *3*, 30-36.

[16] Tomic, Drago. & Nemec, Predrag. (2012). *Volleyball in Theory and Practice*. Belgrade: SIA.

[17] Ivancevic, Vladimior. & Ivancevic, Tamara. (2006). *Natural Biodynamics*. Singapore: World Scientific.

[18] Milosevic, Milenko. & Milosevic, Milos. (2010). *Physical Preparation of Elite Athletes: Standardization of Management Processes*. Belgrade: APP.

[19] Milosevic, Milenko. & Milosevic, Milos. (2014). *Special Physical Education: Textbook on the Management of the Construction of the Physical Integrity and Capacity of Police Officers*. Saarbrücken: Lambert Academic Publishing.

[20] Milosevic, Milenko. & Milosevic, Milos. (2014). *Special Physical Education: Scientific Basis*. Belgrade: CEDIP.

[21] Kovacic, Zlatko. (2014). *Multivariate Analysis*. Belgrade: ČIP Štampa.

[22] Zatsiorsky, Vladimir. & Kramer, William. (2006). *Science and Practice of Strength Training*. Champaign: Human Kinetics.

[23] Bobbert, Maarten., Karin, Gerritsen., Nicolle, Litjens., Knoek, Van Soest. (1996). "Why is countermovement jump height greater than squat jump height?" *Medicine and Science in Sports and Exercise*, *28*, 1402-1412. doi:10.1097/00005768-199611000-00009.

[24] Gavrilovic, Predrag. (1992). "*Comparative Analysis of Transitional Regime of Force Development in Athletes Competing in Different Sports with Willing Contractions and Dynamic Muscle Work*." PhD diss., University of Belgrade.

[25] Friedebold, Gunter., Wolfganf, Niussgen. & Hans, Stoboy. (1957). "Die Veranderung der Elektrischen Aktivitat der Skelettmuskulatur Under den Bedingungen eines Isometrischen Trainings." [The change in the electrical activity of the skeletal muscles under the conditions of an isometric training]. *Experimental Medicine*, *129*, 401-411.

[26] Hans, Stoboy., Wolfgang, Niussgen. & Gunter, Friedebold. (1959). "Das Verhalten der motorrischen Einheiten unter den Bedingungen eines isometrichen Trainings." [The behavior of the motor units under the conditions of isometric training]. *Internationale Zeitschrift für angewandte Physiologie einschliesslich Arbeitsphysiologie*, *17*, 391-399.

[27] Duntsch, Günther. & Hans, Stoboy. (1966). "Das Verhalten von Kraft und Ausdauer wahrend eines isometrischen Trainigs in Abhangigheit von der Muskelmasse." [The behavior of strength and endurance during isometric training depending on the muscle mass.] *Sportarzt Sportmedizin*, 10, 499-504.

[28] Rodacki, Andrew., Neil, Fowler. & Simon, Bennett. (2002). "Vertical Jump Coordination: Fatigue Effects." *Medicine & Science in Sports & Exercise*, *34*, 105-16. doi:10.1097/00005768-200201000-00017.

[29] Sheppard, Jeremy., Emily, Nolen. & Robert, Newton. (2012). "Changes in Strength and Power Qualities over Two Years in Volleyball Players Transitioning from Junior to Senior National Team." *Journal of Strength and Conditioning Research*, *26*, 152-157. doi: 10.1519/JSC.0b013e31821e4d5b.

[30] Furandzijev, Vassil. & Ivan, Abadzijev. (2003). *Basis of preparation of elite and young athletes: The adptacija of cell and molecular level.* Sofia: Tip-top pres.

In: An Essential Guide to Sports Performance ISBN: 978-1-53617-608-7
Editors: Daniel Castillo Alvira et al. © 2020 Nova Science Publishers, Inc.

Chapter 8

MINDFUL COMPASSION AND PSYCHOLOGICAL FLEXIBILITY BASED INTERVENTIONS TO SPORT PERFORMANCE

Bruno Carraça*[1,*]*, António Rosado*[1]*, Cátia Magalhães*[2]*,
***Vitor Ferreira*[1] *and Sidónio Serpa*[1]**

[1]Faculdade Motricidade Humana, Universidade de Lisboa,
Lisboa, Portugal

[2]Instituto Politécnico de Viseu-ESEV; CI&DEI; ISAMB,
Viseu, Portugal

ABSTRACT

This chapter focuses on the increasing interest in mindfulness-based interventions in sport psychology as a way to improve the performance of elite athletes and also in interventions more closely based on compassion, acceptance and commitment approach that want that athletes have a different perspective on their thoughts and feelings, resist attempts to

---

* Corresponding Author's Email: drcarracaclinics@gmx.com.

control or suppress them, and engage in behaviour's consistent with desired sport performance and efforts. This approach encourages mindful present- moment acceptance and willingness to be in contact with internal experience, self-compassion, and full engagement of attention and behaviour on valued activities. Overall findings indicate positive and promising results of a Mindful-Compassion and psychological flexibility-based interventions in increasing the dispositional flow state (indirect measure of performance evaluation), and relief from psychological distress associated with competitive tasks and periods of high workload. These approaches appear to be effective in increasing perceived performance measured directly by the athletes and their coaches.

Keywords: mindfulness, self-compassion, psychological flexibility, performance, interventions/programs, athletes

Introduction

Literature suggests that conventional methods of performance optimization demonstrate reduced effectiveness, so alternative strategies must be considered (Gardner and Moore 2006; Mosewich, Crocker, and Kowalski 2013; Neff and Germer 2013; Palmi, Planas and Solé 2018; Solé et al. 2014). However, psychology has increasingly become interested in the study and training of mindfulness and compassion. Mindfulness practice has deep roots in Buddhist tradition. More than 2,600 years ago, and again in the late 1970s, mindfulness began to be studied by psychologists and researchers, especially regarding stress reduction. More recently, so-called 'third wave' cognitive and behavioural therapies represent a new generation of psychological therapies that are increasingly being used in the treatment of several challenges and psychological problems and also foucus on the interplay of mindfulness, compassion and psychological flexibility, namely the ACT Model. The importance of psychological skills training (PST) in the development of athletic performance is widely recognized. Therefore, psychological skills are posited as effective for attaining optimal athletic performance, and the benefit of PST is widely reported. Although considerable scientific evidence is available regarding the efficacy of traditional psychological performance enhancement methods, some authors claim that sport psychology interventions have not been critically examined, and most studies investigating the efficacy of PST do not meet the criteria for evidence based empirical support. Hence why interest in mindfulness-based interventions has increased in sport psychology as a way to improve the performance of elite athletes (Gardner and Moore 2017; Kabat-Zinn 2003; Kaufman, Glass, and Pineau 2018). Therefore, the combination of Mindfulness-Based Stress Reduction practice (Kabat-Zinn 2003) with interventions focused on compassion and psychological flexibility, offer evidence-based alternatives that promote performance improved and sport injuries prevention in high performance context (Gardner and Moore 2017; Kaufman, Glass, and Pineau 2018; Mosewich, Crocker, and Kowalski 2013; Solé et al. 2014). Hence, this chapter shows as main objective to adapt and evaluate the effectiveness of a mindfulness-based program (MBSoccerP) in sport context. Additionally, it was intended to study the attributes that are involved in the performance of high competition, especially in team sports, in order to understand if strategies based on mindfulness, psychological flexibility and self-compassion promote optimal performance states, reduction of psychopathological symptoms (anxiety) and though suppression. Hence, a first literature review was conducted with the purpose of synthesizing the empirical results that portray the effectiveness of mindfulness-based programs in performance optimization in elite athletes. The purpose of this chapter is to summarize the empirical findings on the effectiveness of mindfulness-based programs to enhance soccer elite athletes performance. In a second moment, another objective is developing the questions about implement and effectiveness of the implementation of the Mindfulness-based program (MBSoccerP) to optimize the sport performance, based on mindfulness evidence based programs developed in sport context. "Mindful Sport Performance Enhancement" (MSPE) (Kaufman, Glass, and Pineau 2018); "Applying Self-Compassion in Sport" (Gilbert 2010; Mosewich et al. 2013; Tirch 2010); "Mindful Athlete" (Mumford 2015); "Mindfulness-Acceptance-Commitment Appraoch" (MAC) (Gardner and Moore 2007, 2012);

Mindfulness-Based Stress Reduction (MBSR) (KabatZinn 1985, 2003). The MBSoccerP program will be described in detail.

The difference between success and failure has become increasingly smaller in sport. A "third wave" approach in sport psychology has been used recently to increase the performance level of the elite athletes with very well-defined programs. (Birrer 2012, Gardner and Moore 2007; Gross et al. 2016). Study findings yielded that high-level athlete's meta-awareness and effective refocusing training by mindfulness-based programs were identified as important factors on performance training and competition (Carraça et al. 2018). Explore the conceptualization and implementation of the Mindfulness-Based Soccer Program (MBSoccerP) to optimize mindfulness, compassion in the elite soccer performance. This chapter allowed documenting advantages in participating in the Mindfulness- Based Soccer Program (MBSoccerP).

Mindfulness, Compassion and Psychological Flexibility

Contemporary psychology describes the concept of mindfulness as central to understanding mental health and well-being, and is conceptualized according to: (1) nonreactivity to internal experience; (2) observation of sensations, thoughts, emotions; (3) action with awareness, concentration and not distraction; (4) word description or label of the event; (5) and the non-judgment of experience (Segal et al. 2002). In this way it allows for a state of mindfulness, a form of non-elaborate, non-judgmental, and present-centered consciousness in which every thought, emotion, or sensation is noted and accepted as it arises (Kabat-Zinn 2003). In this context, emerge mindfulness-based studies on athlete characteristics and consequent performance - such as MBSR / MAC (Gardner and Moore 2004; Gross et al. 2016; Hyland 2011; Kabat-Zinn 2003; Schwanheusser 2009).

Compassion allows one to understand personal suffering as inherent in human life, thus maintaining a sense of connection with others. An individual with a high level of compassion does not suppress his most negative feelings but feels compassion for his experience and adopts a more balanced mental perspective - mindfulness (Kabat-Zinn 2003). Compassion is considered a fundamental positive emotional regulation strategy, characterized by negative and painful feelings that are not avoided, but rather are viewed with openness, warmth and kindness and a feeling of shared humanity.

Compassion is not just a feeling state, its not even a feeling state (which is argued in some models) so we must have the two components which is the stimulus engagement function which every motivation must have and the appropriate response function which every motivation must have. Humans however have cognitive abilities that allow them to work on both. So, a paper I often send round on sympathy and empathy highlights the fact that we can actually be compassion out of logic and moral choice and not feeling. We may want to be vengeful to somebody but are compassionate intent prevents us from acting on that and not causing harm.

Gilbert (2010) and Tirch, Schoendorff, and Silberstein (2014) conceptualizes compassion in evolutionary terms, arguing that compassion is an evolved motivational system designed to regulate negative affect, where compassion is seen to have originated from the same capacities that primates evolved to form attachment bonds and engage in affiliative and cooperative behaviors for group survival. He defines compassion as: "A deep awareness of the suffering of another coupled with the wish to relieve it" (Gilbert and Choden 2013). Gilbert (2010) and Tirch, Schoendorff, and Silberstein (2014) sees compassion as consisting of six 'attributes': sensitivity, sympathy, empathy, compassionate motivation, distress tolerance and non-judgement. 'Sensitivity' involves being responsive to other people's emotions and perceiving when they need help, 'Sympathy' (defined as showing concern for the other person's suffering); 'empathy' (defined as putting yourself in their shoes); 'compassionate motivation' involved the motivation to approach suffering with a specific intent and engage in helpful activity to help alleviate or prevent it.

Distress tolerance is defined as the ability to tolerate difficult emotions in oneself when confronted with someone else's suffering without becoming overwhelmed by them. Gilbert (2010) argues that this is important because if we over-identify with a person's suffering, we may feel a need to get away from them or reduce our awareness of their distress, preventing a compassionate response. This suggests that, although compassion is about 'suffering with' another person, if we feel such extreme personal distress in the face of another's suffering that we become too focused on our own discomfort, this may hinder our ability to help. The final element of Gilbert's model – 'nonjudgement' – is defined as the ability to remain accepting of and tolerant towards another person even when their condition, or response to it, gives rise to difficult feelings in oneself, such as frustration, anger, fear or disgust.

Compassion thus represents a balanced integration between preoccupation with self and preoccupation with others, which researchers recognize as essential to optimal functioning (Neff 2004). In this sense, self-compassion is closely related to the mindfulness concept. Both are conceptions of the narrative of human suffering and how to deal with it. The relationship between mindfulness and self-compassion has been described throughout several studies (Kabat-Zinn 2003; Neff 2009). According to Kabat-Zinn (2013), mindful attention "includes the quality of compassionate affection, self-righteousness, a sense of friendly presence towards oneself and others." Thus, self-compassion is clearly an adaptive way for the athlete to relate to his self and is associated with various characteristics of psychological well-being. Mindfulness training can promote increased self-compassion and consequently may be associated with improved well-being and optimal performance of athletes (Mosewich et al. 2011).

The three components of self-compassion are: kindness, common humanity, and mindfulness. These components combine and mutually interact to create a self-compassionate frame of mind.

Self-kindness is one component that means we are supportive and understanding toward ourselves. Our inner dialogues are gentle and encouraging rather than harsh and belittling. This means that instead of continually punishing ourselves for not being good enough, we kindly acknowledge that we're doing the best we can. Similarly, when external life circumstances are challenging and difficult to bear, we soothe and nurture ourselves. We are moved by our own distress so that warm feelings and the desire to ameliorate our suffering emerge.

Other component is *common humanity* that involves recognizing that everyone fails, makes mistakes, and gets it wrong sometimes. We do not always get what we want and are often disappointed – either in ourselves or in our life circumstances. This is part of the human experience, a basic fact of life shared with everyone else on the planet.

The third component is *mindfulness* that means that self-compassion entails mindful awareness of our negative thoughts and emotions so that they are approached with balance and equanimity. When we are mindful, we are experientially open to the reality of the present moment without judgment, avoidance, or repression (Bishop et al. 2004). Mindfulness of our negative thoughts and feelings means that we do not become "overidentified" (Neff 2003) with them, getting caught up and swept away by our aversive reactions (Bishop et al. 2004).

Finally, the concept of psychological flexibility complements the definition of mindfulness and self-compassion by taking into account the dynamic nature of behavior that unfolds over time. More specifically, psychological flexibility refers to "the ability to be more fully in the present moment as a conscious human being, and to change or persist in behavior when it serves valued ends" (Hayes et al. 2004). This ability can be reflected, for example, in how a person adapts to changing situational demands, reconfigures mental resources, shifts perspectives, and balances life's desires, needs, and goals (Kashdan and Rottenberg 2010). Thus, the definition of psychological flexibility also relates to people's behavior in their different environmental contexts. So, next we decrive the last components to enhance compassionate psychological flexibility in sport context.

- *Cognitive Defusion:* Cognitive fusion and awareness techniques are intended to alter the undesirable functions of thoughts or other intimate events, rather than to change their form, frequency, and situational sensitivity (Hayes et al. 2004). These procedures aim to reduce the literal quality of thinking, weakening the tendency to treat it more as a reference (e.g., "I'm not fine") than as a direct impression (e.g., thinking about not being well). The result of the defusion is usually a drop in belief or attachment to intimate events, not an immediate change in their frequency.

- *Be present:* promotion of constant, non-value contact with psychological and environmental events as they occur. The goal is to experience the world more directly so that their behavior becomes more exible and their actions more consistent with their values.
- *Self as Context:* due to relational frames such as Me vs. You, Now vs. Before, Here vs. there, human language generates a concept of itself as a place or perspective, giving a transcendental and spiritual facet to normal human speakers. The self as a context is partly important from this point of view, since the individual may be aware of his or her experience stream without necessarily being bound by it or an onslaught in which particular experiences occur, thus inciting defusion and acceptance.
- *Values:* Values are qualities chosen for the purpose that they can never exist as objects, but as examples to be reached step by step. In COMPACT approach, acceptance, defusion, and being present do not have an end in themselves but are the most effective means for a life of more consistent and crucial values.
- *Commitment action:* encouragement of the development of broader standards of effective action linked to the values chosen. On the other hand, these attempts lead the individual into contact with psychological barriers addressed through other ACT processes (acceptance, defusion, etc.).

MINDFUL-COMPASSION AND PSYCHOLOGICAL FLEXIBILITY APPROACH ON ELITE SOCCER

The purpose of this chapter is to summarize the empirical findings on the effectiveness of mindful compassion and psychological flexibility-based programs to enhance elite athletes sport performance. More specifically a Mindfulness-based program for soccer athletes.

Despite methodological limitations in the research design, the literature shows MAC (Gardner and Moore 2007, 2012), MSPE (Kaufman, Glass, and Pineau 2018) and MBSoccerP (Carraça et al. 2018, 2019b) programs as effective on enhancing elite athlete's sports performance. To confirm these preliminary results, further research, with improved experimental designs, is recommended. Findings yielded mindfulness programs as an important factor on elite sport performance.

The MBSoccerP to optimize the sport performance is based on mindfulness evidence-based programs developed in sport context: *Mindful Sport Performance Enhancement*" (MSPE)(Kaufman, Glass, & Pineau 2018); "*Applying Self-Compassion in Sport*" (ASCS) (Mosewich, Crocker, Kowalski, & DeLongis 2013; Gilbert 2010; Tirch 2010); "*Mindful Athlete*" (MA) (Mumford 2015); "*Mindfulness-Acceptance-Commitment Appraoch*" (MAC) (Gardner, & Moore 2012, 2007); "*Mindfulness-Based Stress Reduction*" (MBSR) (Kabat-Zinn 2003; Kabat-Zinn, Lipworth, & Burney 1985). The MBSoccerP program will be described in detail.

The difference between success and failure has become increasingly smaller in sport. A "third wave" approach in sport psychology has been used recently to increase the performance level of the elite athletes with very well-defined programs (Gardner and Moore 2007; Gross et al. 2016).

Study findings yielded that high-level athlete's meta-awareness and effective refocusing training by mindfulness-based programs were identified as important factors on performance training and competition (Carraça et al. 2018).

Explore the conceptualization and implementation of the MBSoccerP to optimize mindfulness, compassion in the elite soccer performance. Secondary aims are: understand the relationship between attributes of mindfulness traits and self-compassion - the impact on the state of sports performance and dispositional flow; the relation between psychological symptoms, experiential avoidance and consequent effect on the level of anxiety and sports performance.

Jon Kabat-Zinn et al. (1985) are the first on record to use mindfulness meditation training within sport. Rowers preparing for the Olympics independently practiced mindfulness meditation (using guided tapes once or twice per day, and for fifteen-minute sessions) for two to seven weeks prior to the Olympic Games. Once per week group meditation training sessions were also provided. Kabat-Zinn et al. (1985) reported that some of the U.S. Olympic team rowers who medaled reported the usefulness of mindfulness meditation in helping them optimize performance when racing. More recently, another group of researchers reported initial beneficial findings from mindfulness meditation for sport intervention (Thompson et al. 2011). Recently, mindfulness training has gained traction as a viable alternate approach to prepare athletes for optimal performance (Carraça et al. 2018; De Petrillo et al. 2009; Gardner and Moore 2012).

A mindfulness emphasis includes accepting psycho-emotional experience. Conceptually, mindfulness is about paying attention in a particular way, on purpose, non-judgmentally, in the present moment. Being in the present, which means not dwelling on the past participating future events such as winning or losing. In fact, when athletes describe being in the zone, they often describe a sense of being fully aware and on the present moment.

Mindfulness-based interventions teach tolerance and acceptance of negative thoughts, feelings and emotions. This differs from the traditional implementation of psychological skills training in sport psychology, with the main skills including goal setting, arousal regulation, visualization, and self-talk. Such cognitive behavioral interventions are focused primarily on intentionally controlling one's thoughts, feelings and behaviors, and not regulate them as a mind mode of being.

Mindful individuals perceive barriers or distractions as less relevant or bothering. Moreover, mindful student athletes have a high sense of control and use positive self-talk (Kee and Wang 2008). Relationships between behavior-related cognitions and exercise may become stronger among mindful athletes (Hagger and Chatzisarantes 2007). Taking part in mindfulness training was found to influence a sense of control among athletes (Aherne, Moran, and Lonsdale 2011). Mindfulness reflects a rather general tendency to respond in an insightful and open manner and it may constitute one of the personal resources promoting stronger self-efficacy, and therefore, may indirectly predict sport outcomes (Carraça et al. 2019; Walach et al. 2006). According to the models explaining sport performance there is a relation between self-regulatory beliefs, such as self-efficacy, and mindfulness. Mindfulness is likely to prompt self-regulatory cognitions. Furthermore, dispositional mindfulness (described as the tendency to be mindful in everyday life) is directly related to sport performance (Demarzo et al. 2015; Sole et al. 2014).

Crucial traits of mindfulness are nonjudgmental acceptance, openness to experiences and insight. Mindfulness contributes to both high levels of awareness and acceptance of in the moment reality (Hayes et al. 2004). Aligned with the core tenant of mindfulness is the concept of acceptance, which can be conceptualized as "taking a stance of nonjudgmental awareness and actively embracing the experience of thoughts, feelings and bodily sensations as they occur" (Kabat-Zinn 2013).

The hypothesized link between mindfulness, compassion and performance may refer to the altering perceptions of barriers and sense of control over oneself and the environment. Conceptually, self-compassion aids in changing maladaptive thoughts, feelings and behaviors by allowing and individual to evaluate the self without self-condemnation, promoting more accurate perceptions of the situation. Research in psychology show that self-compassion may play an important role in emotion regulation, and also show associations with a variety of adaptive outcomes, including life satisfaction, happiness, positive affect, mastery goals, and negative associations to self-criticism, anxiety, depression, rumination, perfectionism (Mosewich et al. 2013). Despite the dearth of self-compassion literature and interventions research in sport, there are some studies inside and outside the sport context that have examined the effectiveness and impact of self-compassion interventions. Overall, the evidence suggest that self-compassion may protect against negative cognitions, emotions and behaviors, positioning it strongly for consideration in terms of potential application in sport domain. For example, studies have found that self-compassion was negatively related to shame proneness, social physique anxiety, fear of failure and fear of negative evaluation and support the idea that self-compassion could be particularly useful for athletes dealing with dysfunctional self-conscious emotions and self-evaluative thoughts and behaviors related to appearance and performance (Kilham et al. 2018). Also was found that self-compassion was negatively related to negative affect and several perfectionism components such as concern over mistakes, doubts about actions, and perceived coach pressure (Kowalski, and Ferguson 2014). Taken all together, mindfulness and self-compassion have potential to be applied to different sport areas and domains, where athletes seem to have difficulties with coping, dealing with negative emotions and cognitions, self-criticism, rumination.

Hence, we will present the MBSoccerP and its potential for enhance performance on elite soccer athletes. The protocol presented here comprehend nine 90-120-minute sessions, delivered weekly to groups of soccer athletes. The protocol is presented in its entirety, and no background in psychology, mindfulness, compassion, or on sport sciences is required to benefit from the content. However, when implementing MBSoccerP, trainers can use their knowledge in sport performance, clinical and sport psychology, mindfulness, compassion and experiential acceptance models, and the people they are training to tailor the intervention to participants 'unique competition needs.

Many sport psychology programs provide a basic outline of various mental skills that elite athletes can use to improve their sports work and help their team goals; however, the MBSoccerP links mental skills with the concept of flow awareness, mindfulness, compassion, and psychological flexibility as a change skill, which is the tool that allows on the game a quick mental decisions to be add that radically change a thought process to enhance performance. The MBSoccerP try to be a powerful vehicle for soccer players change because, at list, brings the athlete to the only crucial game moment of importance- the present moment they play on the pitch, and also try to fit both a way of being or living and it is also a tool on can use to build compassion flow and mental flexibility.

MBSoccerP training athletes to look at a range of possibilities and then choosing the best mental approach or decision for their game situation. Hence, MBSoccerP training optimize mindful-compassion key steps that needs to be used by soccer players to experience most of the traditional psychological skills tools like positive and negative thinking, flow, self talk, goal setting, imagery and recovery.

A Specific Mindful-Compassion and Psychological Flexibility Intervention for Soccer Athletes / A Specific Program Approach: MBSoccerP

The MBSoccerP program was developed for elite soccer athletes. This study represents a first step to establish the role of MBSoccerP training as a tool for improve peak performance in sport (Carraça et al. 2018; Kabat-Zinn 2013; Kowalski and Ferguson 2014; Serpa 2017), and sport injury rehabilitation (Mosewich et al. 2014; Sole et al. 2014) and to evaluate the impact of the program. The MBSoccerP has 9 sessions, once weekly for 90/120 minutes, during 8 weeks. The content for each session was developed based on the modified MBSR (Kabat-Zinn 2013), Mindfulness Acceptance and Commitment Program (Gardner and Moore 2012), and Compassion Mind Training (Gilbert 2018; Tirch et al. 2014) material.

Main sessions have the following sequence: review previous session, homework and overall MBSoccerP; centering exercise; short introduction to the topic of the present session task focused exercise; hatha yoga/ stretching exercises (e.g., centering, breath meditation, compassion imagery, defusion metaphors, values and goals, action plans, body scan and mindfulness meditation) role plays, fill worksheets exercises and short talks and group discussion regarding their own reflections and experiences that were related to session's topic plan for future practice; at the end of each session, the participants are given homework assignment that was given presently or sent electronically to each player's e-mail address; mindful-compassion meditation. A more detailed MBSSoccerP content of the nine main topics covered in each session of the program is outlined in Table 1.

Table 1. Mindfulness-Based Soccer Program Structure – MBSoccerP (obtained and adapted from Carraça et al. 2018, 2019)

	Key concepts/Learning Goals	Experiential and Psycho-educational Training	After-Session Assignment
1- Introduction to MBSoccerP Mindfulness and sports	-Definition of Mindfulness; -Definition of Flow -Stress:Responding *vs.* Reacting to Stimulus; -Awareness the best mental tool; - Attention; - The mindful athlete	-3 Minutes meditation - Mindful breathing - Mindful eating	- Breath Meditation - STOP technique - Check in to informal and formal practice - Selected pre, match and post match worksheets - Simple Awareness and/or Mindful Eating
2 - Mindfulness of the Body and mind-self-talk	- Body as an anchor to present/conduit for experience; - Pleasant & Unpleasant *vs.* mindfulness and positive & negative thinking experiences; - Automatic pilot and sport mechanics	- Body Scan - Raisin exercise - The mindfulness solution: Aware, Accept and Action mindfulness and self talk: red thoughts mean stop; yellow is neutral and green is go ("I can do it"); - Metaphor feed the tiger/unwelcome party guest	- Body Scan -Selected Readings/worksheets Remember and repete: Aware, Accept and Action -Body Scan, Sitting Meditation. - Pleasant Events Calendar
3 - Mindfulness and Goal Setting versus Process Goals	- How mind hold the body back; -Goals and Values; - Performance values	-Process goals exercise- ARMS: Action oriented, Realistic, measurable; sequential Performance values and value-driven behavior: Mind is not your friend, and thank your mind, the voice in my head. Mindful yoga Smart Goals: Soothing-Supportive; Specific; Meaningful; accountable/attach/Associate; resources; Time.	- Kindness Meditation - Meditation on Smart Phone App/ email audio exercise -Selected Readings/Worksheets /defusion rate form Mindful Yoga (Yoga 1), Body Scan, Sitting. - Unpleasant Events Calendar

Sessions	Key concepts/Learning Goals	Experiential and Psycho-educational Training	After-Session Assignment
		- Introducing mindful yoga for beginners	
4 - Building a Mindfulness Practice-Thoughts	- Formal *vs.* informal practice -Integrating practice and competition -Finding a home in the body - Helpful practice for athletes Commitment -Content and physically experienced processes; - Removing judgment and self-criticism; Cognitive fusion -Methods of experiencing thought (timing, counting, listening, thought process visualizations)	-Mindfulness of thoughts - Mindful yoga	-Noting Meditation -Relax, Ground, and Clear Meditation -Mediation on thoughts, Smart Phone App/ email audio exercise -Selected Readings/ Worksheets STOP: The One Minute Breathing Space Mindful Yoga (Yoga 2) and Sitting
5 - Emotions, meaning in sports life. Radical acceptance	-What are emotions and physical sensations; -No Bad or shameful emotions -Identifying/ labeling to mitigate impact; Experiential avoidance - Emotion lifespan; - Mindfulness of emotions pre, match, post match	- Finding a home in the body Mindful yoga -Values and committed action Importance of acceptance versus resignation Letting go RAIN four step process: Recognize, Allow, Investigate, and Non-Identification	-Finding a home in the body -Creating a Practising committed action Everything is perfect as it is -Ongoing formal and informal practice
6 - Mindfulness and imagery	Flow Exposure Sport mindfulness Common problems Focus on the task	Mindful yoga Imagery as a tool to. Recall success; Rehearse a game plan; remain focused; remind your goal Compassion imagery exercise on sport context. Awareness of your best performance. Review of 3 A´s of mindfulness: Aware, Accept and Action	Ongoing practice Compassion imagery Remember and repeat: Aware, Accept and Action Selected pre, match and post match worksheets Body Scan, Sitting, Yoga *(+ Mountain or Lake Med.)*

Table 1. (Continued)

Sessions	Key concepts/Learning Goals	Experiential and Psycho-educational Training	After-Session Assignment
6a - Silent mindful running and self compassion		Silent Mindful Walking/mindful running in nature (90-120 minutes) The compassionate letters	Ongoing practice - Mindfulness in breathing one minute meditation - Mindful walking - Body scan Receiving affection from friends, strangers and enemies - Metta (to others and oneself)
7 - Mindfulness Acceptance and Compassion-Body connection & athlete recovery	Ways of training compassion: receiving compassion, showing compassion to oneself and to others Fear of compassion. Shame	Mindfulness of emotions Mindful yoga Loving Kindness Exercise/compassion flow/imagery The compassionate letters experience review	Ongoing practice Breathing practice - 3-minute breathing space in pairs - Closing meta Body Scan, Sitting, Yoga *(+ Lovingkindness)* Mindful Eating, STOP, etc.
8 - Ending MBSoccerP		Body scan review Compassion sport imagery Defusion, values, flow and acceptance review. Mindful yoga	Enhance ongoing MBSoccerP practice

Several specific interventions were used. For example, Mindful Walking and Mindful Breathing are meditations that involve focusing on a specific action or experience of the body in he present moment. The STOP exercises connect emotions and thoughts to the body when experiencing stress; Body Scan involves concentration on specific areas of the body; and Self Compassion Letters and Loving Kindness is a meditation on positive wishes and intention for one's self. Each session also contained a meditation to complete throughout the week and self-guided readings. Additionally, worksheets and email audio applications were introduced to participants could track their mindful compassion training, performance and complete corresponding meditations between each session.

Here are a few key components of practicing mindfulness, compassion and acepptance that key we have identified, set in the context of soccer:

1. At the beginning of the game, on the beginning of second half: Pay close attention to your breathing, especially when you're feeling intense emotions, nerves or frustration. Use the breath as an anchor to come out of your mind and into the body. Re-centre yourself on the present. Decide to accept the feelings you have, let them go, don't judge or rebuke yourself. Once you do this you will be able to smile and enjoy the situation you find yourself in - embrace the challenge.
2. When about to hit a corner, free kick or on a penalty kicks: Notice - really notice - what you're sensing in a given moment, the texture of the pitch below you, the sound of the ball, and the smells that ordinarily slip by without reaching your conscious awareness. - At finals: Recognise that your thoughts and emotions are fleeting and do not define you. Accept they will happen and let them go. Having this insight can free you from negative thought patterns. Try focus into your body's physical sensations, from the cool breeze on your skin to the way your feet feel against the ground when you feed in a ball.
3. When dealing with a confrontational coach, president club or another player when faced with a tense and difficult conversation, imagine a divider between the situation and yourself; give yourself space. This space provided will give you room to focus on your body and relax the areas that are tense or tight. Do this while staying present in the situation i.e., don't rush ahead and compose your response or argument, simply breathe and stay with the moment. Get out of your own head and listen intently to the player or club president while still keeping on eye on your body's reactions. Accept the emotions you are feeling as normal. Take time with your response and be empathetic so as not to let the situation escalate. Finally, when a player is nervous before an important match out a match focus on your breath (or any part of your body that you feel most natural to focus on). Use this focus to bring you back into the present. Your breath is controllable, this

point, focus on what is controllable and gently guide your attention back to this. Use it tactically on the flow game situations.

MBSoccerP Program Evaluation, Treatment Fidelity and Compliance

Pre and post-test evaluation are purpose and design for the program and in the last session the participants are asked to complete a brief written evaluation of the program where they answered open-ended questions about if and how they perceived that the program changed the ways they act or think inside the soccer. To maintain the fidelity to the contents and program consistency of the program and protocol the first author of the current study led the intervention and conduct the sessions. He is a clinic and sport psychologist and an experienced mindfulness-based practitioner and had received training in Mindfulness-based interventions and 3° CBT wave interventions on health, clinical and sport settings. Participation in session was recorded. In addition, in their weekly workbooks participants were asked to complete a record of minutes meditated immediately after each home-meditation session. The main purpose of the interception forms was to encourage reflection on awareness of body sensations, but these forms also provided some information regarding adherence to mindfulness-compassion training through representing internalization of aspects of mindfulness and compassion (Demarzo et al. 2015). Compliance is measured by noting class attendance and assessing the frequency and duration of formal mindfulness practice and the frequency of informal mindfulness practice (i.e., breath awareness and daily life mindfulness).

Overall, literature and studies point out that athletes who train psychological skills based on psychological flexibility, self-pity and mindfulness exhibit higher levels of flow state and sports performance (Gardner, Moore 2017; Kabat-Zinn 2005; Kaufman, Glass, and Pineau 2018; Palmi and Planas 2018; Solé et al. 2014). The results further suggest that the MBSoccerP program seems to function as a buffer for the suppression of thoughts, athlete anxiety and high-performance psychological symptoms, mainly determined by the attributes of self-compassion and mindfulness facets.

PRACTICAL IMPLICATIONS OF THE PROGRAM

The literature suggest that the development of attentional skills, self-compassion and psychological flexibility seem to be an aspect that deserves consideration when it comes to intervention and work with elite athletes. Thus, relevant benefits were achieved and of practical significance.

The MBSoccerP program design shows potential to be successfully replicated among athletes of different sports and can be a good intervention tool to be requested by coaches, sport staff and even used by clinical and sports psychologists. This program also intends to address the need for integration of clinical and sport psychologists in technical teams and/or medical departments, assisting and promoting evidence-based mental coaching.

Also we can point out practical implications for athletes and coaches. Firstly, the results of studies suggest that MBSoccerP-focused performance optimization strategies increase mindfulness and result in implications for experiential living during sporting tasks, as well as aspects of your personal, family and personal life. relational (Jackson 2016; Kaufman, Glass, and Pineau 2018; Palmi and Riera 2017, Palmi, Planas, and Solé 2018). The 2nd practical application refers to the factors that need to be considered when implementing mindfulness-based interventions with high performance athletes. Given the stringent demands of high competition and its context, it has been found that the implementation of the MBSoccerP program meets the literature, which recommends brief, flexible and practical mindfulness interventions in the sports context (Balztell and Akhtar 2014; Humphrey, Yow and Bowden 2000; Ivarsson et al. 2015; Moore and Gardner 2014).

Third, when considering the "optimal dosage" of each session, researchers, MBSoccerP program trainers (e.g., clinical and sports psychologists, sports medicine specialists, and other professionals with previous training in the program) need be aware of the demanding nature of high performance, and remain flexible and attentive to the use of "sporting time" where pressure for results is high, where athletes' schedules are tight, and where sudden scheduling changes may occur.

As a result, this can lead to non-consecutive session ordering or sudden changes in session duration, so the adaptation and minimum criteria of evidence-based programs must always be met for program effectiveness. In most cases, the coach determines that these changes need to be implemented to best meet the team's needs. MBSoccerP trainers may need a pre-implementation plan, which, while flexible, is negotiated with the coaching team to meet and understand the reality of the competitive context.

Alternatively and as a complement to the sessions, athletes should be encouraged to practice mindfulness, compassion and small exercises of psychological flexibility between sessions, becoming a habit of athletes' daily lives. However, given the sporting demands that athletes face, it is suggested to practice minimalistic practice (e.g., mindfulness exercise in one-minute STOP) so as not to result in lack of adherence to the practice.

Finally, the importance of contributing to the scientific robustness and evaluation of the program and in this area of intervention based on mindfulness, compassion and psychological flexibility, ie both field professionals and researchers, may consider data collection (pre- and post-implementation of the program) using mixed methods tools for better insight into the effectiveness of the intervention.

Overall, the contribution to the practical implications stems from the positive and promising results of mindfulness-based interventions, and specifically from MBSoccerP, in increasing the dispositional flow state (indirect measure of performance evaluation); and relief from psychological distress and anxiety associated with competitive tasks and periods of high workload.

MBSoccerP was also effective in perceiving increased performance measured directly by program participants and their coaches. Increasing the mindfulness, self-pity and psychological flexibility traits worked within the program increase the potential for competitive success of athletes and their teams. These results are still important because they translate a set of useful strategies for the protection of physical and mental fatigue and the respective sports performance crises caused by the high competitive frequency.

CONCLUSION

The Mindfulness- Based Soccer Program (MBSoccerP) seems to have impact in increasing the attributes of mindfulness, compassion, psychological flexibility, and in which terms that mediates dispositional flow and peak performance on elite soccer players. This program seems to work as a stress and suppression thoughts buffer.

MBSoccerP is unique being one of the first mindful-compassion based intervention programs available that was developed especially for elite soccer athletes. Is at the end, a step-by step program in cultivating fundamental mindfulness, compassion and psychological flexibility (ACT) skills and then executing those skills within their athletic endeavours. Research (Carraça et al. 2018, 2019) and experiences with the program have made us quite excited about its sport performance enhancement. Worthwhile change is rarely easy, so engagement on MBSoccerP training try to be a new way of approaching Elite soccer sport.

Birrer et al. (2012) and Gardner and Moore (2012) ssuggested that increase in mindfulness may modify the nature of the experience of emotions and cognitions such as anxiety and rumination rather than lessen them. The results of the study have practical implications for athletes and coaches. Together with findings of previous research, the results suggest that training athletes in MBSoccerP increases their mindfulness, experimental acceptance, self-compassion, flow and peak performance. Increasing athletes' mindfulness, compassion and psychological flexibility has implications for athletes' experience during sporting events as well as aspects of their life outside of sport.

In summary, despite the scarcity of literature and studies in this area, the findings provided initial evidence supporting the potential of mindfulness, self-compassion and psychological flexibility training in professional soccer athletes, can be positive or effective. For exemple, the MBSoccerP program not only demonstrates effectiveness in the sports context, as well as promoting the improvement of mindfulness, body awareness, dispositional flow state, self-pity, psychological flexibility and a decrease in psychological distress (anxiety) and suppression of thought, in line with the literature (Kaufman, Glass, and Pineau 2018; Palmi and Solé 2016; Solé et al. 2014).

It is also noteworthy that in order to legitimize the dissemination of these constructs and implement the respective interventions in the sports context, it is crucial to promote interest in practices and interventions based on mindfulness traits, deep living in the present moment, compassionate attributes of relief from psychological suffering, and in defining a life purpose, taking into account the transience of each and every sporting experience. Thus, the importance of preserving and cultivating the habit of regular practice of mindfulness and self-compassion during and after the conclusion of the intervention is the implementation of the MBSoccerP program (Carraça et al. 2018, 2019; Palmi and Riera 2017; Palmi, Planas, and Solé 2018; Solé et al. 2014). Also represents a first step in the introduction and incorporation of interventions based on third generation cognitive behavioral models, in the context of high competition football in Portugal, by presenting the elaboration of a program with the theoretical assumptions and practices explained. Throughout the thesis, specifically the MBSoccerP program.

References

Aherne, Cian, Aidan M. Moran, and Chris Lonsdale. 2011. "The Effect of Mindfulness Training on Athletes' Flow: An Initial Investigation." *The Sport Psychologist* 25: 177–189. doi: 10.3389/fnbeh.2015.00229.

Baltzell, Amy, and Vanessa L. Akhtar. 2014. "Mindfulness Meditation Training for Sport (MMTS) Intervention: Impact of MMTS with Division I Female Athletes." *The Journal of Happiness and Well-being* 2: 160-173.

Bishop, Scott R., Mark A. Lau, Shauna Shapiro, Linda Carlson, Nicole D. Anderson, James Carmody, Zindel Segal, Susan Abbey, Michael Speca, Drew Velting, and Gerald Devins. 2004. "Mindfulness: A Proposed Operational Definition." *Clinical Psychology: Science and Practice* 11: 230-241.

Carraça, Bruno, Sidónio Serpa, António F. Rosado, and Joan Palmi. 2018. "A Pilot Study of a Mindfulness-Based Program (MBSoccerP): The Potential Role of Mindfulness, Self-Compassion and Psychological Flexibility on Flow and Elite Performance in Soccer Athletes." *Latin-American Journal of Exercise and Sports Psychology* 14: 33-39.

Carraça, Bruno, Sidónio Serpa, Joan Palmi, and António F. Rosado. 2018. "Enhance Sport Performance of Elite Athletes: The Mindfulness-Based Interventions." *Cuadernos de Psicología del Deporte* 18: 79-109.

Carraça, Bruno, Sidónio Serpa, António F. Rosado, and Joan Palmi. 2018. "The Mindfulness – Based Soccer Program (MBSoccerP): Effects on Elite Athletes." *Cuadernos de Psicología del Deporte* 18: 62-85.

Carraça, Bruno, Sidónio Serpa, António F. Rosado, and Joan Palmi. 2019. "Mindful-Compassion Strategies in Optimizing Performance of Elite Soccer Players: A Mindfulness-Based Soccer Program (MBSoccerP)." *Biomedical Journal of Scientific & Technical Research* 14: 1-7.

Carraça, Bruno, Sidónio Serpa, António F. Rosado, and Joan Palmi. 2019. "Mindful Compassion Training on Elite Soccer: Effects, Roles and Associations on Flow, Psychological Distress and Thought Suppression." *Latin-American Journal of Exercise and Sports Psychology* 14: 137-145.

Demarzo, Marcelo, Ricardo M. de Oliveira, Daniela F. Silva, Isadora Lessa-Moreno, Luiz C. de Abreu, Alberto Barceló, and Javier Garcia-Campayo. 2015. "Mindfulness Applied to High Performance Athletes: A Case Report." *Actas Espanholas de Psiquiatria* 43: 1-90.

De Petrillo Lillian A., Keith Kaufman, Carol R. Glass, and Diane B. Arnkoff. 2009. "Mindfulness for Long-Distance Runners: An Open Trial Using Mindful Sport Performance Enhancement (MSPE)." *Journal of Clinical Sport Psychology* 3: 357-376.

Gardner, Frank L., and Zella E. Moore. 2004. "A Mindfulness-Acceptance-Commitment Based Approach to Performance Enhancement: Theoretical Considerations." *Behavior Therapy* 35: 707-723.

Gardner, Frank L., and Zella E. Moore. 2006. *Clinical Sport Psychology*. Champaign, IL: Human Kinetics.

Gardner, Frank L., and Zella E. Moore. 2017. "Mindfulness- and Acceptance-Based Interventions in Sport and Performance Contexts." *Current Opinion in Psychology* 16: 180-184. doi: 10.1016/j.copsyc. 2017.06.001.

Gardner, Frank L., and Zella E. Moore. 2012. "Mindfulness and Acceptance Models in Sport Psychology: A Decade of Basic and Applied Scientific Advancements." *Canadian Psychology/Psychologie Canadienne* 53: 309-318.

Gardner, Frank L., and Zella E. Moore. 2007. *The Psychology of Enhancing Human Performance: The Mindfulness-Acceptance-Commitment (MAC) Approach*. New York: Springer.

Gilbert, Paul. 2010. *Compassion Focused Therapy. Distinctive Features*. London: Routledge.

Gilbert, Paul, and Choden. 2013. *Mindful Compassion*. London: Constable and Robinson.

Gilbert, Paul. 2009. *The Compassionate Mind: A New Approach to Life's Challenges*. London: Constable Robinson.

Gross, Mike, Zella E. Moore, Frank L. Gardner, Andrew T. Wolanin, Rachel Pess, and Donald R. Marks. 2016. "An Empirical Examination Comparing the Mindfulness-Acceptance-Commitment Approach and

Psychological Skills Training for the Mental Health and Sport Performance of Female Student Athletes." *International Journal of Sport and Exercise Psychology*. doi: 10.1080/1612197X.2016. 1250802.

Hagger, Martin S., and Nikos N. L. Chatzisarantis. 2007. *Intrinsic Motivation and Self-Determination in Exercise and Sport*. Human Kinetics: Champaign.

Haase, Lori, April C. May, Maryam Falahpour, Sara Isakovic, Alan N. Simmons, Steven D. Hickman, Thomas T. Liu, and Martin P. Paulus. 2015. "A Pilot Study Investigating Changes in Neural Processing After Mindfulness Training in Elite Athletes." *Front Behavior Neuroscience* 9: 229. doi: 10.3389/fnbeh.2015.00229.

Hayes, Steven C., Kirk Strosahl, Kelly G. Wilson, Richard T. Bissett, Jaqueline Pistorello, Dosheen Toarmino, Melissa A. Polusny, Thane A. Dykstra, Sonja V. Batten, John Bergan, Sherry H. Stewart, Michael J. Zvolensky, Georg H. Eifert, Frank W. Bond, John P. Forsyth, Maria Karekla, and Susan McCurry. 2004. "Measuring Experiential Avoidance: A Preliminary Test of a Working Model." *Psychological Record* 54: 553-578.

Humphrey, James H., Deborah A. Yow, and William W. Bowden. 2000. *Stress in college athletics: Causes, consequences, coping*. Binghamton, NY: The Haworth Half-Court Press.

Hyland, Terry. 2011. *Mindfulness and Learning: Celebrating the Affective Dimension of Education*. New York: Springer.

Ivarsson, Andreas, Urban Johnson, Mark B. Andersen, Johan Fallby, and Mats Altemyr. 2015. "It Pays to Pay Attention: A Mindfulness-Based Program for Injury Prevention with Soccer Players." *Journal of Applied Sport Psychology* 27: 319-334. doi:10.1080/10413200. 2015.1008.

Kabat-Zinn, Jon. 2013. *Full catastrophe living: Using the wisdom of your body and mind to face stress, pain and illness*. New York: Bantam/Random House.

Kabat-Zinn, Jon, Louis Lipworth, and Ronald Burney. 1985. "The Clinical Use of Mindfulness Meditation for the Self-Regulation of Chronic Pain." *Journal of Behavioral Medicine* 8:163-190.

Kabat-Zinn, Jon. 2003. "Mindfulness-Based Interventions in Context: Past, Present, and Future." *Clinical Psychology: Science and Practice* 10: 144-156.

Kabat-Zinn, Jon. 2005. *Coming to our Senses: Healing ourselves and the World through Mindfulness.* New York: Hyperion.

Kashdan, Todd B., and Jonathan Rottenberg. 2010. "Psychological Flexibility as a Fundamental Aspect of Health." *Clinical Psychology Review* 30: 865-878.

Kauffman, Keith, Carol R. Glass, and Diane B. Arnkoff. 2009. "Evaluation of Mindful Sport Performance Enhancement (MSPE): A New Approach to Promote Flow in Athletes." *Journal of Clinical Sports Psychology* 4: 334-356.

Kauffman, Keith, Carol R. Glass, and Timothy R. Pineau. 2018. *Mindful Sport Performance Enhancement. Mental Training for Athletes and Coaches.* Washington, DC: American Psychological Association.

Kee, Ying H., and John C. K. Wang. 2008. "Relationships between Mindfulness, Flow Dispositions and Mental Skills Adoption: A Cluster Analytic Approach." *Psychology of Sport and Exercise* 9: 393-411.

Kowalski, Kent, and Leah J. Fergunson. 2014. "Self-Compassion." In *Encyclopedia of Sport and Exercise Psychology,* edited by Robert C. Eklund, and Gershon Tenenbaum, 622-624. Thousand Oaks, CA: Sage.

Leary, Mark, Eleanor Tate, Claire Adams, Ashley B. Allen, and Jessica Hancock. 2007. "Self-Compassion and Reactions to Unpleasant Self-Relevant Events: The Implications of Treating Oneself Kindly." *Journal Personal Social Psychology* 92: 887-904.

Mosewich, Amber D., Peter R. Crocker, Kent C. Kowalski, and Anita Delongis. 2013. "Applying Selfcompassion in Sport: An Intervention with Women Athletes." *Journal of Sport & Exercise Psychology* 35: 514-524. doi: 10.1123/jsep.35.5.51.

Mosewich, Amber D., Kent C. Kowalski, Catherine M. Sabiston, Whitney A. Sedgwick, and Jessica L. Tracy. 2011. "Self-Compassion: a Potential Resource for Young Women Athletes." *Journal of Sport & Exercise Psychology* 33: 103-123.

Mumford, George. 2015. *The Mindful Athlete. Secrets to Peak Performance*. Berkeley, CA: Parallax press.

Neff, Kristin D. 2003. "The Development and Validation of a Scale to Measure Self-Compassion." *Self and Identify* 2: 223-250.

Neff, Kristin D. 2004. "Self-Compassion and Psychological Well-Being." *Constructivism in the Human Sciences* 9: 27-37.

Neff, Kristin D. 2009. "Self-Compassion." In *Handbook of Individual Differences in Social Behaviour.* Edited by Mark R. Leary and Rick H. Hoyle, 561-573. NY: Guilford.

Neff, Kristin D., and Christopher K. Germer. 2013. "A Pilot Study and Randomized Control Trial of the Mindful Self-Compassion Program." *Journal of Clinical Psychology* 69: 28-44.

Neff, Kristin D., Kristin L. Kirkpatrick, and Stephanie S. Rude. 2007. "Self-Compassion and Adaptive Psychological Functioning." *Journal of Research in Personality* 41: 139-154.

Palmi, Joan, Antoni Planas, and Silvia Solé. 2018. "Intervención Mindfulness de Rehabilitación de un Deportista Lesionado: Caso en Fútbol Profesional." [Rehabilitation Mindfulness Intervention of an Injured Athlete: Case in Professional Soccer.] *Revista de Psicologia del Deporte* 27: 115-122.

Palmi, Joan, and Joan Riera. 2017. "Las Competencias del Deportista para el Rendimento." [Athlete's Competencies for Performance.] *Cuadernos de Psicología del Deporte* 17: 13-18.

Schwanhausser, Lori A. 2009. "Application of the Mindfulness-Acceptance-Commitment (MAC) Protocol with an Adolescent Springboard Diver: The Case of Steve." *Journal of Clinical Sports Psychology* 3: 377-396.

Segal, Zindel V., Mark G. Williams, and John D. Teasdale. 2002. *Mindfulness-Based Cognitive Therapy for Depression*. New York: Guilford Press.

Serpa, Sidonio. 2018. Treinador e Atleta: a Relação Sagrada. In *Psicologia aplicada ao treinador esportivo,* edited by Benno Becker, pp. 18-67. Rio Grande do Sul: Editora Freevale.

Solé, Silvia, Bruno Carraça, Sidonio Serpa, and Joan Palmi. 2014. "Aplicaciones del Mindfulness (Conciencia Plena) en Lesión Deportiva." [Applications of Mindfulness (Full Consciousness) in Sports Injur.] *Revista de Psicología del Deporte* 23: 501-508.

Thompson, Rachel W., Keith A. Kaufman, Lilian A. De Petrillo, Carol R. Glass, and Diane B. Arnkoff. 2011. "One Year Follow-Up of Mindful Sport Performance Enhancement (MSPE) with Archers, Golfers, and Runners." *Journal of Clinical Sport Psychology* 5: 99-116. doi: 10.1123/jcsp.5.2.99.

Tirch, Dennis. 2010. "Mindfulness as a Context for the Cultivation for Compassion." *International Journal of Cognitive Psychotherapy* 3: 113-123.

Tirch, Dennis, Benjamin Schoendorff, and Laura R. Silberstein. 2014. *The ACT Practitioner's Guide to the Science of Compassion: Tools for Fostering Psychological Flexibility*. Oakland, CA: New Harbinger Publications.

Walach Harald, Nina Buchheld, Valentin Buttenmuller V, Norman Kleinknecht, and Stefan Schmidt. 2006. "Measuring Mindfulness - The Freiburg Mindfulness Inventory." *Personality and Individual Differences* 40: 1543-1555.

In: An Essential Guide to Sports Performance ISBN: 978-1-53617-608-7
Editors: Daniel Castillo Alvira et al. © 2020 Nova Science Publishers, Inc.

Chapter 9

WOMEN'S PARTICIPATION IN LEISURE CYCLING: A SCOTTISH PERSPECTIVE

Peigi Rodan, Andrew Martin*[*] *and Robert Nash
Creative and Cultural Business, Robert Gordon University, Aberdeen, Scotland

ABSTRACT

This paper aims to investigate overriding factors that prevent female participation in leisure cycling. There has been little written about the influence of individual attitudes and perceptions of bicycle use and even less has been written about female attitudes (Sener, Eluru and Bhat 2009). There is a general gap in research in terms of cycle tourism (for exceptions see Sheng 2015; Zovko 2013; Lumsdon 2000; Beanland 2013; Faulks, Richie and Dodd 2008; Heesch, Sahlqvist and Garrard 2012). However, there is even less research that looks at issues related to female constraints in leisure cycling. Shaw (1994) recognized the need to "remove constraints and to encourage increased opportunities for participation," in terms of LTPA (Shaw 1994 pp12). This research

[*] Corresponding Author's Email: a.martin@rgu.ac.uk.

combines literature on LTPA gender constraints, cycle tourism and cycling in general to contribute to the limited existing knowledge concerning female cycling constraints. Moreover, in contrast to other papers it considers personal attitudes, as well as objective constraints that previous research has been lacking (Raymore 2002). This paper intends to expose constraints in leisure cycling to better prepare governments and organizations to serve the female market that has a desire to cycle for leisure.

Keywords: leisure cycling; women's participation; constraints; Scotland

1. Introduction

1.1. Current Cycling Market

Cycle tourism is a popular leisure time physical activity (LTPA) and is a growing niche market, with cycling breaks growing by 10-15% in the UK (Mintel 2015). A huge increase has been noted in the utilization of the National Cycle Network (NCN) that joins bike paths throughout the UK. Sustrans is a UK charity that works to get fewer people driving and more people walking and cycling. They recorded a 170% increase in the usage of the NCN between 2003 and 2010 (Zovko 2013). Growth in cycling has been driven by the National Cycle Network (NCN) (Beanland 2013; Zovko 2013; Sustrans Scotland 2014), the Olympic games (Grous 2011) and cycling groups that provide social support (Fullagar and Pavlidis 2012).

Cycling takes many forms from competitive cycling to utility cycling and leisure cycling. Leisure cycling has been interpreted as both cycle tourism (Lumsdon 1996) and recreational cycling (Ritchie 1998). The economic value of this niche market in Europe is approximately 44 Billion Euros per annum (Adventure Cycling Association, 2012). Most of this is generated within countries where cycling is more popular than the UK such as Germany and the Netherlands (Beanlands 2013). British interest in cycle tourism is small in comparison with just 7% of adults taking up leisure cycling in the UK (Mintel 2015). However, this is not to say the industry is not contributing significantly to the British economy. Scotland alone generates between £106 – £108 million in direct expenditure every year (Zovko 2013). Indeed, cycling is the 4th most popular recreational activity in the UK (Fullagar 2012) and 45% of the utilization of the National Cycle Network is for leisure purposes (Sustrans 2012).

1.2. Gender Constraints

There is an existing gender gap in participation in cycling in the UK, both in terms of utility (for commuting or transport use) and for leisure, recreation and physical activity (Heesch 2012; Mintel 2015; Sheng 2015; Dalton 2010). However, most of the research on gender imbalance is heavily concentrated on the limits that females face in utility cycling and often disregards leisure cycling barriers (Privitera 2013; Pucher, Buehler and Seinen 2011; Gatersleben and Haddad 2010; Pojani et al. 2017). These barriers appear to be particularly prominent in the UK, Australasia and North America with females typically cycling more in the Netherlands, Germany, Denmark and Switzerland (Gòmez et al. 2005; Heesch 2012). There are also good levels of research into the subject area of gender and leisure as well as the constraints females face in society in terms of their approach to leisure activities. It suggests that in high school, physical activity is not only gendered but is also primarily aimed at males, creating a culture of apathy amongst females (Allender, Cowburn and Foster 2006; Flintoff and Scraton 2001; Flintoff 2008). Moreover, it is evident that females prefer to participate in female only sports and are deterred from activities that include male participants (Lloyd and Little 2010). Cycling is not known to be gender specific and it remains unclear why females in some countries participate less in the activity even though it can be pursued without males.

1.3. Benefits of Leisure Cycling and Female Participation

The invention of the modern bicycle contributed to the emancipation of females and the design where wheels are of equal size was created to cater for female dress (Dando 2007). The bicycle gave females liberty and a new found freedom to travel greater distances. The bicycle has gained in popularity, with bicycle output quadrupling internationally since the 1970's (Fullagar 2012). This popularity could be in part due to people's desire to use motorized vehicles less due to cost saving and environmental concerns (Lumsdon, 2000, Privitera, 2013, Sener, Eluru and Bhat 2009). Dalton (2010) discusses women's willingness to adapt behavior as a means of protecting the environment, suggesting openness to change in the right circumstances. Social benefits of cycle tourism have also been recognized (Faulks, Ritchie and Dodd 2008; Fullagar, and Pavlidis 2012). In fact, it was found that women perceived environmental and social factors as key motivators in their desire to participate in cycling (Heesch, Sahlqvist and Garrard 2012). With these factors, along with the economic benefits cycling can bring a nation (Grous 2011), it seems worthwhile to try and understand societal and personal factors that lead to constraints in female involvement, despite clear desire to participate. Evidence also suggests that in places where female cycling is more prominent and the gender gap is considerably smaller, overall cycling participation and frequency is higher (Emond, Tang and Handy 2009).

2. Literature Review

2.1. Leisure Cycling Gender-Gap

Literature contains multiple definitions of "leisure cycling." This paper adopts the definition from Faulks, Ritchie and Dodd (2008) who recognize leisure cycling and recreational cycling as interchangeable including day trips close to and away from the home as well as long distance and overnight trips on bicycles. This definition has been adopted because day trips are the most common type of leisure cycling, which makes it the most obvious choice from a research perspective (Zovko 2013). Females are generally less likely to partake in leisure and tourism cycling than males in countries such as the UK, Canada, the USA and Australia (Fullagar and Pavlidis 2012; Heesch, Sahlqvist and Garrard 2012; Putcher, Buehler and Seinen 2011). Both Faulks Ritchie and Dodd (2008) and Heesch, Sahlqvist and Garrard's (2012) papers used quantitative data to generate information on cyclists. The fact that their feedback was primarily from men (over two thirds in both) highlights the underrepresentation of women in leisure cycling. However, it should be noted that both research papers were carried out in Australia but, it is clear the UK is also subject to under representation of women. Women are 50% less likely than men to exhibit interest in cycling holidays (Mintel 2015). In countries such as the Netherlands, Germany and Denmark, where the leisure cycle industry is much larger (Beanland 2013) the proportion of females that cycle for leisure is similar to that of males (Heesch, Sahlqvist and Garrard 2012). Although the UK is falling behind in female participation in comparison to its European neighbors, it is advancing in that the gender gap is slowly decreasing (Figure 1) and it's cycling culture is greater than in some other developing countries. Gómez (2000) discusses the cycling culture in Lima Peru. In Peru woman's usage of a bicycle is referred to as exceptional due to its rarity. Gómez et al. (2005) also discusses the gender gap in cycling in Bogotá, Columbia suggesting that females cycle less than males. Although cycling in western societies such as the UK is increasing with a 6% rise from 2013 to 2015 (Mintel 2016) a gender gap is undeniable.

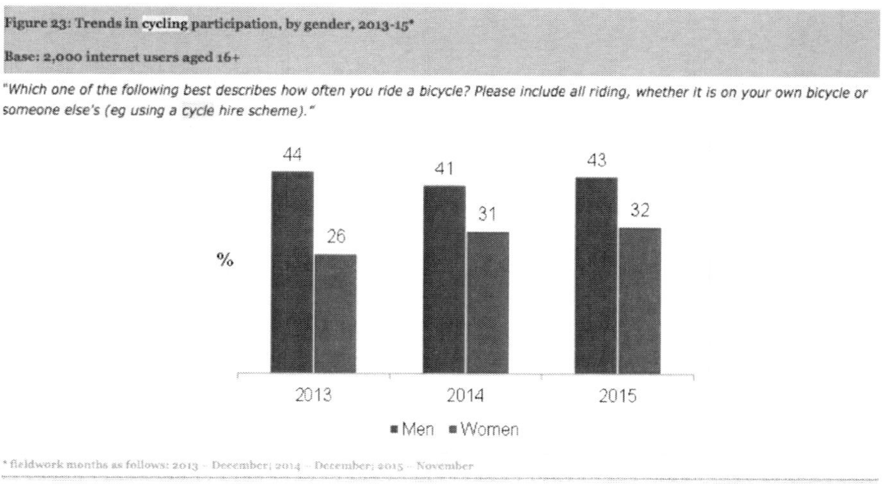

Figure 1. (Mintel 2016).

2.2. Implications of Cycling for Females

It is estimated that cycling saves the Scottish NHS £4 million a year (Zovko 2013) and saves the British economy £128m (Grous 2011) per year. Conversely however, one should also consider the health risks of cycling. A review by Hartog et al. (2010) found that because cyclists are doing exercise they inhale a higher volume of air than drivers. Consequently, cycling could have a detrimental effect on participants' health, although this could be more constraining to the utility cyclist than the leisure cyclist. The literature does not specify that leisure cycling is city bound, and Christmas et al. (2010) found leisure cycling to be more prominent on types of terrain uncommon for utility cyclists such as: forest's, parks, bike tracks rail trails and beaches. Therefore, one cannot simply rule out the detrimental effects air pollution may have on cyclists however, it should be considered a larger threat to utility cyclists than to leisure cyclists.

According to the World Health Organization (WHO) obesity is one of the top-ten health risks people face today (World Health Organization 2000). Only 25% of British females are meeting the recommended benchmark of physical activity compared with 44% of men (British Heart Foundation 2015). LTPA can be seen as difficult, however walking and cycling are recognized as activities that can help women meet the recommended amount of aerobic exercise (Hartog et al. 2010). This is due to the availability and access (Pucher et al. 2010) of cycling as well as the cyclist's primary motivation of enjoyment (Pojani et al. 2017). If more females took up leisure cycling, they could reap the benefits which would both empower them and allow them to enjoy the great outdoors (Henderson 2013).

2.3. Implications of Leisure Cycling in the Tourism Industry

Cycling tourism has the potential to contribute to both the tourism industry and overall GDP of a nation (Beanland 2013; Zovko 2013; Privitera 2013.) Moreover, leisure cyclists spend 9% more than utility cyclists (Rajè and Saffrey 2016) and 20% more than tourists traveling in a vehicle (Belter, Harten and Sorof 2012). Although the cycle market does bring considerable revenue to the UK, cycling levels are still relatively low, making up 2% of overall transport (Department of Transport 2014). Moreover, it is noted that by increasing female participation, cycling overall would grow due to the creation of a cycling culture (Emond, Tang and Handy 2009). This is the case in the Netherlands, where the economic benefit is so high due to the culture being so strong amongst females, who make up a larger population of cyclists than males (Heesch, Sahlqvist and Garrard 2012). From a tourism perspective touring cyclists, cycling event participants and spectators are important (Faulks, Richie and Dodd 2008). However, indirect expenditure is also important with the purchases of food as well as spending associated with visiting other tourism destinations (Beanland 2013). Cycle tourism is also important for its ability to strengthen rural areas that struggle economically (Belter, Harten and Sorof 2012). A final observation is the potential for the growth of leisure cycling to be used as a tool to encourage more overall cycling in the UK. Christmas et al. (2010) discuss commuter cyclist's tendencies leading to increased participation in leisure cycling. In transforming non-leisure cyclists into leisure cyclists, the overall cycling industry could see growth in utility cyclists due to the confidence people can gain from leisure cycling.

2.4. Constraint Theory

Little has been done in regards to female leisure cycling constraints. Much of the current literature concentrates heavily on the gender gap in LTPA, but seldom considers cycling as a specific activity (Shaw 1994; Henderson and Gibson 2003; Lloyd and Little 2010; Buckworth et al. 2007; Flintoff 2008 and Allender, Cowburn and Foster 2006). However, the theories used throughout the literature can be applied to constraints in leisure cycling. A recurring theory that is common in gender and leisure is Constraint Theory. Researchers approach constraints in different ways according to leisure activities. These can vary from systematic groupings of constraints, for example Reid (1998) grouped constraints according to economic system delivery and psychological constraints.

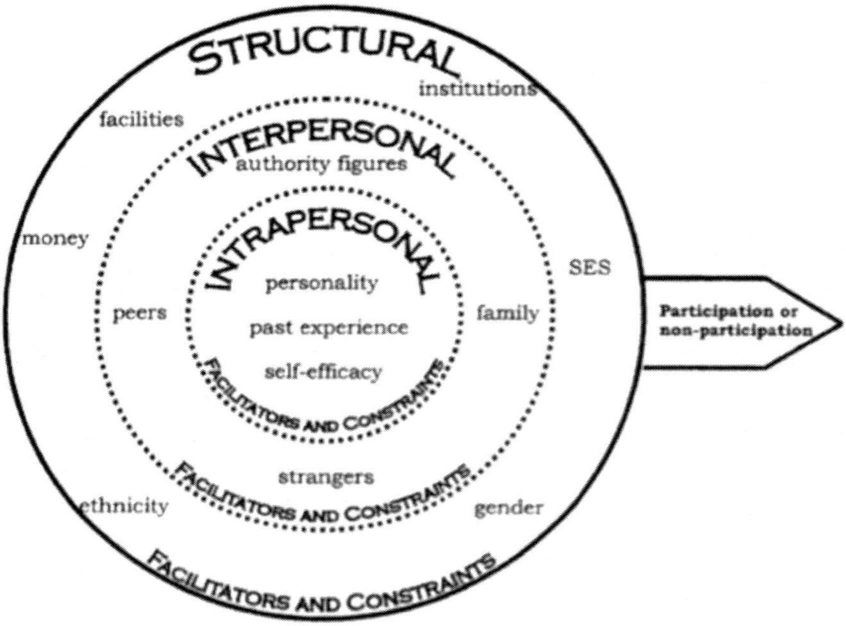

Figure 2. Raymore (2002). An ecological approach to understanding influences on participation.

Others have approached the discussion without grouping constraints to get an overall understanding of general barriers (Jackson 1993). Shaw (1994) views females as disadvantaged in leisure due to oppression in society. She classifies constraints into objective and subjective constraints. Jackson (1993) realized the validity in placing constraints into groups and classifications and came to oppose generalizations of single item barriers. However, it is noted the difficulty in factoring constraints into specific groups due to the extensive forms of barriers that exist in leisure participation (Jackson 1993; Henderson 1997). Raymore's 2002 theory looks at the intrapersonal, interpersonal and structural factors that can lead to participation or non-participation in leisure structures (Figure 2). Raymore (2002) created the model because he believed that the most common constraints theory (Jackson 1993) was heavily based on individual constraints. Henderson and Bialescheki (2005) suggest that Raymore's theory is forward thinking and allows for a better understanding of what disables participation. Schipperijn et al. (2010) chose Raymore's theorys because of its socio-ecological approach in understanding human behavior.

This paper adopts Raymore's (2002) approach to constraints considering structural, interpersonal and intrapersonal constraints. It should be noted that some constraints could be placed in multiple categories therefore this paper aims to put constraints into the most applicable category.

2.5. Structural Constraints

2.5.1. Infrastructure, Safety and Marketing Initiatives

Much of the literature focuses on the empirical evidence that concerns about safety discourage women from cycling. Faulks, Ritchie and Dodd (2008) use motivational theories including Danns (1977) 'push' and 'pull' factors and Moslow's (1943) hierarchy of needs. In using these models along with in-depth interviews, the authors conclude that women consider safety as the most important condition for enabling participation in leisure cycling. It should be noted the research was conducted in New Zealand, where although cycle patterns are similar (Sheng 2015) attitude and facilities may differ. Fullagar and Palvidis's (2012) paper makes apparent women's desire to feel safe when pursuing physical challenges. It is noted that men are more likely to cycle for the purpose of transport (Heesch, Sahlqvist and Garrard 2012) and that women are more inclined to partake in cycling for recreational purposes (Mintel 2015). Sener, Eluru, and Bhat (2009) found that this was due to commuter cyclist's likelihood to cycle during peak traffic times, which poses a bigger threat and plays into the safety consideration for women. One of the most recent attempts to improve safety in the UK is the National Cycle Network (NCN), which aims to promote safer cycling and increase numbers. Although there has been a 7% increase in cyclists (between 2012 and 2013) (Sustrans 2014) it is evident that the gender gap still exists with just a quarter of NCN users being female (Sustrans 2012).

Heesch, Sahlqvist and Garrard (2012) found safety to be a major barrier for both genders however, they considered it more problematic for females. Garrard, Rose and Lo (2008) ethnographic study found females were less inclined to cycle without complete separation paths and that males were more willing to cycle amongst vehicles, suggested that the cause of this may be due to the fact that women are more risk averse than men (Byrnes, Miller and

Schafer 1999). Steep hills are also considered an issue for females (Sener, Eluru and Bhat 2009) which could suggest why female participation is higher in places like the Netherlands where the land is flatter. The anticipation of encountering steep hills along with women's concerns about their own fitness levels (Heesch, Sahlqvist and Garrard 2012) could be affecting their confidence to cycle.

Beanland (2013) and Dalton (2010) recognize the need for stronger marketing towards females. Cycling has often been criticized as being gender biased. An example of this problem is the national infrastructure design guides cover showcasing a young male cycling on a main road with traffic in the background (Aldred, Woodcock, Goodman 2016). This could be both intimidating and off-putting for female cyclists. Shaw (1994) considered television marketing's role in stereotyping males and females into societal roles, the males being more powerful, and women having an idealized thin body type without muscles.

2.5.2. Time and Money

Time is a factor that is often mentioned as the reason that females do not cycle (Fullagar and Pavlidis 2012; Shaw 1994 Sener, Eluru, and Bhat 2009; Gomez et al. 2005). Women who do participate in recreational cycling are primarily in part-time employment and not living with children (Heesch, Sahlqvist and Garrard 2012). However, time is an accepted constraint for both genders, with a 2009 study stating that 40% of adults who did not participate in sport blamed the absence of time (Seddon 2011). Shaw (1994) suggested women's lack of economic power made them less capable of affording their preferred leisure activities. Dalton (2010), Gomez (2000) and Zovko (2013) also consider the price of cycling as constraining. Zovko (2013) in considering cycling events observed that funding of highly competitive cycling events was such that a female demographic would find it harder to afford. It is noted that the females that do participate in leisure cycling tend to be middle class (Heesch, Sahlqvist and Garrard 2012; Shaw 1994; Crone-Grant and Smith 2001). Interestingly though Pojani et al. (2017) noted that in Albania and Kosovo women who cycled were often stereotyped as being poor.

2.6. Interpersonal Constraints

2.6.1. Gender Roles

Both Shaw (1994) and Lloyd and Little (2011) discuss female's ethic of care in their papers concerning gender and leisure. They found that the females desire to take care of loved ones overrides their own personal needs and desires, thus neglecting their own leisure activity requirements. Although it is questionable if females` ethic of care is applicable in terms of cycling constraints. Faulks Ritchie Dodd (2008, 23) paper commends leisure cycling as a way in which "cyclists [can] spend time with family, friends, and other like-minded people," in turn allowing for females to enjoy time with and care for their loved ones. However, the overriding theme here of 'gender roles' does not just relate to the female desire to care for others. Being a housewife has been recognized as a reason to refrain from leisure cycling (Gomez et al. 2005). This can be due to time constraints or the fact that married women should not be "exposed to the eyes of other men" (Pojani et al. 2017 pg 41). More commonly female's responsibility for their children poses as a barrier to cycling (Pojani et al. 2017; Aldred, Woodcock and Goodman 2016). Females' need for social interaction in their leisure time, and males' competitive nature in leisure and sport participation are both considered as gender roles (Allender, Cowburn and Foster 2006; Fullagar and Pavlidis 2012). This suggests females may be deterred from cycling because of possible intimidation by machismo competitiveness and the lack of social interaction due to the individuality of the sport.

2.6.2. Culture and Trends

The UK is considered to have a low cycling culture with Britons making only 2% of their trips by bike (Department of Transport 2014). The Netherlands, Germany and Denmark are all considered to have stronger cycling cultures with ten times more participation than in the UK (Pucher and Buehler 2008). Female participation in these countries tends to be higher than or equivalent to that of males (Heesch, Sahlqvist and Garrard 2012). Gomez (2000) discusses gender in different cultures and the social expectations that are placed on females. The paper discussed the lack of "culture favorable to the use of bicycles as a means of transport, especially by women." (Gomez

2000, 45). The acronym MAMIL (middle aged men in lycra) was introduced in a 2012 Mintel report on the bicycle retail market (Mintel 2012). The report discusses the rising popularity of cycling for men. The weak cycling culture and prevalence of males over females, highlights a gendered culture in the UK. Females have been reported as having more interest in a LTPA in a female only environment (Lloyd and Little 2011; Flintoff and Scraton 2009; Fullagar and Pavlidis 2012), suggesting the MAMIL culture may function as a barrier. Policy makers have stressed the need for not building for the stereotypical MAMIL (Greater London Authority 2013) and to create an unsegregated cycling culture (Aldred, Woodcock and Goodman 2016).

2.7. Intrapersonal Constraints

2.7.1. Appearance

Leisure activities have been identified as a means of challenging gender constraints like body image and appearance (Fullagar and Pavlidis 2012; Henderson 2003). Although literature suggests that many females still feel that their perception of appearance discourages participation (Wolf 1991). High school appeared to be the age that most gave up cycling (Dill and McNeil 2012), because it is a time that females begin to care more about their appearance. A study done by Allender, Cowburn and Foster (2006) on high school PE participation found that girls considered body image and appearance a reason for their negative attitude towards LTPA. The girls felt that being active could cause sweat and have people view them as unattractive and unfeminine. Additionally, the paper also found that "Concerns about body shape and weight management were the main reasons for the participation of young girls." (Allender, Cowburn and Foster 2006, 830). Dalton (2010) argued that cycling specifically, over other LTPAs, engenders concerns about appearance. In common with this view Gomez (2000), who found that females were unable to wear attire such as skirts and heals when cycling which would affect their desire to cycle. It seems cycling for some is a means of being fit and empowered but conversely others may feel 'unfeminine' in the pursuit of the LTPA (Shaw 1994).

3. Methodology

3.1. Research Approach

The philosophy adopted in this research was interpretivism. Orlikowski and Baroudi (1991) describe the aim of interpretivism as seeking to understand how social groups, through participation in social process, create realities and give them meaning, in turn revealing how these meanings help shape their social actions. An inductive approach with phenomenology theory was adopted due to its ability to contribute to a deeper understanding through experiences (Starks and Trinidad 2007). The research outcome does not claim to constitute a theory, but rather to gain 'empirical generalizations' relating to the nature of the research being qualitative with outcomes seldom being hard facts (Bryman and Bell 2013). The research has no pre-assumed hypothesis and endeavors to expand a theory based on a pre-existent body of knowledge.

3.2. Research Strategy

A mono-method qualitative strategy is the most appropriate owing to its inductive view of the relationship between theory and knowledge (Bryman and Bell 2013). Qualitative interviews were adopted because of their capacity for better understanding of human behavior and because qualitative data has been commended and utilized frequently within the realms of feminist research. Bryman and Bell (2003) advocate this citing its "non-hierarchal relationship" and the fact that it realizes the "perspective of the woman that is being interviewed" (Bryman and Bell pp 503). Feminist research focuses on issues that females face, however the researcher must remain cautious and not create strong relationships with the female participants because this may increase the likelihood of bias (Bryman and Bell 2015). This was the case in Trethewy's (1999) research in which she became friends with the participants. Although it breaks down boundaries making relationships more equal, it is likely to affect the outcome of the research. Qualitative research has also been widely used in leisure and tourism research. Scott and Godbey's (1990) paper discuss its ability to reveal leisure behavior as a formative process allowing it to unveil leisure involvement over time in this ever-changing world, coinciding with the objectives of this research. Often qualitative interviews are critiqued because of difficulties in replicating the research and they can be prone to bias due to the small-scale samples however, it does provide deeper meaning (Lloyd and Little 2010). Qualitative research is the preferred approach and is widely used in studies concerning both gender and leisure studies (Christmas, et al. 2010; Fullagar and Pavlidis 2012; Faulks, Ritchie and Dodd 2008; Henderson and Gibson 2013; Lloyd and Little 2010).

The semi-structured interview has been selected because of its interest in the participant's point of view and its capacity to produce richer data. (Bryman and Bell 2003). The primary questions were generally restricted to an inductive format and then focused on the themes identified from the literature. In Henderson and Gibson's (2013) review of women and leisure research they found that semi-structured and in-depth interviews were the primary methods being used in 38% of the research papers that they analyzed. This method was preferred over focus groups, which can suffer from a dominating participant, or from the fact that individual's opinions may be altered due to social pressure (Smithson 2000). In using individual semi-structured interviews opinions and views will rely solely on the female as an individual.

3.3. Pilot Study

A pilot study was carried out in order to strengthen the research. Pilot studies are commonly conducted as a means of testing research questions in order to detect weakness in design and instrumentation (Cooper and Schindler 2003). However, the pilot study has also been recognized as a tool to extract information from an expert in a field of interest of who can subsequently provide informed feedback on the subject of interest (Collis and Hussey 2014). This research used a pilot study for the latter reason as a means of gaining further information on problems of female cycling participation. An interview was conducted using an adaptation of the questionnaire to identify the recurring constraints that women face. One pilot study was carried out with a volunteer from Women's Cycling Forum, an online platform for females who wish to cycle. The participant had a breadth of knowledge of overriding and common issues that women face in their ability and desire to cycle. The interview proved useful in better forming the questions to pinpoint varying reasons why females do not cycle as well as supporting collected secondary data.

3.4. Sampling

Judgment sampling, a type of purposive sampling, was used because the research aims to reveal female constraints. Judgment sampling is used to conform to some criterion (Cooper and Schindler 2003), in this case, active females who don't cycle. The paper looks to specifically identify constraints in cycling, therefore it will only interview females that pursue other LTPA. Purposive sampling is often regarded as preferable in phenomenologist studies (Starks and Trinidad 2007). Judgement sampling was carried out by approaching women in leisure centers, which enhances the chances of the participants being currently active, although they were also asked what LTPA they participated in to ensure high activity levels.

Geography was also adopted as a type of purposive sampling. Henninik, Hutler and Bailey (2011) discuss sampling in terms of a rural and urban sample. This technique was also adopted for this paper in order to get a wider spectrum of views. Seven interviews were conducted in Aberdeen, a coastal Scottish city. The following seven interviews were conducted in Comrie, a village in the center of Scotland. An equal number of participants is deemed important in each geographical location to reduce bias and reveal more equal results (Cooper and Schindler 2003). A total of 14 interviews were carried out over periods between 8 and 20 minutes. This was due to the time constraints faced in women being approached during their leisure time. The locations differ in size which allows for more varied feedback although the feedback does not aim to be representative of a nation, simply to identify deeper understanding into overall female constraints in leisure cycling. It is important to state here that the study only claims to represent the versions of the females 'stories' and that it is not claiming any empirical truth. Although the sample size is small other research into leisure studies have used a similar sample size (Loyed and Little 2010) and Starks and Trinidad (2007) recognized small numbers as being more useful in phenomenology in unraveling deeper experiences of people. No incentives were provided for participation. The questions were open-ended and created based on the recurring themes of constraints through the literature and through the pilot study.

4. Analysis and Discussion

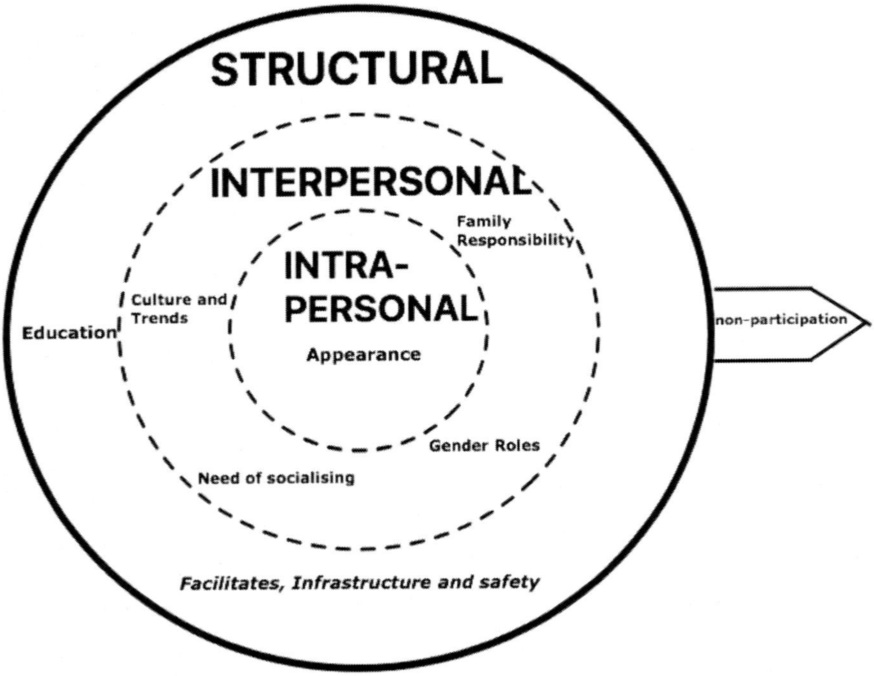

Figure 3. Facilitators for non-participation in leisure cycling.

All of the women interviewed were Caucasian and didn't disclose their sexual orientation. Participants ranged in age from 17 to 60, however most were under the age of 30. All the participants had cycled at an earlier stage in their life but they were currently not participating in cycling in everyday life or as a leisure activity. Although the research took place in two separate Scottish locations females were living in several different locations around Scotland ranging from major cities (Aberdeen, Edinburgh, Dundee) to rural communities (Comrie, Crieff, Bernary, Ellon). It is important to note that although there are similarities shared between women (because of their gender), this paper does not consider the term 'women' as homogenous and opinions do range. There were seven main themes that were identified throughout the research that coincide with the constraint theory, two of which are structural, four are interpersonal and one intrapersonal constraint (Figure 3). For confidentiality purposes each participant has been identified as P* (Participant Number). According to the Scottish Government (2013) evidence suggests the main problem facing females is the issue of safety, which was indeed an unequivocal theme however, other themes strongly emerged including issues of gender expectations.

4.1. Structural Constraints

4.1.1. Facilities, Infrastructure and Safety

The issue of safety was important to a most of participants, with many noting this as the "most important" (P10) constraint. This agrees with Garrard, Rose and Lo's (2008) paper which found that females were particularly sensitive to perceived traffic danger. It seems that most participants also agreed with Garrard (2003) in that cycling would be unacceptable until there are completely separate roads that are only accessed by bicycles and are not shared with parking spaces or buses. P2 stated that: "If there was more cycle lanes or cycle paths where there's no traffic, I would probably feel a lot more comfortable." P4 made direct references to the intimidation of sharing lanes with buses: "There are a lot of lanes but again it's the bus and cyclist lanes and they don't go together, especially in a city which is very bus dominated. I wouldn't feel comfortable being in the bus lane." This highlights why female cycling levels are so high in countries such as the Netherlands, Germany and the Denmark which have many more kilometers of bike paths than the UK (Pucher and Buehler 2008). Moreover, participant's concerns are justified because insufficient separate cycle lanes do cause cycling fatalities. In fact, although cycling levels are much lower in countries such as the UK and USA, fatalities are much higher (Pucher and Buehler 2008). Furthermore, in 2015 between the months of January and July in London six of nine bicycle fatalities were female even though they make up just 26% of London cyclists (Transport for London 2016).

The National Cycle Network have worked to create accessible and safe roads with either no, or minimal traffic across the UK for cyclists (Sustrans 2015), it seems that they still have a long way to go in order to persuade females to join their 'quiet roads.' P9 accused the national cycle network as being misleading:

> "Well to tell you the truth I have some reservations about the route through the Western Isles because it's the main thoroughfare of the local people and I think cyclists might get a shock when they come" she then goes onto say that "I think I could be quite stressed if I was cycling by myself if the roads were busy." In order to increase the female usage of the NCN from one quarter (Sustrans 2012) it seems that a bigger effort must be made to make the paths traffic free. Moreover, only 3 participants were actually aware of the NCN.

Some of the participants living in the city stated that they were "nervous to cycle in the city" (P12) because traffic is "just crazy" (P4). Interestingly five out of the seven participants interviewed in Aberdeen discussed how "Cycling in the countryside, [is] good" (P4) and that they would be more likely to cycle in rural areas and "sleepy villages" (P3). However, some of those who resided in rural areas had the same concerns about "busy roads." P10 discussed how dangerous rural roads can be:

> "It's not very safe for bikes on small rural roads with lots of bends and traffic. People who maybe don't know the road with traffic travelling too fast, there have been accidents, there have been deaths on roads I have travelled on."

It seems many of the participants had a 'grass is greener on the other side' perception of cycling and that in fact, even in considering different locations females are deterred away from roads. The research agrees with Sheng (2015) who discussed women's consideration of safety being of the utmost importance and that males are more motivated by action and adventure in their leisure time and do not share such safety concerns.

Other facilities as well as road infrastructure were noted as being insufficient. Three participants wished for more bike borrowing schemes which could reduce the dedication needed for investing in a bike. P2 also discussed the lack of cycle racks making it difficult to own a bicycle in the city. Finally, P14 who travelled frequently found her bike difficult to transport: "I don't genuinely feel like my bike is something that is transportable." Sener Eluru and Bhat (2009) note the importance of facilities such as bike racks in public places and transport as improving the overall experience of cycling.

4.1.2. Education

It seems that participants felt that there was insufficient education around cycling. Education relates not only to teaching people how to ride bikes correctly, but also how to maintain them and to better educate drivers on sharing the roads with cyclists. P5 said she was more likely to cycle if drivers were given: "more education into cycling." P13 refers to her unwillingness to use her bike because she was not taught how to do it properly in school: "there was no teaching when we were in school of how to safely do it" (P13). Similarly, P12 also felt unprepared to cycle on the roads, moreover her inability was exacerbated because she never sat a driving test, she admitted to feeling scared: "because I don't drive in and around the city."

Even if the women knew how to ride a bike some were concerned about mechanical aspects of a bike, especially if something was to go wrong. It could create difficulties, a view held by P11: "I've had a go with blowing up tires and that seems a bit of a faff as well. You know there are different kinds of valves and things and yeah I think if you've got the wrong one then you can blow your bike up… ." Lack of mechanical and cycling knowledge was noted in Fullagar and Pavlidis' (2012) research in making females feel inadequate when considering cycling. The lack of education is indicative as to why levels of cycling are low. Countries with higher cycling participation offer extensive education for both cyclists and drivers (Pucher and Buehler 2008).

4.2. Interpersonal

4.2.1. Family Responsibility

Although leisure cycling appears attractive to families and children the research revealed that women not only face difficulties associated with utility cycling (due to children), but also in relation to cycling for leisure purposes (Smart et al. 2014; Dill and McNeil 2012. The pilot study that there may be an issue associated with mothers feeling unable to justify going out for a cycle due to their parental responsibilities. Both P9 and P10 stated how they are more capable of cycling now, but in the past, it would have been too difficult with young children. P10 stated that: "time would restrict people who have got young families and got that full-on timetable which I don't have anymore." P9 said that she was in "full time work" whist bringing up a family, which made cycling too difficult. This was something that Heesch, Sahlqvist and Garrard (2012) also found. Women who did cycle were not living with children and were only working part-time. That said, even mothers that were unemployed may have reservations about cycling, P15, an unemployed mother thought that taking a child out on a bike is simply too dangerous: "I wouldn't be comfortable, I don't like having him on the same bicycle as me, or behind me and not knowing what he is up to." This reflects mothers' worries about taking small children on the back of their bike.

Even as children grow older it can be hard to motivate children to cycle as a family activity. Both P9 and P11 expressed their desires to cycle as a family however their children showed little interest. Female roles in childcare, according to Smart et al. (2014) competes with other constraints because so much of female time is spent taking care of children. This suggests that even if the roads were made better, society may need to adapt to give women more time and share childcare roles, such as they do in the Nordic countries.

4.2.2. Gender Roles

It appeared that simply being a female made cycling unacceptable for some participants. In recent years there has been more recognition of issues such as catcalling and sexual assault (Sanghani 2015), and it continues to be an issue with females on a bicycle. P3 and P7 had particularly unpleasant experiences around sexual harassment. P3 recalled a time she was on a bicycle and was catcalled: "catcalled and like… I've had people say 'f**king ride that bike'" and P7 had bad experiences when jogging: "sexual harassment often happens when I go running" which appears to deter her from cycling "that's probably why I wouldn't go out I don't like cycling by myself." This concurs with Gomez (2000) who highlights the issue of female's constant fear of being sexually harassed.

An extension of the machismo culture around cycling has led many participants to feel intimidated about taking part. During the pilot study it was made clear that the patronizing and masculine nature of cycling runs through the cycling world from bike shops to cycle clubs. Eight of the participants commented on how intimidating cycling can be to approach as a non-cyclist. Some participants suggested their lack of confidence related back to their early education that was highly gendered and orientated towards competitive activities. Allender, Cowburn and Foster (2006) found that children's participation in recreational activities was more active and enjoyable when they were not competitive.

Participants 6 and 13 both mentioned cycling as being "unfeminine" which again aligns with Gomez (2000) who's paper discusses Peruvian citizens surprise towards female cyclists as appearing disrespectful and unfeminine. It comes as a surprise that there are some similarities between participants in this research (carried out in Scotland) and the findings from Gomez's research that was carried out in Peru. Both countries are very different but share a somewhat old-fashioned view on women.

4.2.3. Culture and Trends

The saying 'safety in numbers' appeared to resonate with many of the women who all appeared to be much more willing to cycle if they saw more other women doing it. P6 said that she stopped cycling because "it didn't seem cool anymore, most of my friends stopped doing it and I didn't want to be considered a weirdo" which agrees with P7 who stated that "I think because more people do it you'd feel like a bit less weird because in Scotland you're not really seeing that many people on bikes."

It may seem that participants are simply wishing to 'follow the crowd', however, research shows that the greater the number of cyclists, the safer it becomes (Bauman 2008). High levels of cycling have low levels of fatalities (Jacobsen 2003). Cultural normalization (increasing the number of female cyclists), would help make cycling more acceptable to females (Zovko 2013; Emond, Tang and Handy 2009). Every participant admitted that they would be likely to participate if they lived in a country with a large cycling culture, where it was trendy.

4.2.4. Importance of Socializing

A recurring theme was female's perception of cycling being boring or isolating. It appears that females preferred more social activities that allowed for more interaction. P12 thought that one of the main reasons she didn't cycle was because she didn't "have any girlfriends who were cycling" and P5 seemed to think that "It's quite an isolated sport, you can't do it in a group". This perception of cycling being unsocial as a constraint aligns with Allender, Cowburn and Foster's (2006) findings that females look for social interaction during their leisure time.

It was noted throughout the literature that females prefer to be in an 'all female environment' (Lloyd and Little 2011; Flintoff and Scraton 2001; Fullagar and Pavlidis 2012) when taking part in LTPA's. This suggests that all female cycle groups would encourage more females to cycle. P7 said that: "If they did organize some more… all girls cycling or whatever that would be quite good." However interestingly, a large group, even if they are all women could be intimidating. P8 discusses her lack of confidence in approaching sports in particular social circumstances and states that she would "rather go with a friend." Sheng (2015) noted female's tendencies to have higher social anxiety in approaching particular group sports.

It seems that although cycling alone seems unsocial for many women, they still feel intimidated about joining cycling groups. However, other participants saw the positive side in cycling with just a few close friends and the joy it could bring: "If I ever entered cycling it would be probably with a female friend" (P9) and P11 talked about her friend that cycled "I've got a friend that cycles a lot and she talks about cake and coffee all the time so that sounds pretty good." Fullagar (2008) recognizes leisure cycling's ability to form new friendships. Moreover, during the pilot study P1 identified the ability of cycling to create friendship groups and cycle to places that serve coffee. Despite this, many females appear to interpret cycling as either completely independent or in overly large competitive groups.

4.3. Intrapersonal Constraints

4.3.1. Appearance

All participants claimed to have cycled at a young age. P3 was perplexed at the concept of young children not riding a bike concluding that as a child it was "the funniest thing." However, the pattern of participants giving up in high school was undeniable. When asked why they stopped in high school participants seemed unsure at first. However, further discussion identified the issues as their self-consciousness and desire to fit in. P3 claimed to be "very self-conscious as a kid" and P12 was "concerned with what I looked like and fitting in as well."

This was a subject area that was rarely touched on in the literature despite, the overriding evidence of the problems it can cause. Dill and McNeil (2012) found that adults who currently cycle were continuing it on from a younger age. This suggests that males are more comfortable on a bike due to their continuation of the activity from high school, something that many girls clearly don't experience.

Another notable element of females' concern about their appearance in association with cycling was their negative attitude towards cycling attire. Eight of the participants made references to the unappealing look of lycra for which cycling now appears to be famous for, with the growth of MAMILS. P10 discussed the "perceived macho element to the lycra clad men going around in bunches" and that she "wasn't prepared to go around in tights or lycra." P3 stated that: "I think lycra isn't cool." The questionnaire did not ask any questions relating to lycra but it seemed participants were interpreting recreational cycling as something serious, in which lycra had to be worn. Some participants discussed how unappealing helmets could be, although they recognized how important they were. Interestingly, Pucher and Buehler (2008) interviewed Dutch cycling experts and planners, who predominantly opposed bicycle helmet laws because it made cycling less convenient, less comfortable and less fashionable. A view that the participants seemed to share, P14 thought that they made her "look daft." Helmets are putting women off cycling even though they might not be as useful as perceived and can give people a false sense of safety (Wardlaw 2000).

5. Conclusion, Limitations and Recommendations

5.1. Conclusion

This paper explored reasons that prevent females from participating in leisure cycling. This is important because previous literature had concentrated on utility cycling. The paper identified constraints that women faced. A review of the literature suggested that safety and a lack of a cycling culture appeared to be the most recurring themes that prevented female participation. In this research Constraint Theory helped clearly segregate constraints allowing for a more straightforward research design and discussion.

The research concurred with the literature to a certain extent, in that most of the participants' main concerns were the lack of infrastructure and facilities to improve safety. Another emerging theme was women's fear of being in a minority of females that cycled, something that is more resonant in leisure cycling than utility cycling. It seemed that in order to have a larger representation of women cycling, a strong culture of female cyclists would have to be built up so that women can be inspired by peers to cycle alongside one another. It seems the intimidation of the MAMIL trend made some females feel intimidated. Although culture can seem ingrained in a society and hard to change, growing trends can contribute to the growth of a culture (Pucher and Buehler 2008).

Time was only really an issue for women that had children. All other participants felt they had time for leisure activities, and it was merely a choice of how they wished to spend their leisure time. Although cycling is often viewed as a family leisure activity, parents found it hard to motivate their children towards cycling or felt insecure carrying their child on their bikes due to the unsafe road conditions. However, Smart et al. (2013) found that it was not necessarily children that stopped women from being able to cycle. They suggested that time constraints allowed women little time to participate due to a lack of maternity leave given to males to enable a sharing of parental responsibilities. The research agreed with Shaw (1994) in that mothers could not justify taking sufficient leisure time for themselves due to their ethic of care, overriding desires for leisure time. In terms of cost it most participants felt that bikes were an investment and did not hinder them from participation.

This paper is important in highlighting that there is a willingness amongst women to participate in leisure cycling with only one constraint being intrapersonal. Interpersonal constrains were more frequent, highlighting the importance of the influence of peers as well as females need to socialize in a non-competitive atmosphere during their leisure time. The research shows that some changes would need to be made in order to encourage more females from non-participants into participants. This paper provides a better understanding of why females are constrained from cycling, it allows for communities and governments to adopt policies to encourage female cyclists.

5.2. Recommendations

It is clear how beneficial cycling can be to the economy and the tourism industry. Marketers need to take advantage of the growing trend in cycling and target females to foster a cycling culture, as suggested by Aldred, Woodcock, Goodman (2016). Arguably no major change will take place until there is a huge effort to segregate cycle paths from roads with traffic on them. Although Sustrans is making progress in their growth of paths and path usage, more needs to be done to keep traffic separate. There needs to be more promotion of the cycle paths to increase awareness of their existence. A good place to advertise the current cycle paths would be in leisure centers in an effort to target females that have a current interest in leisure sports but who may be unaware of the outdoor opportunities outdoors.

Other facilities such as adapting public transport for cyclists need attention. Buses could have racks attached to the front or back which could hold bikes, allowing people to reach destinations for leisure cycling more easily. These are utilized extensively in parts of the US as well as in Vancouver and are popular to help the transportation of bicycles (Figure 4).

Moreover, tourism destinations should offer facilities for cyclists, such as stands and pumps to attract more cyclists (this is more common in Australia). In considering the views expressed in the pilot study that the cycle world is often seen as a 'man's world,' more females could be at the forefront of cycling. This may include cycling outlets making a bigger effort to hire more females to better culturally normalize cycling for females and greater inclusion of women when advertising cycling.

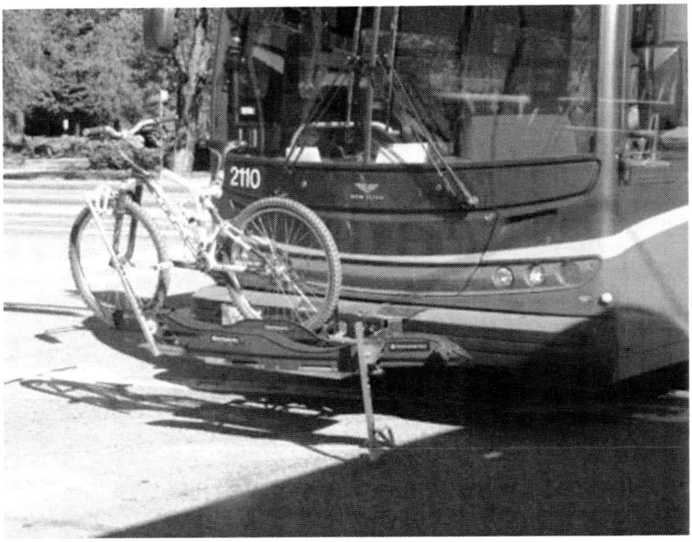

Figure 4. Photograph by Cycle City Tours (2016) Highlighting the Facilities Offered to Cyclists in Vancouver.

Greater efforts should be made in education to ensure that cycle proficiency is a legal requirement in every school and there ought to be a greater emphasis on vehicle driving etiquette in association with cyclists during driving tests and lessons. Cycling activities during high school time may reduce the perception of cycling as masculine or 'uncool'. Flintoff (2008) discusses the issues of sports being highly competitive in high school. By integrating cycling as an activity, it would reduce the issues of females being segregated due to overly competitive male culture. This would also increase the chances of females continuing to cycle into adulthood. At present the continuation of cycling from high school is primarily recurrent in the male demography (Zovko 2013).

Inspiration can be taken from European leaders by adopting laws making car drivers responsible for the safety of cyclists and having roads created to prioritize cyclists. This would help encourage participation due to heightened perceptions of security (Pucher and Buehler 2008). An elevated tax on car usage and making parking more difficult in town centers will encourage people to use a bike over a car and access the city center in a more leisurely manner on their bicycles. Another option is the introduction of bike hire systems which have been a huge success in cities such as Cambridge, where the gender gap is almost non-existent (Aldred, Woodcock and Goodman 2016). A borrow bike system in major cities would be a great tourist attraction and increase revenue options for Governments and councils through advertisement and customer payments (Collinson 2017).

Finally, in an effort to reduce the intimidation women feel about starting up cycling, gym groups such as spin classes which already have an established relationship with females, should offer outdoor cycling sessions to ease them into outdoor cycling. If such policies and provisions are adopted it could allow for a cycling culture to grow and the gender gap to reduce. This research can be useful to local governments and national tourism agents if they are looking for mechanisms which would help shrink the gender gap. Further research could be carried out over a period as roads begin to improve, to see if female attitudes towards cycling become more positive. Research could also be conducted into demography's in terms of religion, ethnicity and income which may reveal more specific reasons for constraints.

5.3. Limitations

Due to time and money constraints interviews were only carried out in two locations, which led to some location specific views and opinions. Because the participants were approached, without prior organization of meetings, participants had little time to consider their answers and also could not participate in interviews for a long period of time. Arguably however, participants not having prior knowledge of the interview could lead them to have more honest answers. The study was small scale revealing the opinions of a small population however, it should be noted that this research was exploratory. The research is based on a particular sample who were largely middle-class, Caucasian, young Scottish females. Hence, the research does not claim to be representative of all women. Finally, interviews could only be undertaken in two locations in Scotland despite the researches ambition to give insight into constraints women may face in the UK and other countries with an existent gender gap.

References

Adventure Cycle Association, 2012. "*Nine new indicators that bicycle travel and tourism are booming.*" Accessed November 24, 2012. https://www.adventurecycling.org/about-us/media/press-releases/9-new-indicators-that-bicycle-travel-and-tourism-are-booming.html.

Aldred, Rachel, James Woodcock, and Anna Goodman, 2016. "Does more cycling mean more diversity in cycling?" *Transport Reviews*, 36(1); 28-44.

Allender, Steven, Gill Cowburn, and Charlie Foster, 2006. "Understanding participation in sport and physical activity among children and adults: a review of qualitative studies". *Health education research*, 21(6);826-835.

Bauman, Adrian E, Chris Rissel, Jan Garrard, Ian Ker, Rosemarie Speidel, and Elliot Fishman, 2008. "Cycling: Getting Australia Moving: Barriers, facilitators and interventions to get more Australians physically active through cycling". *Melbourne, Australia: Department of Health and Ageing*; 593-601.

Beanland, Andy, 2013. *Cycle tourism for sustainable rural development: Understanding and interpreting lessons from Europe*, 52 London: Winston Churchill Fellowship.

Belter, Torsten, Maike Von Harten, and Sandra Sorof, 2012. *Costs and Benefits of cycling*, 99. EnercitEE.

British Heart Foundation, 2015. *Physical Activity Statistics*. London. The British Heart Foundation.

Bryman, Alan, and Emma Bell, 2013. *Business Research Methods*. 4th ed. Oxford: University Press.

Buckworth, Janet, Rebecca Lee, Gail Regan, Lori Schneider, and Carlo Diclemente, 2007. "Decomposing intrinsic and extrinsic motivation for exercise: Application to stages of motivational readiness". *Psychology of Sport and Exercise*, 8(4); 441-461.

Byrnes, James, David Miller, and William Schafer, 1999. "Gender differences in risk taking: a meta-analysis". *Psychol. Bull.* 125 (3); 367–383.

Cycle City Tours, 2016. "*10 Things to Know About Biking in Vancouver*". Accessed 12 April, 2016. http://cyclevancouver.com/10-things-to-know-about-biking-in-vancouver/.html.

Christmas, Simon, Shaun Helman, Sue Buttress, Celia Newman, and Rebecca Hutchins, 2010. *Cycling, safety and sharing the road: Qualitative research with cyclists and other road users*. London: Department for Transport.

Collinson, Patrick, 2017. *On your bike: the best and the worst of city cycle schemes.* The Guardian. Accessed 16 April, 2017. https://www.theguardian.com/money/2017/feb/25/best-and-worst-city-cycle-schemes-bike-sharing-london/.html.

Collis, Jill, and Roger Hussey, 2014. *Business Research: a practical guide for Business Research Methods. 8th ed*, 144-145. New York, McGraw-Hill.

Dalton, Anja, 2010. "*Cycling circles: gender perspectives and social influence in UK cycling*." MA Thesis, University of West England, Bristol.

Dando, Christina. E., 2007. "Riding the wheel: selling American women mobility and geographic knowledge". *ACME: An International Journal for Critical Geographies*, *6*(2); 174-210.

Department of Transport, 2014. "*National Travel Survey*." Accessed November 24, 2014. https://www.gov.uk/government/uploads/system/uploads/attachment_data/file/457752/nts2014-01.pdf.

Dill, Jennifer, and Nathan McNeil, 2012. "*Four Types of Cyclists? Testing a typology to better understand bicycling behavior and potential*". PhD thesis. Portland State University.

Emond, Catherine R., Wei Tang, and Susan Handy, 2009. "Explaining Gender Differences in Bicycling Behaviour" *Paper presented at*

Women's Issues in Transportation, TRB 2009, New Orleans, Louisiana, August 21-24.

Faulks, Pamela, John Dodd and Brent Ritchie, 2008. "Bicycle tourism as an opportunity for re-creation and restoration? Investigating the motivations of bike ride participants". *Paper presented at New Zealand Tourism and Hospitality Research Conference*, Hanmer Springs, New Zealand, August 14-18.

Flintoff, Anne, and Sheila, Scraton, 2001. "Stepping into active leisure? Young women's perceptions of active lifestyles and their experiences of school physical education". *Sport, education and society*, 6(1); 5-21.

Flintoff, Anne, 2008. "Targeting Mr Average: participation, gender equity and school sport partnerships". *Sport, education and society*, 13(4); 393-411. Vancouver.

Fullagar, Simone, and Adele, Pavlidis, 2012. ""It's all about the journey": women and cycling events". *International Journal of Event and Festival Management,* 3(2); 149-170.

Fullagar, Simone, 2008. "Leisure practices as counter-depressants: Emotion-work and emotion-play within women's recovery from depression". *Leisure Sciences*, 30(1); 35-52.

Garrard, Jan, 2003. "Healthy revolutions: promoting cycling among women". *Health Promotion Journal of Australia*, 14(3); 213-215.

Garrard, Jan, Geoffrey Rose, and Sing Kai Lo, 2008. "Promoting transportation cycling for women: the role of bicycle infrastructure". *Preventive medicine*, *46*(1); 55-59.

Gatersleben, Birgitta, and Hebba Haddad, 2010. "Who is the typical bicyclist?" *Transportation research part F: traffic psychology and behavior*, 13(1); 41-48.

Gomez, L., 2000. *Gender Analysis of Two Components of the World Bank Transport Projects in Lima, Peru: Bikepaths and Busways. World Bank Internal Report,* Washington: World Bank.

Gomez, Luis. F., Olga Sarmiento, Diego Lucimi, Gladys Espinosa, Roberto Forero and Adrian Bauman, 2005. "Prevalence and factors associated with walking and bicycling for transport among young adults in two low-income localities of Bogotá, Colombia". *Journal of Physical Activity and Health*, 2(4); 445-459.

Greater London Authority, 2013. "*The mayor's vision for cycling in London*" Accessed March 2, 2013. https://www.london.gov.uk/sites/default/files/cycling_vision_gla_template_final.pdf.

Grous, Alexander, 2011. *The British Cycling Economy: 'Gross Cycling Product'*. Accessed February 22, 2011. http://eprints.lse.ac.uk/38063/html.

Heesch, Kristian, C., Shannon Sahlqvist and Jan Garrard, 2012. "Gender differences in recreational and transport cycling: a cross-sectional mixed-methods comparison of cycling patterns, motivators, and constraints". *International Journal of Behavioral Nutrition and Physical Activity,* 9(1); 1.

Henderson, Karla. A., and Debborah M. Bialescheki, 2005. "Leisure and Active Lifestyles: Research reflections". *Leisure Sciences.* 27 (5); 255-365

Henderson, Karla A. and H. J. Gibson, 2013. "An integrative review of women, gender, and leisure: Increasing complexities". *Journal of Leisure Research*, 45(2); 11.

Henderson, Karla. A. 1997. "A critique of constraints theory: A response". *Journal of Leisure Research*, 29(4); 453-458.

Jackson, Edgar L.m 1993. "Recognizing patterns of leisure constraints: Results from alternative analyses". *Journal of leisure research*, 25(2); 129.

Jacobsen, Peter, 2003. "Safety in numbers: more walkers and bicyclists, safer walking and bicycling". *Injury Prevention*, 9; 205–209.

Lloyd, Kathy, and Donna E. Little, 2010. "Self-determination theory as a framework for understanding women's psychological well-being outcomes from leisure-time physical activity". *Leisure Sciences*, 32(4); 369-385.

Lumsdon, Les, 2000. "Transport and tourism: cycle tourism–a model for sustainable development?" *Journal of Sustainable Tourism*, 8(5); 361-377.

Lumsdon, Les, 1996. Cycle Tourism in Britain. *Insights,* March, 27-32. London: English Tourist Board.

Mintel. *Bicycles – UK – June.* London: Mintel Group Limited, 2012.

Mintel. *Walking and cycling holidays taken in the past 5 years.* London. Mintel Group Limited, 2015.

Mintel. *Walking and cycling holidays taken in the past 5 years.* London: Mintel Group Limited, 2016.

Mintel. *Domestic Holiday Activities.* London: Mintel Group Limited, 2017.

Mintel. *Cycling behaviors and experiences.* London: Mintel Group Limited, 2017.

Orlikowski, Wanda J., and Jack Baroudi, 1991. "Studying information technology in organizations: Research approaches and assumptions". *Information Systems Research*, *2*(1);1-28.

Pojani, Dorina, Dukagjin Bakija, Entela Shkreli, Jonathan Corcoran, and Iderlina Mateo-Babiano, 2017. Do Northwestern and Southeastern Europe Share a Common "Cycling Mindset"? Comparative Analysis of Beliefs toward Cycling in the Netherlands and the Balkans. *EJTIR*, 17(1); 25-45.

Privitera, Donatella, 2013. "Sustainable Transport and Quality of Life Analysis of Cycling Impact in Italy". *Sustainable Technologies, Policies, and Constraints in the Green Economy;* 251.

Pucher, John, and Ralph Buehler, 2008. "Making cycling irresistible: lessons from the Netherlands, Denmark and Germany". *Transport Reviews*, 28(4); 495-528.

Pucher, John, Ralph Buehler and Mark Seinen, 2011. "Bicycling renaissance in North America? An update and re-appraisal of cycling trends and policies". *Transportation research part A: policy and practice,* 45(6); 451-475.

Pucher, John, Ralph Buehler, David R. Bassett, and Andrew L. Dannenberg, 2010. "Walking and cycling to health: a comparative analysis of city, state, and international data". *American journal of public health*, *100*(10); 1986-1992.

Raymore, Leslie A., 2002. "Facilitators to leisure". *Journal of Leisure Research*, 34(1); 37.

Reid, Donlad. G., 1988. "The needs of the unemployed and the ability of leisure providers to respond". *Loisir et* Société/*Society and Leisure*, 11(1); 117-127.

Ritchie, Brent, 1998. "Bicycle tourism in the South Island of New Zealand: planning and management issues". *Tourism Management*, 19(6); 567-582.

Sanghani, Radhika, 2015. "*Catcalling happens to most women between the ages of 11 and 17*". Accessed April 12, 2015. http://www.telegraph.co.uk/women/womens-life/11637697/Catcalling-Women-sexually-harassed-on-the-street-from-puberty.html.

Schipperijn, Jasper, Ulrika K. Stigsdotter, Thomas B. Randrup and Jens Troelsen, 2010. "Influences on the use of urban green space–A case study in Odense, Denmark". *Urban Forestry & Urban Greening*, 9(1); 25-32.

Scott, David, and Geoffrey C. Godbey, 1990. "Reorienting leisure research—The case for qualitative methods". *Loisir et Société/Society and Leisure*, *13*(1); 189-205.

Scottish Government 2013. "*Equality Outcomes: Gender Evidence Review*". Accessed March 15, 2015. http://www.gov.scot/resource/0042/00421042.pdf .

Seddon, Carla, 2011. *Lifestyles and Social Participation*. Office for National Statistics. *Social Trends* 41. London: Crown.

Sener, Ipek, Naveen Eluru, and Chandra R. Bhat, 2009. "Who are bicyclists? Why and how much are they bicycling?" *Transportation Research Record: Journal of the Transportation Research Board*, (2134); 63-72.

Shaw, Susan M., 1994. "Gender, leisure, and constraint: Towards a framework for the analysis of women's leisure". *Journal of leisure research*, 26(1); 8.

Sheng, Ying, 2015. "*Understanding the motivations of bicycle tourism in New Zealand: the case of the Hauraki Rail Trail*" PhD dissertation, Auckland University of Technology.

Smart, Michael J., Kelcie M. Ralph, Brian D. Taylor, Carole Turley and Anne E. Brown, 2014. "*Honey can you pick-up groceries on your way home? analyzing activities and travel among students and in non-traditional households.*" PhD Dissertation. University of California transportation center.

Smithson, Janet, 2000. "Using and analysing focus groups: limitations and possibilities". *International journal of social research methodology, 3*(2); 103-119.

Starks, Helene, and Susan Brown Trinidad. 2007. "Choose your method: A comparison of phenomenology, discourse analysis, and grounded theory". *Qualitative health research*, 17(10);1372-1380.

Sustrans, 2012. "*The real cycling revolution: How the face of cycling is changing*". Accessed March 2, 2012. http://www.sustrans.org.uk/sites/default/files/file_content_type/real-cycling-revolution.pdf.

Sustrans 2015. "*About the National Cycle Network*". Accessed February 2, 2015. http://www.sustrans.org.uk/ncn/map/national-cycle-network/about-network.html.

Sustrans Scotland, 2014. "*Walking and Cycling Outcomes.*" Accessed March 2, 2014.http://www.sustrans.org.uk/sites/default/files/images/files/scotland/policy/Sustrans-Scotland-walking-and-cycling-outcomes-report-September-2014-optimised.pdf.

Transport for London, (2016). "*Casualties in Greater London during 2015*". Mayor of London: London.

Trethewey, Angela, 1999. 'Disciplined bodies: Women's embodied identities at Work,' *Organization Studies,* 20 (3); 423-50.

Wardlaw, Malcolm J., 2000. "*Three lessons for a better cycling future*". British Medical Journal.14; 582-1585.

Wolf, Naomi, 1991. *The beauty myth: how images of beauty are used against women.* New York: William Morrow.

World Health Organization, 2000. *Obesity: Preventing and Managing the Global epidemic*. World Health Organisation: Geneva.

Zovko, Ivan, 2013. The Value of Cycle Tourism. *Opportunities for the Scottish Economy. Scotland.* Scottish Enterprise: Glasgow.

In: An Essential Guide to Sports Performance ISBN: 978-1-53617-608-7
Editors: Daniel Castillo Alvira et al. © 2020 Nova Science Publishers, Inc.

Chapter 10

SADDLE HEIGHT CONFIGURATION BASED ON MEASUREMENT OF DYNAMIC KNEE FLEXION ANGLE LEADS TO GREATER SELF-REPORTED CYCLING COMFORT IN RECREATIONAL CYCLISTS

***David Jiménez-Sutil and Ángel Lago-Rodríguez**, PhD**
Faculty of Health Sciences, Universidad Isabel I, Burgos, Spain

ABSTRACT

The aim of this work was to compare self-reported cycling comfort in recreational cyclists pedaling under three different saddle height configurations. Ten recreational cyclists (age: 38.1 ± 6.6 years), with no prior experience on cycling posture biomechanical analysis, were asked to self-report their comfort after pedaling under four different saddle height configurations defined by: i) cyclists' self-selected saddle height

* Corresponding Author's Email: angellagorodriguez @gmail.com.

(Self-selected); ii) anthropometric measures (Anthropometric), iii) static measurement of knee flexion angle (Static); iv) dynamic measurement of knee flexion angle (Dynamic). Self-reported cycling comfort was measured using a visual analog scale (VAS). The highest self-reported comfort was found to be paired with pedaling under saddle height configured based on a dynamic measurement of knee flexion angle. Moreover, comfort reported for pedaling under self-selected saddle height was significantly larger than for Anthropometric and Static conditions. Interestingly, saddle height was found similar for Dynamic and Self-selected conditions, which were significantly different to saddle height from Anthropometric and Static conditions. Based on the positive association reported for pedaling discomfort and musculoskeletal problems, our results lead to the suggestion that recreational cyclists should configure their bicycle's saddle height based on dynamic measurement of knee flexion angle in order to avoid injuries.

Keywords: saddle height; cycling comfort; biomechanical analysis.

INTRODUCTION

An optimal bicycle configuration is crucial to maximize performance and minimize injury risks for both recreational and elite cyclists (Callaghan 2005; Silberman et al., 2005; Wishv-Roth 2009). It has been shown that an incorrect position on the bicycle may lead to overuse injuries (Bini, Hume, and Croft 2011). Furthermore, changes in body position resulting from adjustments made in bicycle configuration have been reported to lead to adaptations at different performance levels: i) muscular activation (Diefenthaeler et al., 2008; de Moura et al., 2017; Peveler et al., 2012); ii) force applied to pedals (Bini, Hume, and Croft 2011; Verma et al., 2016); iii) lower limb kinematics (Nordeen-Snyder 1977); and iv) oxygen consumption (Nordeen-Snyder 1977; Peveler 2008).

Saddle height is one of the crucial parameters that need to be correctly adjusted for an appropriate bicycle configuration (Dorel et al., 2009; Ferrer-Roca et al., 2014, 2012; Peveler et al., 2012; Wanich et al., 2007). It has been shown that small saddle height manipulations affect cyclists' biomechanical, physiological and perceptual responses to pedaling, as well as their adherence to cycling (Kruschewsky et al., 2018). Moreover, cyclists reported discomfort while pedaling under incorrect saddle height adjustments (Priego Quesada et al., 2017), which has been further associated with musculoskeletal problems (Bressel et al., 2009; Dettori and Norvell 2006; Kotler, Babu, and Robidoux 2016; Silberman 2013). Therefore, cyclists should take special attention on a correct adjustment of their bicycle's saddle height.

Despite the crucial role that bicycle configuration plays on cycling performance, there is yet disagreement within the scientific community regarding the optimal bicycle configuration; being saddle height one of the most controversial aspects of the bicycle configuration process (Bini, Hume, and Croft 2011). Two main groups of methods for accurate saddle height configuration can be found in the literature. First, methods based on anthropometric measurements from the lower leg, such as percentage of trochanteric length or inseam leg length (Ericson et al., 1986; Hamley and Thomas 1967; Nordeen-Snyder 1977; Shennum 1976). Second, methods based on measurement of knee flexion angle, which can be assessed through static (Holmes, Pruitt, and Whalen 1994) or dynamic analysis (Burke 2002). As previously stated by Bini et al., (2011), there is still not enough valid and reliable scientific data allowing us to determine which saddle height configuration method is more appropriate. Several attempts have been previously made though (Peveler et al., 2005; Peveler and Green 2011), leading to the suggestion that methods based on the analysis of knee flexion angle are better than the anthropometric methods for reducing injury risk and improving performance, since the former account for inter-individual differences in leg kinematics (Bini, Hume, and Croft 2011). However, further research is needed in order to compare the effects of different saddle height configuration methods over cycling performance and pedaling comfort.

Athletes' self-perceived comfort is crucial for sport performance, since it has been associated with injury prevention and performance enhancement in running (Lucas-Cuevas et al., 2014; Luo et al., 2009) or basketball (Lam, Sterzing, and Cheung 2011). Cyclists' pedaling comfort is influenced by the cycling posture acquired over the bicycle (Priego

Quesada et al., 2017), which is partially determined by saddle height. However, no previous work has compared the level of comfort reported by cyclists pedaling under saddle height configurations based on different methods proposed in the literature. Thus, the aim of this work was to compare self-reported cycling comfort in recreational cyclists pedaling under four different saddle height configurations, which were based on: i) cyclists' self-selected height (Self-selected); ii) anthropometric measures (Anthropometric); iii) static measurement of knee flexion angle (Static); and iv) dynamic measurement of knee flexion angle (Dynamic).

METHODS

Participants

A total of ten subjects (n = 10) were recruited for this study (age: 38.1 ± 6.6 years). All participants were recreational cyclists, with a minimum experience of at least 3 years cycling, and with previous experience competing in amateur cycling championships. None of the individuals had previously participated in a cycling posture biomechanical analysis in order to accurately setup their bicycle, and they did not show any neurological or physical impairment. Participants were informed regarding the aim of the study, and voluntarily signed an informed consent before their participation. This investigation was performed in accordance to the Declaration of Helsinki (2013), and met the ethical standards in Sport and Exercise Science Research (Harriss and Atkinson 2015).

Experimental Design

An intra-individual experimental design was used. Participants were asked to attend one experimental session, in which self-reported pedaling comfort was registered after cycling under four different saddle height configurations: i) cyclists' original self-selected saddle height configuration (Self-selected); ii) saddle height based on anthropometric measures (Anthropometric), iii) saddle height determined by a static measurement of knee flexion angle (Static); and iv) saddle height defined based on a dynamic measurement of knee flexion angle (Dynamic). Self-reported cycling comfort was measured using a visual analog scale (VAS), following indications by Bousie et al., (2018).

Procedures

After participants arrival to the testing room, anthropometric measures (i.e., height, body mass, trochanteric length, and inseam length) were registered, along with the original bicycle saddle height. In order to obtain saddle height based on the anthropometric method, the 88.5% of the inseam length for each participant was calculated. To calculate saddle height based on the static goniometry method, participants were asked to sit on their bicycle, and saddle height was adjusted until participants' knee flexion angle was ~25°. Finally, in order to adjust saddle height based on the dynamic goniometry method, participants were recorded with a camcorder while cycling during 10 s. This record was then analyzed offline using Kinovea motion analysis system (version 0.8.15; www.kinovea.org), and saddle height was adjusted until a ~35° knee flexion angle was obtained during offline analysis.

After four saddle height configurations were determined (i.e., Self-selected, Anthropometric, Static, and Dynamic), participants were asked to perform a standardized warm-up. Following indications from Bousie et al., (2018), during the warm-up period participants were instructed to self-select a gear that would allow them to maintain a comfortable pace for 60-90 min. A value of 12 on a scale of rate of perceived exertion (RPE) based on Borg's 15-point scale (Bousie et al., 2013; Clarsen, Krosshaug, and Bahr 2010; Sanner and O'Halloran 2014; Wilber et al., 1995) was defined as a comfortable cycling pace for each participant (Borg and Noble 1974; Skinner et al., 1973). Thus, cadence and RPE were the primary determinants of participants' performance. As previously stated by Bousie et al., (2018), RPE is sometimes preferred over power output as a performance measure, since it enables researchers to assess cycling intensity independently of the inter-individual variance for power profile (Edwards et al., 1972; Feriche et al., 1998; Pérez-Landaluce et al., 2002), and it allows participants to use their own bicycle, equipment, and setup, conditions which were crucial for the correct development of this study.

After finishing the warm-up, participants started cycling for 10 min at the pace previously self-defined, under saddle height configuration registered at their bicycle when first arrived to the testing room (Self-selected). After finishing this 10 min cycling period, participants were asked to get off the bicycle, and self-report how comfortable they felt during cycling. In order to measure cycling comfortability, a 10 cm VAS was used (Bousie et al., 2018), in which two values were shown: 0 (i.e., "not comfortable at all") and 10 (i.e., "greatest comfort possible"). While participants rated how comfortable they felt during cycling, bicycle's saddle height was adjusted according to one of the three saddle height configurations which remained to be tested (Anthropometric, Static, Dynamic). The order of saddle height evaluation was counterbalanced between participants, and then cycling comfortability for each of them was measured as previously stated for the Self-selected condition.

Statistical Analysis

In order to compare self-reported comfort registered for each experimental condition we performed an analysis of variance for repeated measures (ANOVA-RM), with Configuration method (Self-reported, Anthropometric, Static, Dynamic) as the intra-individual factor. Furthermore, we performed an analysis of variance for repeated measures (ANOVA-RM) for saddle height registered on each experimental condition, introducing Configuration method (Self-reported, Anthropometric, Static, Dynamic) as the intra-individual factor. For both analyses, the assumption of sphericity was tested, and the Greenhouse-Geisser correction was used when this assumption was violated.

Significant results were followed by pairwise comparisons, using Bonferroni corrections. Practical significance for pairwise comparisons was assessed by calculating Cohen's *d* effect size (Lakens 2013). Effect sizes (d) of above 0.8, between 0.8 and 0.5, between 0.5 and 0.2 and lower than 0.2 were considered as large, moderate, small, and trivial, respectively (Cohen 1988). Furthermore, ANOVA-RM effect sizes were estimated using partial eta squared (η2p), with < 0.25, 0.26–0.63 and > 0.63 considered small, medium and large effect sizes respectively (Ferguson 2009; Richardson 2011). Statistical analysis was performed using the Statistical Package for Social Sciences (version 20.0 for Mac, SPSSTM Inc, Chicago, IL, USA). Statistical significance was set at $p < 0.05$.

Results

Summary of participants' anthropometric characteristics, along with their training experience, is shown in Table 1.

Table 1. Summary of personal and anthropometric sample characteristics, along with information regarding training experience

Variable		Mean ± Standard deviation
Age		38.10 ± 6.59
Height		175.20 ± 7.33
Mass		75.70 ± 6.29
Years with bicycle		7.10 ± 2.69
Trochanter height		85.37 ± 7.29
Inseam height		77.02 ± 6.97
Training	Days/week	4.7 ± 0.67
	Km/week	231 ± 58.2
	Hours/session	10.1 ± 2.64

Saddle Height

The ANOVA-RM for saddle height showed a significant effect for bicycle configuration factor ($F_{2.139,\ 19.250} = 103.12$; p-valor < 0.001; η2p = 0.92). Post-hoc analysis revealed that saddle height for Static condition (78.29 ± 7.23) was significantly larger than all three remaining conditions: Self-selected (73.83 ± 6.50; p < 0.001; 95%CI [2.253, 6.673]); Dynamic (73.13 ± 6.31; p < 0.001; 95%CI [4.11, 6.218]); and Anthropometric (68.16 ± 6.15; p < 0.001; 95%CI [7.805, 12.451]). Furthermore, saddle height was found significantly larger for Self-selected and Dynamic conditions, when compared to Anthropometric (73.83 ± 6.50 vs. 68.16 ± 6.15; p < 0.001; 95%CI [3.282, 8.048]; 73.13 ± 6.31 vs. 68.16 ± 6.15; p < 0.001; 95%CI [3.349, 6.579]; respectively).

Cycling Comfort

The ANOVA-RM for cycling comfort revealed a significant effect for bicycle configuration factor ($F_{3,\ 27} = 103.12$; p-valor < 0.001; η2p = 0.88). Post-hoc analysis unveiled significant greater comfort for Dynamic condition (8.55 ± 0.44), when compared to Self-selected (6.85 ± 1.03; p = 0.006; 95%CI [0.519, 2.881]); Static (4.2 ± 0.63; p < 0.001; 95%CI [3.639, 5.061]); and Anthropometric (3.95 ± 1.28; p < 0.001; 95%CI [3.278, 5.922]). Furthermore, significant larger comfort was reported for Self-selected condition (6.85 ± 1.03), compared to Static (4.2 ± 0.63; p = 0.001; 95%CI [1.253, 4.047]) and Anthropometric (3.95 ± 1.28; p < 0.001; 95%CI [1.703, 4.097]) conditions.

DISCUSSION

The aim of this work was to compare self-reported cycling comfort in recreational cyclists pedaling under four different saddle height configurations: i) Self-selected; ii) Anthropometric; iii) Static; and iv)

Dynamic. We found greatest self-reported comfort to be associated with saddle height configured based on a dynamic measure of knee flexion angle (Dynamic), which was significantly greater that comfort reported for Static, Anthropometric, and Self-selected conditions. Furthermore, recreational cyclists were significantly less comfortable when pedaling with saddle height configured based on Anthropometric and Static methods, in comparison with pedaling under the original Self-selected saddle height. Interestingly, saddle height configured based on dynamic measure of knee flexion angle was not significantly different from saddle height self-selected by recreational cyclists.

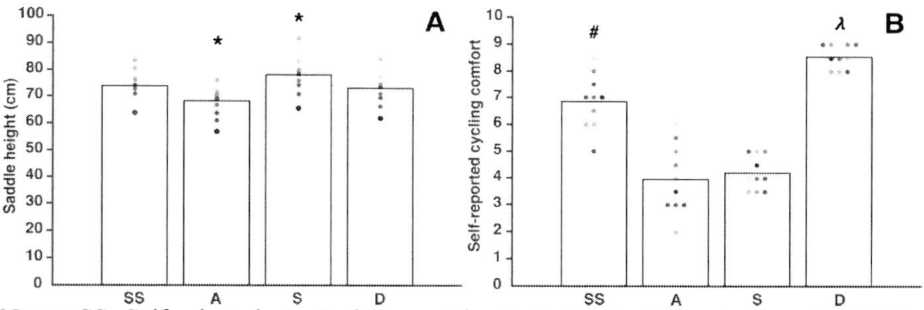

Notes: SS: Self-selected; A: Anthropometric; S: Static; D: Dynamic; * $p < 0.001$ for comparisons with three remaining experimental conditions. **λ** $p < 0.01$ for comparisons with three remaining experimental conditions. # $p \leq 0.001$ for comparisons with Anthropometric and Static conditions.

Figure 1. Panel A represents saddle height for each experimental condition. Panel B shows cyclists' self-reported cycling comfort under each saddle height configuration condition.

We found recreational cyclists to be more comfortable when pedaling under a saddle height configured based on a dynamic measurement of knee flexion angle (~35°), which is in line with previous work suggesting that saddle height should be configured based on measurement of knee flexion angle, since—in contrast with anthropometric methods—it accounts for inter-individual differences in leg kinematics (Bini, Hume, and Croft 2011). The degree of knee flexion angle has been proposed as gold standard for saddle height configuration (Bini, Hume, and Croft 2011; Priego Quesada et al., 2017). It has been recommended that bicycles' configuration should be setup in order to achieve a 25°-30° knee flexion angle during static measurements (Bini, Hume, and Croft 2011; Burke and Pruitt 1996; Peveler, Pounders, and Bishop 2007), whereas during dynamic measures knee flexion angle should get up to 30°-40° (Ferrer-Roca et al., 2012). Based on our results, it is recommended to configure saddle height of recreational cyclists based on a dynamic measurement of knee flexion angle that leads to ~35°, since it would allow them to be more comfortable while pedaling. Previous work found that club-level cyclists were more comfortable while pedaling with saddle height configured within the recommended 25°-30° knee flexion angle measured in static conditions, compared to 20° and 40° knee flexion configurations (Priego Quesada et al., 2017). Thus, it is recommended that future lines of research compare self-reported cycling comfort under saddle height setup based on a broader range of knee flexion angles, both for the static and dynamic configuration protocols, in order to ascertain which configuration leads to the highest comfort possible.

We found that saddle height arranged based on a dynamic measure of knee flexion angle was not significantly different from the height self-selected by recreational cyclists before performing a biomechanical analysis of their cycling posture. Moreover, saddle height for Anthropometric and Static conditions was found significantly different from both Self-selected and Dynamic conditions. Interestingly, self-reported cycling comfort was found significantly greater at Self-selected condition, in comparison with Anthropometric and Static conditions. Altogether, the aforementioned results suggest that recreational cyclists are able to setup their bicycle's saddle height similarly to what would be done when performing a biomechanical pedaling analysis based on a dynamic measurement of knee flexion angle. Accordingly, in line with Bini et al., (2011), our results suggest that recreational cyclists configured their bicycle's saddle height based on cycling comfort, since we found that Self-selected saddle height allows recreational cyclists to be more comfortable during pedaling than saddle height configured based on Anthropometric and Static conditions.

Engagement in physical activity has been associated with high levels of pleasure during exercise (Ekkekakis 2009; Ekkekakis, Parfitt, and Petruzzello 2011; Kwan and Bryan 2010). It has been previously suggested that bicycle configuration partially determines adherence to cycling (Priego Quesada et al., 2017), most likely because perceived discomfort during cycling has been associated with less exercise volume and decreased adherence to physical activity programs (Kwan and Bryan 2010; Rhodes and Kates 2015; Schneider, Dunn, and Cooper 2009). Based on the higher comfort reported in our study for saddle height configured based on Dynamic and Self-selected conditions, compared to Static and Anthropometric, it might be proposed that recreational cyclists should ideally established their bicycle's saddle height through a Dynamic biomechanical analysis of their pedaling posture, or alternatively through self-selected saddle height based on their self-perceived comfort. This recommendation is crucial when we take into account that cyclists' bike perceptions may play a significant role for injury prevention and enhanced cycling performance (Priego Quesada et al., 2017).

Conclusion

In conclusion, it is recommended that recreational cyclists configured their bicycle's saddle height based on a dynamic measurement of their knee flexion angle through a pedaling biomechanical analysis, since it would allow them to be more comfortable while cycling, which would potentially result in more time of practice and lower probability of getting injured.

References

Bini, Rodrigo, Patria A. Hume, and James L. Croft. 2011. "Effects of Bicycle Saddle Height on Knee Injury Risk and Cycling Performance."

Sports Medicine 41: 463-476. doi: 10.2165/11588740-000000000-00000.

Borg, Gunnar A. V. 1974. "Perceived Exertion." *Exercise and Sport Sciences Reviews* 2: 131-153.

Bousie, Jaquelin A., Peter Blanch, Thomas G. McPoil, and Bill Vicenzino. 2013. "Contoured In-Shoe Foot Orthoses Increase Mid-Foot Plantar Contact Area When Compared with a Flat Insert during Cycling." *Journal of Science and Medicine in Sport* 16: 60-64. doi: 10.1016/j.jsams.2012.04.006.

Bousie, Jaquelin A., Bill Vicenzino, Thomas G. McPoil, and Peter Blanch. 2018. "Hardness and Posting of Foot Orthoses Modify Plantar Contact Area, Plantar Pressure, and Perceived Comfort When Cycling." *Journal of Science and Medicine in Sport* 21: 691-696. doi: 10.1016/j.jsams.2017.11.013.

Bressel, Eadric, Jeffrey M. Willardson, Brennan Thompson, and Fabio E. Fontana. 2009. "Effect of Instruction, Surface Stability, and Load Intensity on Trunk Muscle Activity." *Journal of Electromyography and Kinesiology* 19: 500-504. doi: 10.1016/j.jelekin.2008.10.006.

Burke, Edmund R. 2002. *Serious Cycling. 2nd Ed.* Champaign, Ill.: Human Kinetics.

Burke, Edmund R., and Andrew L. Pruitt. 1996. "Body Positioning for Cycling." In *High-Tech Cycling,* edited by Edmund R. Burke, 79-99. Champaign, Ill., Human Kinetics Publishers.

Callaghan, Michael J. 2005. "Lower Body Problems and Injury in Cycling." *Journal of Bodywork and Movement Therapies* 9: 226-236. doi: 10.1016/j.jbmt.2005.01.007.

Clarsen, Benjamin, Tron Krosshaug, and Roald Bahr. 2010. "Overuse Injuries in Professional Road Cyclists." *American Journal of Sports Medicine* 38: 2494-2501. doi: 10.1177/0363546510376816.

Cohen, Jacob. 1988. "Statistical Power Analysis for the Behavioral Sciences." *Technometrics*.

Dettori, Nathan J., and Daniel C. Norvell. 2006. "Non-Traumatic Bicycle Injuries: A Review of the Literature." *Sports Medicine* 36: 7-18. doi: 10.2165/00007256-200636010-00002.

Diefenthaeler, Fernando, Rodrigo R. Bini, Ana P.B. Karolczak, and Felipe P. Carpes. 2008. "Muscle Activation during Pedaling in Different Saddle Position" *Revista Brasileira de Cineantropometria e Desempenho Humano*.

Dorel, Sylvain, Jean M. Drouet, Antoine Couturier, Yvan Champoux, and François Hug. 2009. "Changes of Pedaling Technique and Muscle Coordination during an Exhaustive Exercise." *Medicine and Science in Sports and Exercise* 41: 1277-1286. doi: 10.1249/MSS.0b013e31819825f8.

Edwards, Richardc H.T., Anders Melcher, Carl M. Hesser, Ove Wigertz, and Lars G. Ekelund. 1972. "Physiological Correlates of Perceived Exertion in Continuous and Intermittent Exercise with the Same Average Power Output." *European Journal of Clinical Investigation* 2: 108-114. doi: 10.1111/j.1365-2362.1972.tb00578.x.

Ekkekakis, Panteleimon. 2009. "Let Them Roam Free?: Physiological and Psychological Evidence for the Potential of Self-Selected Exercise Intensity in Public Health." *Sports Medicine* 39: 857:888. doi: 10.2165/11315210-000000000-00000.

Ekkekakis, Panteleimon, Gaynor Parfitt, and Steven J. Petruzzello. 2011. "The Pleasure and Displeasure People Feel When They Exercise at Different Intensities: Decennial Update and Progress towards a Tripartite Rationale for Exercise Intensity Prescription." *Sports Medicine* 41: 641-671. doi: 10.2165/11590680-000000000-00000.

Ericson, Mats O., Ake Bratt, Ralph Nisell, Gunnar Németh, and Jan Ekholm. 1986. "Load Moments about the Hip and Knee Joints during Ergometer Cycling." *Scandinavian Journal of Rehabilitation Medicine* 18: 165-172.

Ferguson, Christopher J. 2009. "An Effect Size Primer: A Guide for Clinicians and Researchers." *Professional Psychology: Research and Practice* 40: 532-538. doi: 10.1037/a0015808.

Feriche, Belén, José L. Chicharro, Almudena F. Vaquero, Margarita Pérez, and Alejandro Lucía. 1998. "The Use of a Fixed Value of RPE during a Ramp Protocol. Comparison with the Ventilatory Threshold." *Journal of Sports Medicine and Physical Fitness* 38: 35-38.

Ferrer-Roca, Ventura, Raúl Bescos, Andreu Roig, Piero Galilea, Oliver Valero, and Juan García-López. 2014. "Acute Effects of Small Changes in Bicycle Saddle Height on Gross Efficiency and Lower Limb Kinematics." *Journal of Strength and Conditioning Research* 28: 784-791. doi: 10.1519/JSC.0b013e3182a1f1a9.

Ferrer-Roca, Ventura, Andreu Roig, Piero Galilea, and Juan García-Lopez. 2012. "Influence of Saddle Height on Lower Limb Kinematics Inwell-Trained Cyclists: Static vs. Dynamic Evaluation in Bike Fitting." *Journal of Strength and Conditioning Research* 26: 3025-3029. doi: 10.1519/JSC.0b013e318245c09d.

Hamley, E. J., and Valorie Thomas. 1967. "Physiological and Postural Factors in the Calibration of the Bicycle Ergometer." *Journal of Physiology* 191: 55-56.

Harriss, David, and Greg Atkinson. 2015. "Ethical Standards in Sport and Exercise Science Research: 2016 Update." *International Journal of Sports Medicine* 36: 1121–1124. doi: 10.1055/s-0035-1565186.

Holmes, James C., Andrew L. Pruitt, and Nina J. Whalen. 1994. "Lower Extremity Overuse in Bicycling." *Clinics in Sports Medicine* 13: 187-205.

Kinovea Association. *Kinovea Website*. http://www.kinovea.org. Published May 2012. Updated 2014. Accessed June 2, 2014.

Kotler, Dana H., Ashwin N. Babu, and Greg Robidoux. 2016. "Prevention, Evaluation, and Rehabilitation of Cycling-Related Injury." *Current Sports Medicine Reports* 15: 199-206. doi: 10.1249/JSR.000000000 0000262.

Kruschewsky, Alberto B., Rodolfo A. Dellagrana, Mateus Rossato, Luiz Fernando P. Ribeiro, Caetano D. Lazzari, and Fernando Diefenthaeler. 2018. "Saddle Height and Cadence Effects on the Physiological, Perceptual, and Affective Responses of Recreational Cyclists." *Perceptual and Motor Skills* 25: 923-938. doi: 10.1177/003151251 8786803.

Kwan, Bethany M., and Angela D. Bryan. 2010. "Affective Response to Exercise as a Component of Exercise Motivation: Attitudes, Norms,

Self-Efficacy, and Temporal Stability of Intentions." *Psychology of Sport and Exercise* 11: 71-79. doi: 10.1016/j.psychsport.2009.05.010.

Lakens, Daniël. 2013. "Calculating and Reporting Effect Sizes to Facilitate Cumulative Science: A Practical Primer for t-Tests and ANOVAs." *Frontiers in Psychology* 26: 863. doi: 10.3389/fpsyg.2013.00863.

Lam, Wing-Kai, Thorsten Sterzing, and Jason T. Cheung. 2011. "Reliability of a Basketball Specific Testing Protocol for Footwear Fit and Comfort Perception." *Footwear Science* 3: 151-158. doi: 10.1080/19424280.2011.630680.

Lucas-Cuevas, Angel G., Pedro Pérez-Soriano, Jose I. Priego-Quesada, and Salvador Llana-Belloch. 2014. "Influence of Foot Orthosis Customisation on Perceived Comfort during Running." *Ergonomics.* 57: 1590-1596. doi: 10.1080/00140139.2014.938129.

Luo, Geng, Pro Stergiou, Jay Worobets, Benno Nigg, and Darren Stefanyshyn. 2009. "Improved Footwear Comfort Reduces Oxygen Consumption during Running." *Footwear Science* 1: 25-29. doi: 10.1080/19424280902993001.

Moura, Bruno M., Vanderson L. Moro, Mateus Rossato, Ricardo D. de Lucas, and Fernando Diefenthaeler. 2017. "Effects of Saddle Height on Performance and Muscular Activity during the Wingate Test." *Journal of Physical Education* 28: e2838. doi: 10.4025/jphyseduc. v28i1.2838.

Nordeen-Snyder, Katherine S. 1977. "The Effect of Bicycle Seat Height Variation upon Oxygen Consumption and Lower Limb Kinematics." *Medicine and Science in Sports and Exercise* 9: 113-117.

Pérez-Landaluce, Javier, Benjamín Fernández-García, Manuel Rodríguez-Alonso, Francisco García-Herrero, Pedro García-Zapico, Ángeles M. Patterson, and Nicolás Terrados. 2002. "Physiological Differences and Rating of Perceived Exertion (RPE) in Professional, Amateur and Young Cyclists." *Journal of Sports Medicine and Physical Fitness* 42: 389-395.

Peveler, Willard W., Phillip Bishop, Joseph Smith, Mark Richardson, and Ed Whitehorn. 2005. "Comparing Methods for Setting Saddle Height in Trained Cyclists." *Journal of Exercise Physiology Online* 8: 51-55.

Peveler, Willard W. 2008. "Effects of Saddle Height on Economy in Cycling." *Journal of Strength and Conditioning Research*. 22: 1355-1359. doi. 10.1519/JSC.0b013e318173dac6.

Peveler, Willard W., Josh D. Pounders, and Phillip A. Bishop. 2007. "Effects of Saddle Height on Anaerobic Power Production in Cycling." *Journal of Strength and Conditioning Research* 21: 1023-1027. doi: 10.1519/R-20316.1.

Peveler, Willard W., and James M. Green. 2011. "Effects of Saddle Height on Economy and Anaerobic Power in Well-Trained Cyclists." *Journal of Strength and Conditioning Research* 25: 629-633. doi: 10.1519/JSC.0b013e3181d09e60.

Peveler, Willard W., Brandy Shew, Samantha Johnson, and Thomas G. Palmer. 2012. "A Kinematic Comparison of Alterations to Knee and Ankle Angles from Resting Measures to Active Pedaling during a Graded Exercise Protocol." *Journal of Strength and Conditioning Research* 26: 3004-3009. doi: 10.1519/JSC.0b013e318243fdcb.

Priego Quesada, Jose I., Pedro Pérez-Soriano, Angel G. Lucas-Cuevas, Rosario S. Palmer, and Rosa M. Cibrián Ortiz de Anda. 2017. "Effect of Bike-Fit in the Perception of Comfort, Fatigue and Pain." *Journal of Sports Sciences* 35: 1459-1465. doi: 10.1080/02640414.2016.1215496.

Rhodes, Ryan E., and Andrew Kates. 2015. "Can the Affective Response to Exercise Predict Future Motives and Physical Activity Behavior? A Systematic Review of Published Evidence." *Annals of Behavioral Medicine* 49: 715-731. doi: 10.1007/s12160-015-9704-5.

Richardson, John T.E. 2011. "Eta Squared and Partial Eta Squared as Measures of Effect Size in Educational Research." *Educational Research Review* 6: 135-147. doi: 10.1016/j.edurev.2010.12.001.

Sanner, William H., and William D. O'Halloran. 2000. "The Biomechanics, Etiology, and Treatment of Cycling Injuries." *Journal of the American Podiatric Medical Association* 90: 354-376. doi: 10.7547/87507315-90-7-354.

Schneider, Margaret, Andrea Dunn, and Daniel Cooper. 2009. "Affect, Exercise, and Physical Activity among Healthy Adolescents." *Journal of Sport and Exercise Psychology* 31: 706-723. doi: 10.1123/jsep. 31.6.706.

Shennum, Paul Lawrence. 1976. "The Effect of Saddle Height on Oxygen Consumption during Bicycle Ergometer Work." *Medicine and Science in Sports and Exercise* 8: 119-121.

Silberman, Marc R. 2013. "Bicycling Injuries." *Current Sports Medicine Reports* 12: 337-345. doi. 10.1249/JSR.0b013e3182a4bab7.

Silberman, Marc R., David Webner, Steven Collina, and Brian J. Shiple. 2005. "Road Bicycle Fit." *Clinical Journal of Sport Medicine : Official Journal of the Canadian Academy of Sport Medicine* 15: 271-276. doi: 10.1097/01.jsm.0000171255.70156.da.

Skinner, James S., Ron Hutsler, Viktor Bergsteinova, and Edmon. R. Buskirk. 1973. "The Validity and Reliability of a Rating Scale of Perceived Exertion." *Medicine & Science in Sports & Exercise* 5: 94-96. doi: 10.1249/00005768-197300520-00018.

Verma, Rachita, Ernst A. Hansen, Mark de Zee, and Pascal Madeleine. 2016. "Effect of Seat Positions on Discomfort, Muscle Activation, Pressure Distribution and Pedal Force during Cycling." *Journal of Electromyography and Kinesiology* 27: 78-86. doi: 10.1016/j.jelekin. 2016.02.003.

Wanich, Tony, Christopher Hodgkins, Jean A. Columbier, Erika Muraski, and John G. Kennedy. 2007. "Cycling Injuries of the Lower Extremity." *Journal of the American Academy of Orthopaedic Surgeons* 15: 748-756. doi: 10.5435/00124635-200712000-00008.

Wilber, C. A., George J. Holland, Ronald E. Madison, and Steven F. Loy. 1995. "An Epidemiological Analysis of Overuse Injuries among Recreational Cyclists." *International Journal of Sports Medicine* 16: 201-206. doi: 10.1055/s-2007-972992.

Wishv-Roth, Trish. 2009. "Assessment of Cycling Biomechanics to Optimise Performance and Minimise Injury." *Journal of Science and Medicine in Sport* 12: S51. doi: 10.1016/j.jsams.2008.12.119.

Worl Medical Association. 2013. "World Medical Association Declaration of Helsinki: Ethical Principles for Medical Research Involving Human Subjects." *JAMA - Journal of the American Medical Association* 310: 2191–2194. doi: 10.1001/jama.2013.281053.

About the Editors

Daniel Castillo, PhD

Editor

Daniel Castillo is a PhD in Sports Sciences, MSc in Physical Activity and Sports Sciences Research, MSc in Teaching Training for Secondary Education and MSc in High Performance in Team Sports. Currently, he is working as a Professor in the Faculty of Health Sciences, Isabel I University of Burgos (Spain), and he is part of the Sport Performance Lab. Current major research topics include: monitoring training and match loads in team sports, soccer small-sided games- and match- related fatigue, physical fitness performance of professional soccer players, physical and physiological performances in soccer referees and cerebral palsy soccer players. He has published around 35 scientific studies indexed in Journal Citation Reports (JCR) and is member of editorial committees and reviewers of Sports Sciences Journals. Additionally, Daniel has worked as Coach in a Professional Soccer Academy during 10 years.

Javier Raya-González, PhD

Co-Editor

Javier Raya-González is PhD in Sport Sciences, MSc in Physical Activity and Health, MSc in Injury Prevention and Rehab in Soccer and MSc in Teaching Training for Secondary Education. Currently, he is working as a Professor in the Faculty of Health Sciences, Isabel I University of Burgos (Spain), and he is part of the Sport Performance Lab. His main field of research is the strength training applied to team sports players to optimizing the performance and to prevent sport injuries, as well as the control and quantification of training and match load in team sports and its relationship with performance and injury prevention. Javier has published around 30 scientific studies in national and international Sports Sciences journals. Additionally, Javier had worked as Strength and Conditioning Coach with professional soccer players.

INDEX

A

B

C

D

E

T

V